Color Atlas of Emergency Trauma

SECOND EDITION

COLOR ATLAS OF
EMERGENCY TRAUMA

SECOND EDITION

Edited by

Demetrios Demetriades, MD, PhD, FACS

Professor of Surgery, University of Southern California's Keck School of Medicine, and Vice-Chairman of Surgery and Director of the Trauma Program and Surgical Intensive Care Unit at the Los Angeles County–USC Medical Center

Edward J. Newton, MD, FACEP, FRCPC

Professor and Chairman of Emergency Medicine, University of Southern California's Keck School of Medicine, and Chairman of the Los Angeles County–USC Medical Center's Department of Emergency Medicine

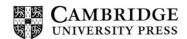

CAMBRIDGE
UNIVERSITY PRESS

CAMBRIDGE UNIVERSITY PRESS
Cambridge, New York, Melbourne, Madrid, Cape Town,
Singapore, São Paulo, Delhi, Tokyo, Mexico City

Cambridge University Press
The Edinburgh Building, Cambridge CB2 8RU, UK

Published in the United States of America by Cambridge University Press, New York

www.cambridge.org
Information on this title: www.cambridge.org/9781107001527

First published 2011

Printed in the United Kingdom at the University Press, Cambridge
A catalogue record for this publication is available from the British Library

Library of Congress Cataloging-in-Publication Data

Demetriades, Demetrios, 1951–
Color atlas of emergency trauma / Demetrios Demetriades, Edward J. Newton. – 2nd ed.
      p.   cm.
Rev. ed. of: Color atlas of emergency trauma / Diku P. Mandavia, Edward J. Newton, Demetrios Demetriades. 2003.
Includes bibliographical references and index.
ISBN 978-1-107-00152-7 (Hardback)
1. Medical emergencies–Atlases.   2. Emergency medical services–Atlases.   3. Wounds and injuries–Atlases.   I. Newton, Edward,
1950– II. Mandavia, Diku P., 1965– Color atlas of emergency trauma.   III. Title.
[DNLM: 1. Wounds and Injuries–Atlases.   2. Emergencies–Atlases.   WO 517]
RC86.7.M3478 2011
616.02′50222–dc22   2011013009

ISBN 978-1-107-00152-7 Hardback

Dedicated with thanks to my family and colleagues. To my students of trauma and emergency care, may the collected experience contained in this atlas assist your pursuit of excellence.

E. Newton

To my parents, my wife Elizabeth, my daughters Alexis and Stefanie, and my son Nicky.

D. Demetriades

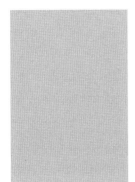

Contents

List of contributors   x
Foreword by David B. Hoyt and Sandra M. Schneider   xi
Preface   xiii
Acknowledgments   xiv

1   HEAD INJURY   1
Demetrios Demetriades and Leslie Kobayashi

1.1	Scalp Injuries	4
1.2	Skull Fractures	4
1.3	Intracranial Hematomas	11
1.4	Penetrating Head Injury	20
1.5	Transtentorial Herniation	24
1.6	Diffuse Cerebral Edema	26
1.7	Pediatric Head Injury	27
1.8	Diffuse Axonal Injury	28

2   FACIAL INJURY   30
Edward J. Newton

2.1	Eye Injuries	33
2.2	Periorbital Lacerations	37
2.3	Facial Fractures	37
2.4	Nasal Injuries	42
2.5	Penetrating Facial Trauma	42
2.6	Complex Oromaxillofacial Trauma	44
2.7	Facial Nerve Injury	47
2.8	Parotid Gland Injury	48

3   NECK INJURY   50
Demetrios Demetriades and Lydia Lam

Penetrating Neck Injuries   52

3.1	Anatomical Zones of the Neck	52
3.2	Epidemiology of Penetrating Neck Trauma	54
3.3	Physical Examination of Penetrating Injuries of the Neck	54
3.4	Protocol for Initial Evaluation and Management of Penetrating Injuries to the Neck	56
3.5	Radiological Investigations for Penetrating Neck Trauma	57
3.6	Evaluation of the Vascular Structures in the Neck	59
3.7	Evaluation of the Aerodigestive Tract in the Neck	63
3.8	Airway Establishment in the Presence of a Neck Hematoma	65
3.9	Bleeding Control in the Emergency Department	66
3.10	Penetrating Trauma to the Carotid Artery	68
3.11	Penetrating Trauma to the Vertebral Artery	69

3.12 Penetrating Trauma to the Subclavian Vessels 70

Blunt Neck Trauma 71

3.13 Vascular Injuries 72
3.14 Blunt Laryngotracheal Trauma 74

4 THORACIC INJURY 75
Demetrios Demetriades and Peep Talving

4.1 Chest Wall, Soft Tissues 78
4.2 Rib Fractures 78
4.3 Hemo-Pneumothorax 81
4.4 Lung Contusion 89
4.5 Subcutaneous Emphysema 90
4.6 Penetrating Cardiac Injury 92
4.7 Blunt Cardiac Trauma 100
4.8 Blunt Thoracic Aortic Injury 101
4.9 Penetrating Thoracic Outlet Injuries 105
4.10 Transmediastinal Gunshot Wounds 107
4.11 Diaphragmatic Injuries 109
4.12 Esophageal Injuries 114
4.13 Thoracic Duct Injury 116
4.14 Traumatic Asphyxia 117
4.15 Impaled Thoracic Foreign Bodies 118

5 ABDOMINAL INJURY 119
Demetrios Demetriades and Kenji Inaba

Blunt Abdominal Trauma 122

5.1 Mechanism of Injury 122
5.2 Diagnosis of Hemoperitoneum 123
5.3 Splenic Injuries 125
5.4 Liver Injuries 127
5.5 Pancreatic Injuries 131
5.6 Renal Injuries 133
5.7 Bladder Injuries 135
5.8 Urethral Injuries 137
5.9 Duodenal Injuries 139
5.10 Small-Bowel Injuries 140
5.11 Colorectal Injuries 141

Penetrating Abdominal Trauma 142

5.12 Mechanism of Injury 142
5.13 Investigations in Penetrating Abdominal Injury 144
5.14 Transpelvic Gunshot Injuries 145
5.15 Penetrating Injuries to the Liver 146
5.16 Penetrating Splenic Injuries 149
5.17 Penetrating Pancreatic Injuries 150
5.18 Penetrating Renal Injuries 150
5.19 Penetrating Colorectal Injuries 152
5.20 Abdominal Vascular Injuries 153
5.21 Abdominal Trauma in Pregnancy 154

6 MUSCULOSKELETAL INJURY 160
Edward J. Newton

6.1 Classification of Fractures 161
6.2 Open Fractures 162
6.3 Mangled Extremity 163
6.4 Open Joint Injury 164
6.5 Epiphyseal Injuries 165
6.6 Torus and Greenstick Fractures 166
6.7 Supracondylar Fracture 167
6.8 Amputations 168
6.9 Tendon Injury 170
6.10 Peripheral Vascular Injury 170
6.11 Peripheral Nerve Injury 174
6.12 Metacarpal Fractures 177
6.13 Scaphoid Fractures 178
6.14 Scapholunate Dislocation 179
6.15 Lunate and Perilunate Dislocation 179
6.16 Wrist Fractures 180
6.17 Forearm Fractures 181
6.18 Elbow Dislocation 183
6.19 Radial Head Fracture 183
6.20 Humeral Fracture 184
6.21 Shoulder Dislocation 185
6.22 Clavicle Fracture 187
6.23 Sternoclavicular Dislocation 188
6.24 Scapula Fracture 188
6.25 Pelvic Fractures 189
6.26 Hip Dislocation 193
6.27 Hip Fractures 195
6.28 Femoral Shaft Fracture 196
6.29 Patellar Fracture 197
6.30 Tibial Plateau Fracture 198
6.31 Knee Dislocation 198
6.32 Maisonneuve Fracture Complex 200
6.33 Ankle Dislocation 201
6.34 Subtalar Dislocation 202
6.35 Lisfranc Fracture 203
6.36 Metatarsal Base Fractures 204
6.37 Calcaneal Fractures 205

7   SPINAL INJURIES   207
Mark J. Spoonamore and Demetrios Demetriades

Spinal Cord Injuries   211
7.1   Complete Spinal Cord Transection   211
7.2   Central Cord Syndrome   213
7.3   Brown-Séquard Syndrome   215
7.4   Anterior Cord Syndrome   216

Upper Cervical Spine Dislocations   216
7.5   Atlanto-Occipital Dislocation   217
7.6   Atlantoaxial Dislocation   218
7.7   Rotatory Subluxation of C-1 on C-2   219
7.8   Ligamentous Injuries   220

Cervical Spine Fractures   222
7.9   C-1 Burst Fracture (Jefferson Fracture)   222
7.10   Odontoid (Dens) Fractures (C-2)   224
7.11   Hangman's Fracture (C-2)   226
7.12   Fractures of the Lower Cervical Spine (C-3–C-7)   228
7.13   Flexion and Extension Teardrop Fracture   229
7.14   Compression or Burst Fracture of the Vertebral Body   231
7.15   Clay Shoveler's Fracture   232
7.16   Fractures of the Pedicles, Laminae, and Lateral Masses   233
7.17   Facet Dislocation   234
7.18   Cervicothoracic Spinal Injury   237

Thoracic Spine Injuries   239

Lumbar Spine Injuries   242
7.19   Lumbar Compression Burst Fractures   242
7.20   Chance Fractures   245
7.21   Fracture-Dislocation of the Lumbar Spine   247

Pediatric Spinal Injury   248

Penetrating Injuries to the Spinal Cord   250

8   BURN INJURIES   253
Andrew Tang, Charity Wip, Warren Garner, and Demetrios Demetriades

Extent of Burn Injury   256
8.1   First-Degree Burn   256
8.2   Second-Degree Burn   257
8.3   Third-Degree Burn   261
8.4   Fourth-Degree Burn   262

Special Considerations of Burn Injury   263
8.5   Inhalation Injury   263
8.6   Abdominal Compartment Syndrome   264
8.7   Circumferential Burn   265
8.8   Scald Burns   266
8.9   Chemical Burns   267
8.10   Electrical Burns   268
8.11   Outcome of Burn Injury   269

9   SOFT TISSUE INJURIES   271
Demetrios Demetriades and Marko Bukur
9.1   Dog Bite Injury   273
9.2   Cat Bite Injury   275
9.3   Human Bite Injury   276
9.4   High-Pressure Injection Injury   278
9.5   Retained Foreign Body   279
9.6   Extremity Compartment Syndrome   280

10   BALLISTICS   284
Ramon Cestero, David Plurad, and Demetrios Demetriades
10.1   Definitions   284
10.2   Low-Velocity Projectiles   286
10.3   High-Velocity Projectiles   288
10.4   Shotgun Injuries   291
10.5   Blast Injuries   295
10.6   Nonlethal Weapons   299
10.7   Myths and Facts about Bullets   300

11   DISASTER MEDICINE   301
Edward J. Newton
11.1   Epidemiology of Injuries in Mass Disasters   301
11.2   Triage   302
11.3   Specific Injuries   304
11.4   Guidelines for Rescue Efforts   306

Index   308

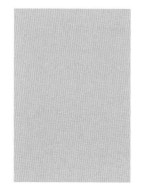

Contributors

Marko Bukur, MD
Fellow in Trauma and Surgical Critical Care,
University of Southern California's Keck School of
Medicine, CA, USA

Ramon Cestero, MD
Fellow in Trauma and Surgical Critical Care,
University of Southern California's Keck School of
Medicine, CA, USA

Demetrios Demetriades, MD, PhD, FACS
Professor of Surgery, University of Southern
California's Keck School of Medicine and
Vice-Chairman of Surgery and Director of the Trauma
Program and Surgical Intensive Care Unit at the
Los Angeles County–USC Medical Center, CA, USA

Warren Garner, MD
Professor of Surgery, University of Southern
California's Keck School of Medicine, CA, USA

David B. Hoyt, MD, FACS
Executive Director, American College of Surgeons

Kenji Inaba, MD, FRCSC, PhD, FACS
Program Director, Surgical Critical Care Fellowship,
University of Southern California's Keck School of
Medicine, CA, USA

Leslie Kobayashi, MD
Fellow in Trauma and Surgical Critical Care,
University of Southern California's Keck School of
Medicine, CA, USA

Lydia Lam, MD
Assistant Professor of Surgery, University of Southern
California's Keck School of Medicine, CA, USA

Edward J. Newton, MD, FACEP, FRCPC
Professor and Chairman of Emergency Medicine,
University of Southern California's Keck
School of Medicine and Chairman of the
Los Angeles County–USC Medical
Center's Department of Emergency Medicine,
CA, USA

David Plurad, MD
Commander in the US Navy; Director,
US Navy Trauma Training Center,
Los Angeles County–USC Medical Center,
CA, USA

Sandra M. Schneider, MD
President, American College of Emergency
Physicians

Mark J. Spoonamore, MD
Assistant Professor, Clinical Orthopedic
Surgery; Medical Director, Center for Spinal Surgery,
University of Southern California's Keck School of
Medicine, CA, USA

Peep Talving, MD, PhD, FACS
Assistant Professor of Surgery, University of
Southern California's Keck School of Medicine,
CA, USA

Andrew Tang, MD
Surgical Critical Care Fellow, University
of Southern California's Keck School of Medicine,
CA, USA

Charity Wip, MD
Burn Unit Fellow, Los Angeles County–USC Trauma
Center, CA, USA

Foreword

The second edition of the *Color Atlas of Emergency Trauma* is a definitive addition to the published works on traumatic injuries. The first edition received critical acclaim from the international trauma community, including a commendation from the British Medical Association. The new edition is more vivid, with more figures and illustrations, and will undoubtedly receive similar praise.

What sets this wonderful text apart from others of its type is the selection of critical images that vibrantly illustrate the steps involved in determining the presence of an injury. The authors have combined succinct text with graphic images, which will help learners retain a visual picture of the relevant details they will need to remember when they encounter injuries in their practices. Each chapter includes an introduction and description of epidemiology, clinical findings, and investigations, all of which are complemented by numerous photographs highlighting the injuries and making each scenario and problem feel real.

The experience this book offers is a great adjunct to traditional texts and to other educational resources. It is visual. It is relevant. It gets right to the point, and it makes learning complex concepts much easier and exciting.

The authors are amongst the most experienced trauma surgeons in the nation. They have written on virtually every topic in clinical trauma and have led our thinking in most aspects of trauma care for more than 20 years. Dr. Demetriades' eye towards important details of each diagnosis is reflected in the photographs and diagnostic images chosen. The reader will enjoy learning about the spectrum of traumatic injuries by using this atlas. The student learning trauma from a traditional textbook, when complemented by the *Color Atlas of Emergency Trauma*, will have a facilitated learning experience. This book should be standard reading for any trauma surgeon or student.

David B. Hoyt, MD, FACS
Executive Director, American College of Surgeons

Trauma is pervasive in our society and as much as any area of medicine, it requires rapid recognition and intervention to preserve life. Trauma care also requires a coordinated and cooperative approach by multiple specialists for optimal outcome. This text is an example of that cooperation. The systematic presentation of physical, radiographic and operative findings makes this a valuable resource for clinicians, teachers, and students.

Sandra M. Schneider, MD
President, American College of Emergency Physicians

Preface

Trauma is very different from other emergency medical conditions. Very often there is no clinical history available and the treatment is given before the definitive diagnosis. The physiological reserves of many trauma victims are limited and small errors can carry a heavy price. The comprehension and intuition required to treat traumatic injury is gained over many years of clinical experience at the bedside of critically injured patients. The aim of this atlas is to share the experience of the authors from one of the largest trauma centers in the United States and provide a solid companion to the many well-written textbooks on trauma management.

This project represents many decades of collective clinical experience. We have assembled one of the largest collections of trauma images to help bring the reader "to the bedside" of the patients. The acquisition and final assembly of this collection of images was a difficult process and they were acquired with the gracious cooperation of our patients. We regularly use these images in our clinical teaching and hope this atlas will supplement other instructional resources in trauma management.

Demetrios Demetriades, MD, PhD
Edward J. Newton, MD

Acknowledgments

The authors greatly acknowledge the major contributions of Dr. Diku Mondavia, co-editor of the first edition of the atlas

Alexis Demetriades
Scientific Illustrator, Illustrations and Image Processing

Robert S. Amaral, MA
Medical Illustrator, Illustrations

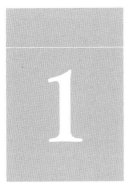

1

Head Injury

Demetrios Demetriades and Leslie Kobayashi

Introduction

Head trauma is the most common cause of death and permanent disability following trauma. Blunt head injury is most commonly the result of motor vehicle crashes, auto versus pedestrian collisions, or falls from significant heights. Gunshot wounds cause the vast majority of penetrating head injuries, although stab wounds and impalement injuries may also be seen.

Clinical Examination

Head injury is classified into mild, moderate, and severe categories, depending on the patient's Glasgow Coma Scale (GCS) (see Table 1.1) at the time of presentation.

Mild head injury patients have a GCS of 14–15. Typically these injuries include concussion or transient loss of consciousness or neurologic function. Concussion does not result in any gross pathologic abnormalities of the brain, but subtle changes have been described using electron microscopy. Although the neurologic examination is usually normal, post-concussive neuropsychiatric symptoms are common. These include amnesia of the event, headache, loss of concentration, dizziness, sleep disturbance, and a host of related symptoms. These symptoms resolve within 2 weeks for the vast majority of patients but may persist for many months in a small percentage. "Hard" neurologic findings such as diplopia, motor weakness, pupillary abnormalities, and other cranial nerve deficits are never due to post-concussive syndrome and demand further investigation.

Moderate head injury (GCS 8–14) and severe head injury (GCS <8) comprise a spectrum of injuries including cerebral contusion, diffuse cerebral edema, axonal shear injury, subarachnoid hemorrhage (SAH), and extra-axial lesions (subdural hematoma and epidural hematoma).

Table 1.1 Glasgow Coma Scale scoring system

EYES (E)		
Open	Spontaneously	4
	To verbal command	3
	To pain	2
	No response	1
BEST VERBAL RESPONSE (V)		
	Oriented and converses	5
	Disoriented and converses	4
	Inappropriate words	3
	Incomprehensible sounds	2
	No response	1
BEST MOTOR RESPONSE (M)		
To verbal stimuli	Obeys	6
To painful stimulus	Localizes pain	5
	Flexion–withdrawal	4
	Abnormal flexion (decorticate rigidity)	3
	Extension (decerebrate rigidity)	2
	No response (flaccid)	1
TOTAL		3–15

The GCS is useful in categorizing patients as to severity of head injury but is not sufficient to determine the presence or absence of neurologic injury, as it does not assess pupils, subtle changes in mentation, cranial nerve injury, or skull fractures. A complete evaluation therefore demands a rapid but thorough examination done prior to administering paralytic agents. The head is inspected for signs of trauma including lacerations, hematomas, areas of skull depression, raccoon eyes, Battle's sign, hemotympanum, rhinorrhea, and otorrhea. The pupils are examined for symmetry and reaction to light; the extraocular movements and other cranial nerve functions are assessed; motor and sensory function is assessed for symmetry.

Patients with increased intracranial pressure (ICP) inevitably have some diminution in their typical level of alertness. As ICP increases further, herniation of the uncus across the tentorium can occur, resulting in compression of the ipsilateral cerebral peduncle and ipsilateral oculomotor nerve. Consequently, ipsilateral ptosis, restricted extraocular movement, and pupillary dilation occur, along with contralateral motor posturing (decorticate, followed by decerebrate, and finally flaccid paralysis). Once this process begins, there is a very brief interval for effecting a reversal by lowering ICP.

Investigations

All patients with GCS persistently <14, or patients with a GCS of 15 with definite loss of consciousness, persistent amnesia, significant mechanism, advanced age, presence of anticoagulation, or post-traumatic seizure require evaluation by head computerized tomography (CT) without contrast. Selected patients may require further investigation by contrast enhanced CT, CT angiography, magnetic resonance imaging (MRI), or, rarely, cerebral angiography. The ability to perform 3-D or multiplanar reconstruction may be particularly helpful in the diagnosis of injuries like basilar skull fracture and posterior fossa intracranial hemorrhages.

Multiple trauma patients may have injuries to the chest or abdomen that require immediate operative intervention which takes precedence over potential head injury. In these cases CT scan may be deferred, although some patients may be stable enough to undergo a CT scan of the head to identify any intracranial hematoma. If one is identified, simultaneous evacuation of the brain hematoma can be done while a laparotomy or thoracotomy is in progress. In patients who are too unstable to undergo CT scan of the head and who show signs of neurologic deterioration, intraoperative burr holes can be placed to evacuate a hematoma.

Skull x-rays are seldom indicated because CT scan is more sensitive in identifying skull fractures and provides much more information regarding any underlying brain injury. Skull x-rays can be useful in locating foreign bodies (e.g., bullet fragments) or intracranial air, and as part of a skeletal survey in suspected child abuse.

Cervical spine injury is frequently associated with blunt head trauma, and the evaluation of the spine is difficult in a patient whose mental status is diminished because of head injury. Consequently, it is essential to immobilize the spine and evaluate the integrity of the spinal column by CT scan in any patient not meeting criteria for clinical clearance. The cervical spine should remain immobilized in unresponsive patients until they are conscious enough to be cleared clinically or until bony and ligamentous injury can be ruled out with CT scan with or without MRI.

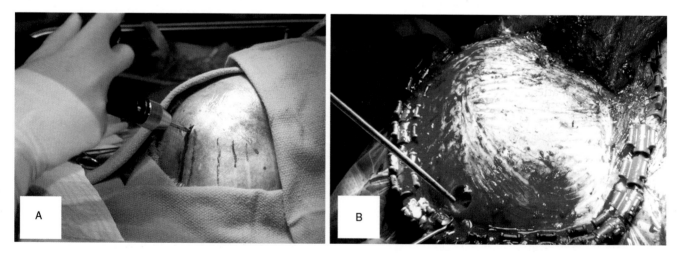

Figure 1.1 Exploratory burr holes may be considered in cases with neurological deterioration if a CT scan is not available. (A) Photograph with scalp prepared and creation of burr hole in progress. (B) Scalp reflected with exposed cranium and drilled burr hole placed in the operating room.

General Management

The goal of cerebral resuscitation in the emergency department (ED) is to prevent secondary injuries to the brain, which are worsened by hypoxia, hypotension, seizures, hyperthermia, and hypercarbia.

Cerebral resuscitation and treatment are performed in the context of overall resuscitation and are guided by advanced trauma life support (ATLS) principles. Patients with severe head injury tend to hypoventilate and are at risk for aspiration of oral secretions. Consequently, securing an airway and ensuring adequate ventilation are the highest priorities. A brief neurologic examination should be performed prior to using paralytic drugs for rapid sequence intubation (RSI) to secure the airway. Patients with a GCS $\leq$ 8 require intubation, although patients with a higher GCS may also need intubation.

Maintaining adequate cerebral perfusion pressure is important in the face of increased ICP to prevent secondary ischemic injury. Consequently, measures to maintain adequate systemic blood pressure are essential and include crystalloid infusion, blood transfusion, thoracotomy, laparotomy, and vasopressive medications as indicated.

For patients with evidence of increased ICP or clinical signs of actual or impending transtentorial herniation, immediate measures to decrease ICP are indicated. The patient should be adequately sedated, and analgesics should be used to control pain. Hyperventilation to reduce pCO_2 to a level of 32–35 mm Hg decreases cerebral blood flow and thus decreases intracranial blood volume, allowing a temporary decrease in ICP. Osmotic diuresis with mannitol and use of loop diuretics such as furosemide dehydrate all tissues including brain, again allowing more space for an expanding hematoma and lowering ICP. These medications must be used with extreme caution if at all in multiply injured patients, as severe systemic hypotension may result; in these cases, consideration should be given to the use of hypertonic saline. Hypertonic saline also functions as an osmotic agent decreasing cerebral edema but without the diuretic effect often seen with mannitol. The neck should be cleared of any binding or restricting devices or ties to improve venous drainage from the head. Positioning the head at 30 degrees elevation can decrease ICP once the spine has been cleared radiographically. Placement of a ventriculostomy to drain cerebrospinal fluid (CSF) has been shown to be effective not only in treating elevated ICP but also in following the progress of the patient's condition. In refractory cases barbiturate coma may be used to decrease cerebral metabolic demand. In extreme cases a decompressive craniectomy or lobectomy may be considered. The patient should not be allowed to become hyperthermic as this significantly increases cerebral metabolism and oxygen demand, the use of ice packs, Tylenol or other antipyretic agents should be considered. Conversely the use of cerebral or systemic mild hypothermia has been shown experimentally to improve outcome from severe head injury.

Definitive treatment for head injury depends on the nature of the lesion. Closed skull fractures require no specific treatment, but open fractures should be irrigated, debrided, and closed. Depressed skull fractures require elevation of the fragment if it is depressed greater than one bone width, and debridement if the wound is grossly contaminated. Basilar skull fractures usually heal uneventfully, but patients with rhinorrhea or otorrhea require careful follow-up to ensure that the fistula closes. Most CSF leaks stop within 2 weeks, but persistent leaks may require a formal dural closure. Most epidural hematomas (EDHs) require surgical evacuation, although those that are <1 cm may be treated by observation and repeat CT scan if the patient is asymptomatic. Larger EDHs require craniotomy for evacuation. Subdural hematoma (SDH) is rarely asymptomatic, and in many cases surgical treatment may be needed to evacuate the hematoma. Subarachnoid hemorrhage is treated with nimodipine (calcium channel blocker) to decrease surrounding vasospasm, and measures to decrease rebleeding are undertaken. Intraventricular hemorrhage may require ventriculostomy to remove blood and CSF, but the prognosis usually remains poor. Patients requiring surgery and those with depressed skull fracture and cerebral contusion should be started on a short course of anticonvulsant medication to decrease early post-traumatic seizure risk.

Common Mistakes and Pitfalls

1. Certain patients are at higher risk for intracranial injury from even relatively minor mechanisms of injury. These include the elderly, chronic alcoholics, infants, patients with cerebral atrophy, and patients on antiplatelet or anticoagulant medications. A low threshold for obtaining a head CT scan should be maintained in these patients.
2. Altered mental status, seizures, and focal neurologic deficits should not be ascribed to intoxication, dementia, or other chronic conditions if there is a history or evidence of head trauma present.
3. Excessive hyperventilation (to a pCO_2 <30 mm Hg) should be avoided because the vasospasm lowers

cerebral blood flow to a point that cerebral ischemia can occur.

4. Delayed presentation of SDH and EDH can occur, often with subtle neurologic signs. Obtaining a repeat CT scan or initial CT scan even weeks after the injury is appropriate in selected cases.

5. Subacute SDH may appear isodense with surrounding brain 5–10 days after the injury. Altering the density values of the CT or use of contrast will demonstrate the lesion.

6. Coagulopathy is common with serious head injury and may result in more severe bleeding, hemorrhage from other noncerebral sites, and disseminated intravascular coagulopathy (DIC). A baseline coagulation profile should be obtained in all patients with serious head injury and repeated periodically during admission. The appropriate blood products should be administered early.

7. Child abuse must be suspected in cases of intracerebral injury or skull fracture in infants and children.

1.1 Scalp Injuries

The scalp is a tough, mobile, multilayered covering of the skull. It is composed of epidermis, dermis and a strong fibrous layer of subdermal tissue, a muscle layer, and the galea or periosteal covering of the skull. The scalp is highly vascular, and vessels are fixed within the scalp and unable to retract and constrict when lacerated. Consequently, scalp wounds frequently bleed profusely and can result in hemorrhagic shock. In scalping type injuries careful attention must be paid to ensuring that there are not also skull fractures associated with the soft tissue injury. A completely avulsed scalp can be replaced and usually heals well because of its extensive vascularity.

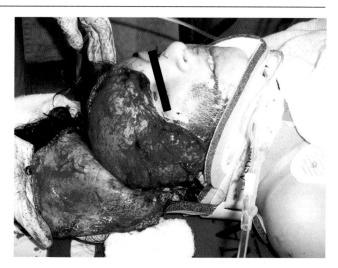

Figure 1.2 Photograph of a patient with major avulsion of the apical scalp.

1.2 Skull Fractures

Skull fractures are common sequelae of both blunt and penetrating head trauma. Although it may be an isolated finding, skull fracture is frequently associated with intracranial injury. Skull fractures are particularly dangerous in certain anatomic locations, such as across the middle meningeal arterial groove, across dural sinuses, or in the occipital area because the intracranial bleeding associated with these fractures may be rapidly life-threatening.

As with fractures of other bones, skull fractures are classified as simple or comminuted, displaced or nondisplaced, and open or closed. Linear fractures are the most common type of skull fracture and generally result from lower energy blunt trauma over a large surface area. In contrast comminuted fractures contain multiple fracture lines, and generally take a larger amount of force to create than linear fractures. Comminution starts at the point of maximal impact and spreads centrifugally along the skull. When found in the occipital region in children, comminuted fractures may suggest abuse. Displaced fractures are a result of a very high energy direct blow to a small surface area; a free piece of bone or a fragment end is driven inward and its edge is found below that of its adjacent fragment. Open fractures which communicate with the skin or mucus membranes may result in direct introduction of contaminants such as hair, skin, or foreign debris into the

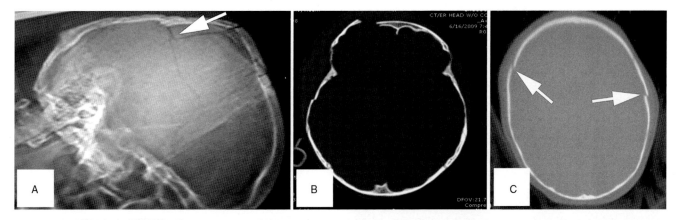

Figure 1.3 Skull fractures. (A) Lateral skull radiograph showing a comminuted fracture of the apex of the skull (arrow). (B) CT scan with bone windows showing a displaced fracture of the skull. (C) CT scan with bone windows showing right frontal and left parietal skull fractures with minimal displacement (arrows).

cranial vault. Subsequent infection can produce meningitis, osteomyelitis, or, more commonly, brain abscess. Consequently, open wounds of the cranium must be carefully debrided, irrigated, and closed to prevent such complications.

Isolated skull fractures may result in headache and local tenderness. Clinical findings with basilar skull fracture depend on which fossa of the cranium is involved. Frontobasilar fractures may present with raccoon eyes, rhinorrhea, and anosmia; middle fossa fractures present with hemotympanum, otorrhea, vertigo, or Battle's sign; posterior fossa fractures may present with ataxia and nystagmus. In children very often significant cephalohematomas are associated with underlying skull fracture; this finding is unfortunately much less specific in adults.

Linear Skull Fracture

Linear is the most common fracture pattern, accounting for approximately 80% of all skull fractures. Linear fractures result from a direct blow to the head, most often after motor vehicle crashes, although the incidence of serious head injury from this source has decreased as a result of the use of motorcycle helmets, seatbelts, and airbags. Other causes of linear skull fractures include falls and assaults. The vast majority (85%) of fractures occur in males.

Skull fractures are relatively common in children in spite of the greater pliability of their skulls. Skull fractures in infants are commonly due to child abuse, and the circumstances surrounding the injury need to be carefully investigated. Skull fractures in neonates can also occur in association with a cephalohematoma as a

result of a difficult delivery and use of forceps. Management of these injuries is generally conservative unless the skull fragments are depressed. A "growing" skull fracture occasionally occurs in children as a result of the interposition of a leptomeningeal cyst between the fracture edges, and it may require surgery. Healing of a skull fracture takes place over many months, so children should be rechecked approximately 6 months following a fracture to ensure that proper healing has occurred; ultrasound is particularly useful in follow-up as an adjunct to clinical examination in this circumstance.

A skull fracture may occasionally become apparent on physical examination while a scalp laceration is explored. It is felt as a step-off of the normally smooth skull surface. These fractures should be treated as any other open fracture with irrigation, and closure of each layer of the scalp, including the galea. A CT scan should be obtained to delineate the extent of the fracture and to determine if intracranial injury has occurred.

Plain radiography of the skull is rarely obtained in the current era as CT scan has largely replaced it. The sensitivity for detection of skull fracture with CT scan is very high; CT scan will reveal a linear fracture as a gap in the skull and has the advantage of demonstrating any underlying injury to the brain. A fracture must be distinguished from suture lines and vascular grooves. Suture lines have a characteristic zigzag appearance and are located in predictable locations. They are of near uniform width throughout their course. Vascular grooves have sequential bifurcations. Fracture lines can cross either of these structures and typically are wider in their center, tapering in width toward either end. The incidence of brain injury in the presence of a skull fracture is as high

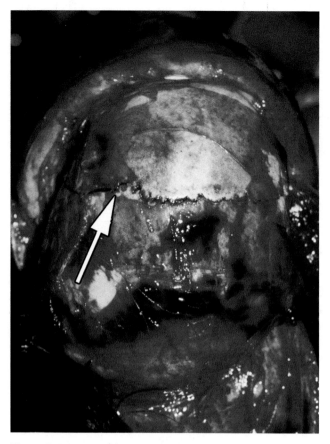

Figure 1.4 Autopsy photograph after retraction of the scalp of a patient with semicircular linear skull fracture (arrow).

as 34%. Fractures across the middle meningeal vascular groove are associated with epidural hematoma in a small percent of cases, but 80% of epidural hematomas are associated with a skull fracture.

Depressed Skull Fracture

The typical depressed skull fracture occurs when a large amount of force is applied to a small area of the skull (e.g., a blow with a hammer) which results in a stellate fracture with a depressed center. Physical examination of the skull may reveal a depression in the skull, but more commonly the fracture is not palpable because of overlying soft tissue swelling. CT scan is highly sensitive and accurate in detecting depressed skull fracture as well as underlying brain injury.

Patients with depressed skull fractures have an increased incidence of post-traumatic seizures because the impact of the fragments on the cortex of the brain results in areas of scarring that ultimately become seizure foci. Consequently, anticonvulsant prophylaxis is begun in the ED and continued for 1 week. Management of a closed depressed skull fracture is controversial. Some advocate conservative treatment for all of these fractures; others recommend surgical elevation of the fragments if the depression

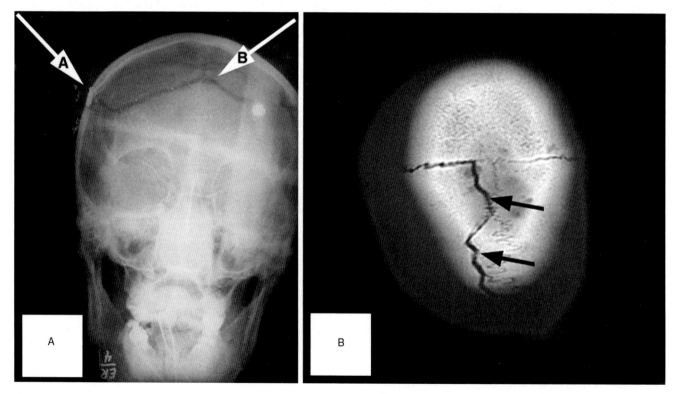

Figure 1.5 Linear skull fractures. (A) Skull radiograph showing linear skull fracture (arrow B) caused by a gunshot wound to the right temporal area (arrow A). (B) CT scan with bone windows showing extensive linear skull fractures.

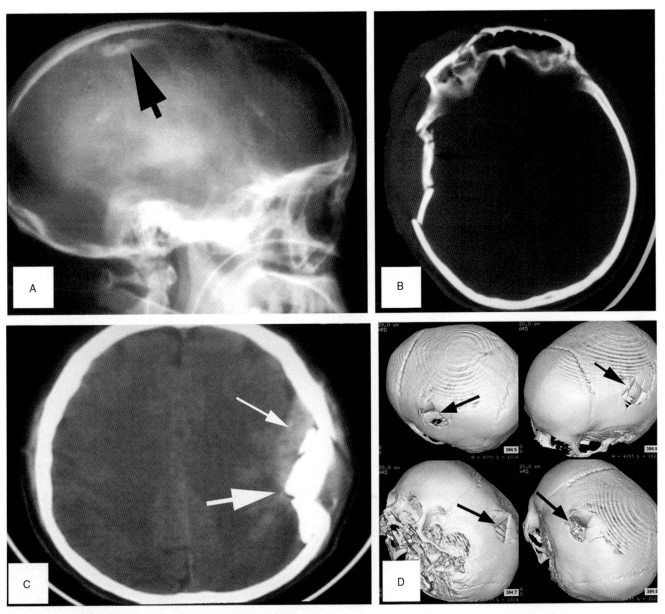

Figure 1.6 Depressed skull fractures. (A) Lateral radiograph of the skull showing hyperdensity due to overlapping bone fragments (arrow) at the apical–parietal skull. (B) CT scan bone windows showing right temporoparietal comminuted depressed fracture (arrow) and associated soft tissue swelling. This patient suffered a concomitant epidural hematoma. (C) CT scan showing depressed fracture of the left parietal bone (large arrow) with underlying epidural hematoma (small arrow). (D) CT scan showing 3-D reconstruction of a skull with left parietal depressed comminuted skull fracture (arrow).

is greater than one bone width (from inner to outer table). Open, contaminated depressed fractures clearly require surgical debridement.

Open Skull Fracture

Open skull fracture can result from penetration of both the scalp and the skull from blunt or penetrating trauma or from fracture of air-filled sinuses that communicate with the intracranial space. Although pneumocephalus can rarely result in a mass effect and displacement of intracranial contents, more commonly its significance is the creation of a communication between the CSF and the environment which often leads to the development of meningitis or brain abscess. Open skull fracture should be treated as any open fracture, with surgical debridement, irrigation, and appropriate parenteral antibiotics.

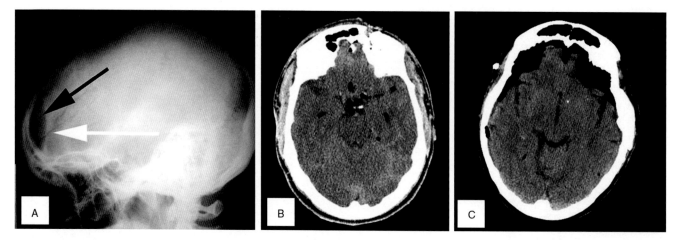

Figure 1.7 Open skull fractures. (A) Lateral radiograph of the skull showing a frontal linear skull fracture (white arrow) and frontal pneumocephalus (black arrow). (B) CT scan of a patient with a skull fracture through the frontal sinus and associated pneumocephalus. (C) CT scan of massive bifrontal pneumocephalus.

Basilar Skull Fracture

The skull base is divided into three compartments, and the clinical presentation differs depending on the location of the fracture. Basilar skull fracture is often a clinical diagnosis based on physical findings of raccoon eyes, Battle's sign, CSF rhinorrhea or otorrhea, and hemotympanum. Injury to cranial nerves that exit the base of the skull is common, and a careful neurologic examination is required to seek out these injuries. CT scan is primarily used to make the diagnosis. The sensitivity of CT scan for basilar skull fractures is lower than for fractures of the rest of the cranium. The presence of an experienced neuroradiologist, multiple physician readers, and the use of high-resolution multiplanar reconstruction, and maximum intensity projection help to increase the sensitivity of CT scans for detection of basilar skull fractures, as do thin dedicated cuts through the temporal bone. The fracture line may be visualized directly or by indirect evidence such as blood in the sphenoid sinus, the mastoid air cells, or the auditory canal or fracture of the posterior wall of the maxillary sinus.

Because fracture fragments often tear the underlying dura, leakage of CSF through the nose (rhinorrhea) or ear canal (otorrhea) is common. If the tympanic membrane remains intact, a hemotympanum may be seen. Battle's sign occurs because of tracking of blood through the mastoid air cells to the skin behind the ear, which appears ecchymotic. This sign is often delayed many hours and may not be

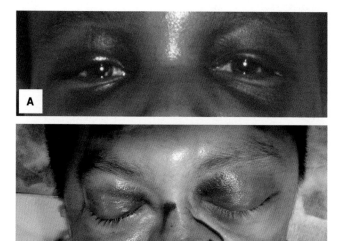

Figure 1.8 Physical exam findings indicative of basilar skull fracture of the anterior cranial fossa. (A) Patient with bilateral periorbital ecchymosis (raccoon eyes), due to fracture of the base of the anterior skull fossa. (B) Bilateral raccoon eyes and massive epistaxis with balloon tamponade in a patient with severe basilar skull fractures, severe traumatic brain injury, and associated coagulopathy.

apparent on initial examination. Similarly, raccoon eyes appear sooner but become increasingly evident with time and may not be apparent on initial examination.

Treatment of a basilar skull fracture is conservative unless cranial nerve injury mandates surgical decompression. In the presence of a basilar fracture in anterior cranial fossa, a nasogastric tube should never be inserted because of the risk of getting into the brain through the fracture. In these cases an orogastric tube is preferable. Although meningitis can ensue from a persistent CSF leak, prophylactic antibiotics are not indicated. About 90% of the dural tears heal within 1 week. Persistent leakage beyond 2 weeks may require operative repair with a dural patch.

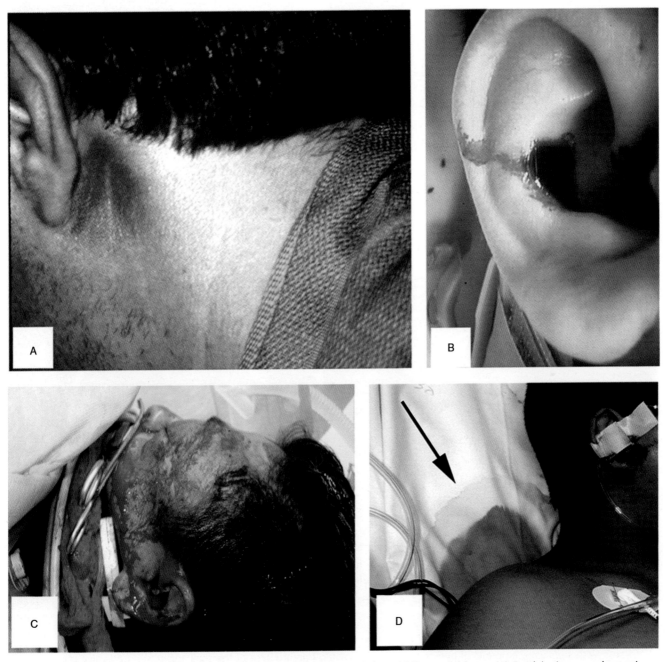

Figure 1.9 Physical exam findings indicative of basilar skull fracture of the middle cranial fossa. (A) Battle's sign – ecchymosis over the mastoid process, indicating basilar fracture and tracking of blood through the mastoid air cells. (B) Bloody otorrhea following basilar skull fracture of the middle cranial fossa with rupture of tympanic membrane. (C) Massive basilar fracture of the anterior and middle cranial fossae with severe epistaxis requiring balloon tamponade and bloody otorrhea. (D) Bloody otorrhea, arrow reveals the "halo effect" or "double ring sign" of CSF separating from blood when applied to the sheet. This sign can also be seen when the bloody drainage is applied to a paper towel or filter paper.

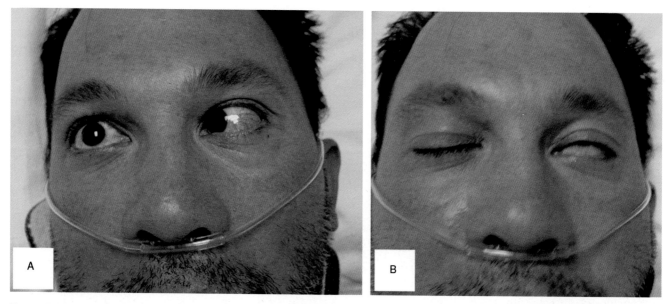

Figure 1.10 Complications in basilar skull fractures. (A) Patient with basilar skull fracture with fixed medial gaze indicative of right cranial nerve VI injury (abducens nerve). (B) The same patient has ptosis indicative of cranial nerve VII (facial nerve) compression.

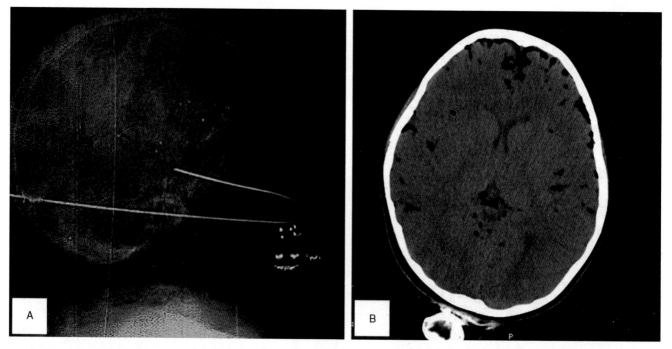

Figure 1.11 Iatrogenic complications in basilar skull fractures. (A) Plain x-ray showing a nasogastric tube inserted in the brain through a fracture of the anterior cranial fossa. In the presence of such fractures, an orogastric tube should be inserted. (B) CT scan with significant amounts of pneumocephalus following fracture base of the skull and use of bag-valve mask by the paramedics.

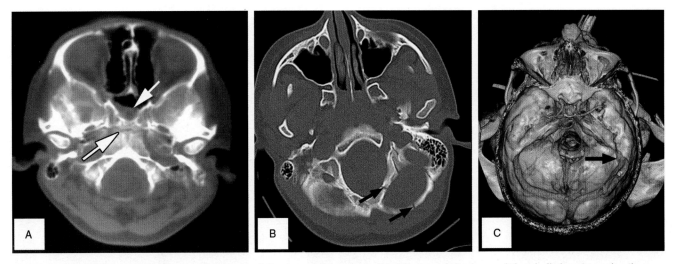

Figure 1.12 Radiological diagnosis of fractures of the base of the skull. (A) CT scan of the base of the skull showing a basilar skull fracture (bottom arrow) and isolated air–fluid level in the sphenoid sinus (top arrow), which is characteristic of basilar skull fracture. (B) CT scan with occipital basilar skull fractures. (C) CT scan showing 3-D reconstruction shows basilar skull fracture (arrow).

1.3 Intracranial Hematomas

Epidural Hematoma

Epidural hematoma (EDH) accounts for approximately 10–15% of severe head injuries, with the peak incidence in young adult males between the ages of 15 and 24. Common etiologies include motor vehicle accidents, auto versus pedestrian accidents, and sports injuries. The typical EDH is unilateral and occurs as a result of a temporoparietal skull fracture that transects the course of the middle meningeal artery. Blood accumulates outside the dura mater, dissecting the dura from the inner table of the skull and compressing underlying brain as it expands under arterial pressure.

The classical pattern is that of an initial head trauma with loss of consciousness due to concussion, followed by a lucid interval as the patient recovers from the concussion, with a subsequent decreased level of consciousness due to mass effect from the accumulating EDH. However, only 30% of patients with EDH demonstrate this classical pattern. The duration of the lucid interval is highly variable, and most patients are not completely asymptomatic during this interval. Because the bleeding is under arterial pressure, it generally accumulates quickly, causing a mass effect with shift of the ipsilateral hemisphere and, eventually, transtentorial herniation. Some small

EDHs never progress to this stage and can be managed conservatively.

The diagnosis of EDH is based on CT scan that reliably demonstrates the typical hyperdense

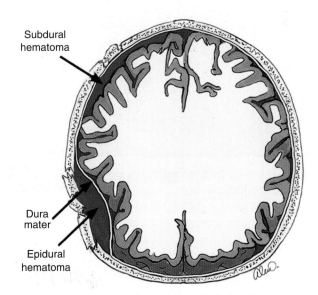

Figure 1.13 Illustration of epidural and subdural hematomas: The epidural hematoma is lenticular in shape located between the skull and the dura mater. The subdural hematoma is crescent-shaped and located between the dura matter and the brain parenchyma.

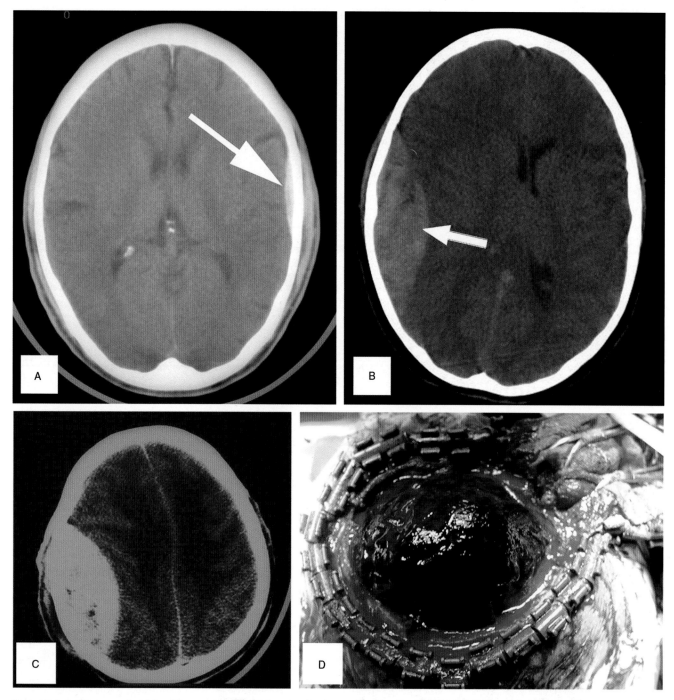

Figure 1.14 CT scans of epidural hemorrhages progressing in size and mass effect. (A) Subtle left parietal EDH without mass effect; arrow reveals lenticular space occupying hyperdense lesion. (B) EDH in the right parietal area (arrow) with narrowing of right ventricle and midline shift. (C) Massive acute right parietal EDH with a mass effect and increased intracranial pressure. (D) Intraoperative appearance of a large EDH. The hematoma is on top of the dura mater.

accumulation of blood in a lenticular shape at the periphery of the cerebrum, indenting the cerebral cortex and brain parenchyma. Outside of the posterior fossa, the hematoma will not cross suture lines, as the dura is tightly adherent at suture lines. CT scan is indicated in patients who have a history of a potentially severe mechanism of head injury with loss of consciousness, evidence of a skull fracture, or a less than normal GCS on initial examination.

The diagnosis may not be apparent on the initial CT scan if the patient suffers from severe anemia (lowering the density of the hematoma on CT scan) or has severe hypotension (which reduces the rate of arterial blood loss), or if the CT scan is obtained too soon after the trauma (before a significant amount of blood has accumulated). Approximately 8% of EDHs are detected after a significant delay. Occasionally EDH may result from tears of venous sinuses or veins, and the accumulation of blood occurs more slowly.

Treatment of EDH is surgical evacuation of the clot and repair of the vessels or dural sinus involved. Patients who are not in coma at the time of presentation usually recover very well, as often there is little underlying brain damage. Mortality ranges from none to 20% in various series.

Subdural Hematoma

Subdural hematoma (SDH) is divided into three categories based on the time elapsed since the injury. These categories are acute SDH (0–24 hours), subacute SDH (1–7 days), and chronic SDH (>7 days). The importance of this distinction is that the appearance of the hemorrhage on CT scan varies with time as it moves from a solid hyperdense clot (acute SDH) to an intermediate or isodense phase in which the hematoma is often indistinguishable from adjacent normal brain tissue (subacute SDH). After approximately 5–10 days a chronic phase begins in which the cellular elements of the hematoma break down and are reabsorbed, leaving a fluid-filled encapsulated hypodense mass

(chronic SDH). Radiographic interpretation has to take these sequential changes into account.

SDH accounts for approximately 40% of cases of severe head injury. It is found in all age groups, but certain populations are at higher risk for SDH, including the elderly, chronic alcoholics, patients who are anticoagulated, and infants (shaken baby syndrome).

Symptoms of SDH depend on multiple variables, including the size and location of the SDH, the rate of accumulation of blood, the degree of underlying brain injury, the extent of cerebral atrophy, and the premorbid level of functioning. Acute SDH results from either a direct blow to the head resulting in cortical brain damage and bleeding or acceleration/deceleration forces causing avulsion of the bridging veins from the dura to the surface of the brain, resulting in accumulation of blood beneath the dura. This collection of blood is seen on CT scan as a hyperdense semilunate (crescent-shaped) hematoma that conforms to the convexity of the cerebral hemisphere. Depending on the size of the hematoma and the degree of underlying cerebral edema, a mass effect will occur with obliteration of the ventricles and cisterns and shift of cerebral structures across the midline that may culminate in transtentorial herniation. Because of underlying cortical damage, patients will often demonstrate contralateral focal neurologic deficits consistent with the location of the SDH. Additional

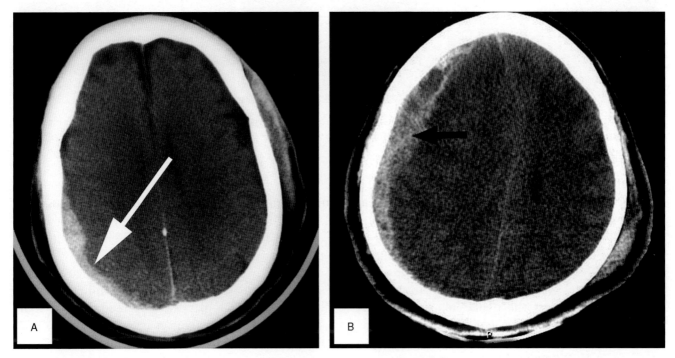

Figure 1.15 Axial CT scans of subdural hemorrhages. (A) Small right parieto-occipital acute SDH without mass effect (arrow). (B) Right SDH (arrow) with left cephalohematoma demonstrating coup–countrecoup injury. Note the significant midline shift.

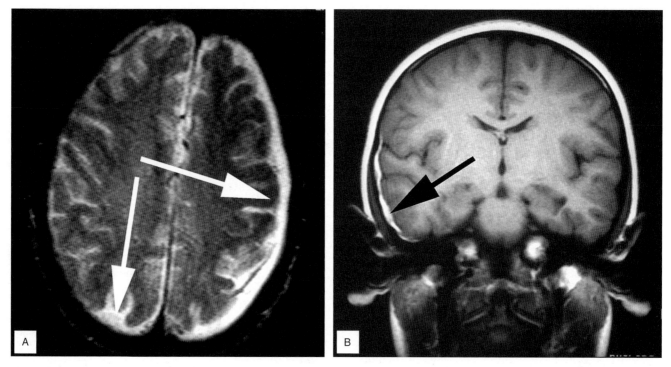

Figure 1.16 MRI appearance of acute subdural hemorrhages. (A) Axial image of a right frontotemporal "rim subdural" (arrow A) and a left parieto-occipital contrecoup contusion (arrow B). (B) Coronal image showing a temporal rim SDH (arrow).

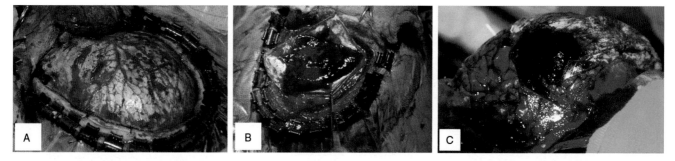

Figure 1.17 Acute subdural hematomas. (A) Intraoperative appearance of a large acute SDH, after removal of the cranium. Note the tense dura with engorged vasculature. (B) Intraoperative appearance of a large acute SDH after opening the dura. (C) Autopsy appearance of a large acute SDH.

symptoms include altered mental state, headache, nausea and vomiting, and other symptoms related to increased intracranial pressure.

As the SDH persists beyond 5–7 days, resorption of cellular elements results in loss of density of the hematoma. At some point (usually from 5–10 days), the density of the hematoma will be very similar to that of the adjacent brain parenchyma, making it difficult to distinguish with standard CT scan exposures. In some cases, only subtle evidence of mass effect such as compression of the ipsilateral ventricle will suggest the presence of an SDH.

Slight differences in density can be magnified by altering the Hounsfield units of the CT scan exposure, and these "subdural windows" may be diagnostic. Alternatively, a contrast-enhanced CT scan can be done in which the isodense hematoma will appear less dense than the contrast-enhanced adjacent brain. MRI may also be used and in some series have an increased sensitivity for intracranial hemorrhage compared to CT scan. Symptoms at this stage include headache, diminished concentration and alertness, and variable focal neurologic deficits.

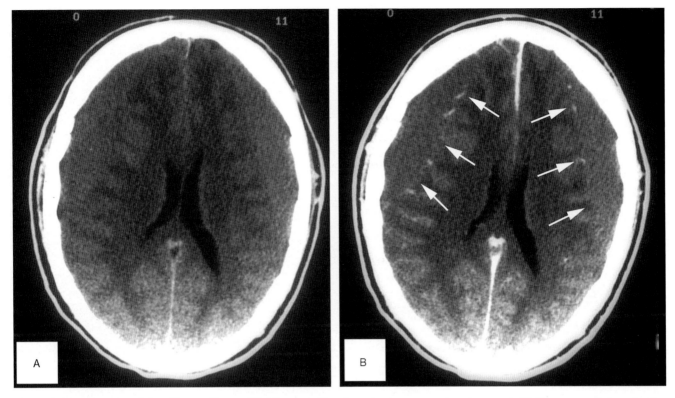

Figure 1.18 Subacute subdural hemorrhage. (A) CT scan without contrast appears almost normal. (B) However, after contrast bilateral isodense SDHs are seen (arrows) with early capsule formation medially and minimal mass effect (compression of right lateral ventricle).

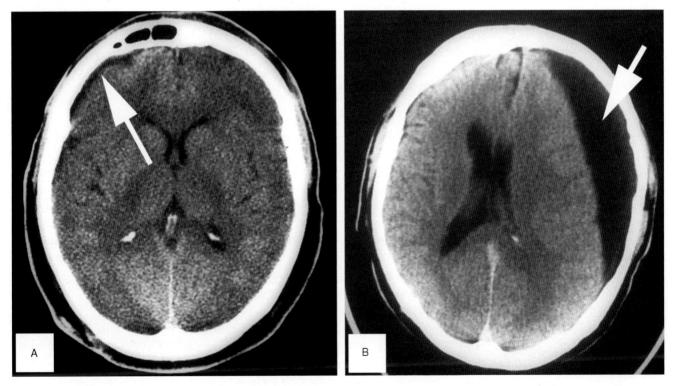

Figure 1.19 Chronic subdural hemorrhages. (A) Axial image of small chronic right frontal SDH (arrow) without mass effect. (B) Large chronic left SDH (arrow) with mass effect and left to right shift.

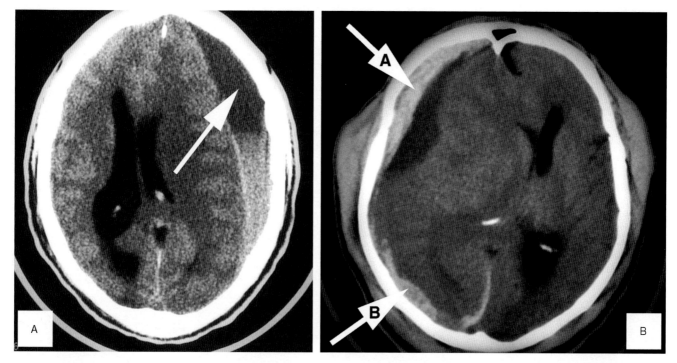

Figure 1.20 Acute on chronic subdural hemorrhage. (A) Axial image of acute on chronic SDH. The acute hemorrhage can be seen in the dependent (lower) aspect of the SDH and the chronic collection at the top (arrow). Note the significant midline shift. (B) Acute rebleeding in a chronic right frontal SDH (arrow A) and occipital areas (arrow B) and midline shift.

As the process of resorption continues beyond 2 weeks, the SDH enters a chronic phase. The SDH releases osmotically active cellular elements as it breaks down that cause the hematoma to expand. Symptoms may be very subtle or may be suggestive of increased intracranial pressure. Chronic SDH occurs more commonly in patients with significant preexisting cerebral atrophy, so that changes in mental state such as increasing confusion, disorientation, lethargy, and depression make SDH difficult to detect. In fact, the original head trauma may have been relatively minor and completely forgotten by the time the patient presents for care. There is a high risk of rebleeding into a chronic SDH so that a sudden decompensation may be the presenting complaint when this occurs. CT scan reveals a hypodense semilunate collection of fluid with a surrounding hyperdense capsule and variable amounts of cellular debris in the dependent portion of the SDH. Rebleeding is seen as a hyperdense collection of blood superimposed on an encapsulated chronic hematoma.

Treatment for a large SDH in the acute or subacute stages is evacuation via craniotomy. Small hematomas can be managed conservatively with close neurologic observation. The decision regarding management of a chronic SDH depends on the premorbid function of the individual, size of the SDH, and current symptoms. Seizure prophylaxis should be provided in all cases for the first week to decrease the incidence of early post-traumatic seizures.

Traumatic Subarachnoid Hemorrhage

Most subarachnoid hemorrhages (SAHs) occur spontaneously as a result of a rupture of an arteriovenous malformation (AVM) or berry aneurysm. However, head trauma can also result in SAH and tends to have a worse outcome than nontraumatic SAH. The SAH appears as a hyperdense collection of blood that tracks along the outer edge of the brain parenchyma beneath the arachnoid membrane. On CT scan it is seen tracking into sulci, usually in the frontal lobes. The CT scan appearance may be very subtle, and the SAH is easily missed. Typically it shows as fingerlike white projections, more obvious in the sylvian fissure. Often SAH is associated with intraventricular, subdural, and intraparenchymal bleeding, as well as with mass lesions such as SDH. The exact patient presentation

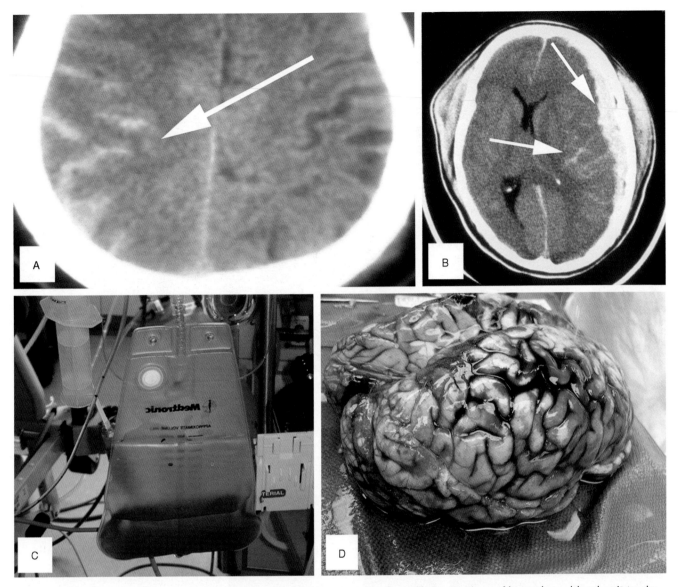

Figure 1.21 Subarachnoid hemorrhage. (A) CT scan of SAH appears like fingerlike projections of hyperdense blood as it tracks along the sulci of the posterior parietal lobe (arrow). (B) CT scan showing left parietal SAH (lower arrow), acute left SDH (upper arrow). Note the effacement of the posterior horn of the left lateral ventricle and midline shift. (C) Bloody CSF drainage from a ventriculostomy catheter in a patient with SAH. (D) Autopsy specimen of a brain with SAH seen here tracking along the sulci of the brain beneath the arachnoid membrane.

depends on the location of the hemorrhage but often includes headache, altered level of consciousness, nausea and vomiting, nuchal rigidity, coma, and, rarely, retinal subhyaloid hemorrhage.

Treatment of an isolated traumatic SAH is conservative. There is less risk of rebleeding than with SAH caused by aneurysm rupture, but trauma patients should be observed for this complication as well. During the acute phase, intense vasospasm caused by subarachnoid blood may worsen symptoms and outcome by causing ischemia in adjacent normal brain. Use of calcium channel blockers has shown some utility in reducing this vasospasm. Long-term sequelae include obstructive hydrocephalus which may require creation of a ventriculoperitoneal shunt for decompression.

Intraventricular Hemorrhage

Hemorrhage into the ventricular system is more common following hypertensive bleeds than

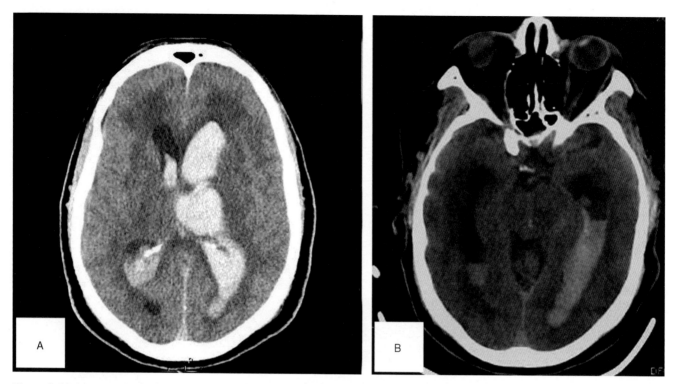

Figure 1.22 Intraventricular hemorrhage. CT scans show massive bilateral intraventricular hemorrhages.

after trauma. Occasionally blood from a traumatic lesion (e.g., SAH) will track into the ventricular system, or lacerations of the brain parenchyma may communicate directly with the ventricles. The prognosis of intraventricular hemorrhage is not as grim as in cases of spontaneous bleeding, and patients may recover well. Complications include obstructive hydrocephalus which may require placement of a ventriculoperitoneal shunt.

Intraparenchymal Hemorrhage

Direct laceration of the brain parenchyma by penetrating wounds or bone fragments may result in

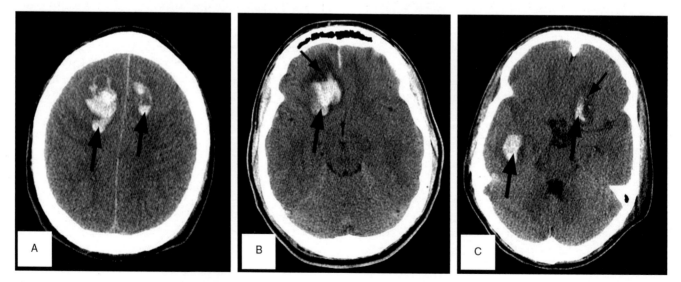

Figure 1.23 Intraparenchymal hemorrhages. (A) CT scan revealing large bilateral intraparenchymal hemorrhages. (B) CT scan of a patient with a large right intraparenchymal hemorrhage (large arrow) with surrounding penumbra of ischemic brain tissue (small arrow). (C) CT scan with two intraparenchymal hemorrhages in the right temporal and left frontal areas (large arrows), the frontal hemorrhage is surrounded by edematous brain tissue (small arrow).

hemorrhage that is relatively confined to the brain parenchyma. Bleeding in these cases is usually tamponaded by surrounding tissue but may become extensive enough to produce a midline shift. Exposure of injured brain thromboplastin to the circulation results in activation of the coagulation cascade and frequently produces DIC, which is a poor prognostic sign. Coagulopathy increases with increasing severity of brain injury, and is particularly common after penetrating injuries. This coagulopathy may be present on admission or may manifest as late as 3–4 days after injury, and as such serial examination of coagulation factors should be performed.

Cerebral Contusion

Cerebral contusion occurs as the brain parenchyma strikes fixed portions of the skull during sudden deceleration or acceleration. It is often associated with a coup–contrecoup injury and may be found relatively distant from the site of head impact. Certain locations are particularly prone to contusion: the frontal lobe striking the anterior skull and the temporal lobe striking the projections of the sphenoid bone are the two most common locations for cerebral contusion.

The clinical presentation depends on the size and location of the contusion. Frontal lobe contusions are characterized by agitation, confusion, perseveration or repetitive questioning, impaired short-term memory, and aggressiveness that often requires physical or chemical restraint.

Initially the contusion is primarily hemorrhagic. Over a period of hours to days, localized cerebral edema develops, causing a mass effect that potentially can result in transtentorial herniation. Management with diuresis and intracranial pressure monitoring is helpful with contusions that develop a mass effect. Glucocorticoids are not helpful because the edema is vasogenic in nature. Eventually the edema regresses and the hematoma reabsorbs completely or liquefies, leaving a cystic fluid-filled structure.

Cerebral contusions, especially frontal or temporal, are also characterized by a high incidence of post-traumatic seizures. Because of this, routine prophylactic treatment with anticonvulsants (e.g., phenytoin) is recommended for approximately 7 days following injury. Short courses of anticonvulsants have been shown to significantly decrease the risk of early post-traumatic seizures; in contrast, extending treatment with anticonvulsants has not been proven to be useful in prevention of delayed onset seizures or risk of post-traumatic epilepsy. Traumatic epilepsy can manifest in a delayed manner with the first reported incidence occurring greater than 1 year from injury in 50% of cases and first incidence occurring greater than 4 years from injury in up to 20% of cases.

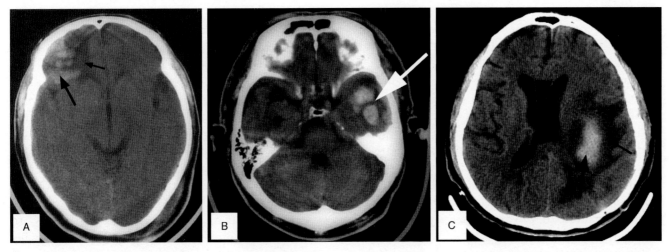

Figure 1.24 Cerebral contusion. (A) CT right frontal lobe contusion (large arrow) with surrounding edema (small arrow). (B) Axial CT scan showing a left temporal lobe contusion (arrow) with surrounding edema. (C) Axial CT scan with large left hemispheric contusion (large arrow) and surrounding edema (small arrow).

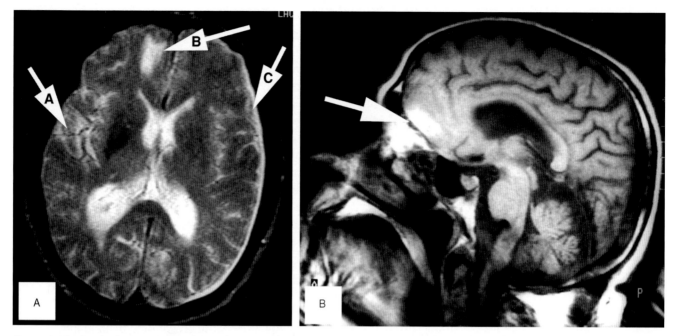

Figure 1.25 Cerebral contusion. (A) MRI images showing right frontal lobe contusion (arrow B), with large rim SDH (arrow C), and contrecoup contusion of the right temporal lobe (arrow A). (B) MRI images showing frontobasilar contusion (arrow) adjacent to frontal and ethmoid bones.

1.4 Penetrating Head Injury

The vast majority of penetrating head wounds involve gunshot wounds. These are devastating injuries that frequently result in death or profound disability in survivors. As a bullet enters the skull, it produces multiple high-velocity fragments (both from shattered skull fragments and from bullet fragmentation) that cause multiple injuries. Although the skull absorbs some kinetic energy, the bullet retains sufficient energy to cause a pressure wave once it enters brain parenchyma. This produces a rapidly expanding cavity and subsequent recoil of brain tissue. The abrupt deformation of brain tissue results in laceration and contusion of brain parenchyma, accumulation of blood in the epidural or subdural spaces, intraparenchymal bleeding, and direct laceration of brain tissue by bullet and bone fragments. Because of the high kinetic energy imparted to the brain, subsequent cerebral edema is common.

Other types of penetrating injuries involve less kinetic energy and have a better prognosis. Stab wounds, impalement injuries, and low-velocity shrapnel wounds can produce all of the same injuries but most commonly result in open skull fracture and direct laceration of brain parenchyma. Impaled

objects result from both accidental trauma and intentional injury. Many different objects may be involved, but knives and metal rods are the most common. A careful physical examination is indicated with stab wounds of the scalp to ensure that the knife blade has not broken off inside the cranium. Wounds associated with these injuries may appear very innocuous and may be missed altogether as they are often covered with matted hair. Surprisingly, many of these patients are relatively asymptomatic and often have a normal neurologic examination in spite of a dramatic presentation. Plain anteroposterior and lateral radiographs of the skull will accurately delineate the location and depth of penetration of radiopaque impaled objects. If the patient can fit into the CT scan gantry without disturbing the impaled object, the CT scan will demonstrate underlying brain injury, although metal artifact may be problematic. Impaled foreign bodies should be removed only after an angiogram to rule out a vascular injury or in the operating room, where prompt vascular control can be obtained once the object is removed.

Management depends on the overall condition of the patient. Frequently, gunshot wound victims have

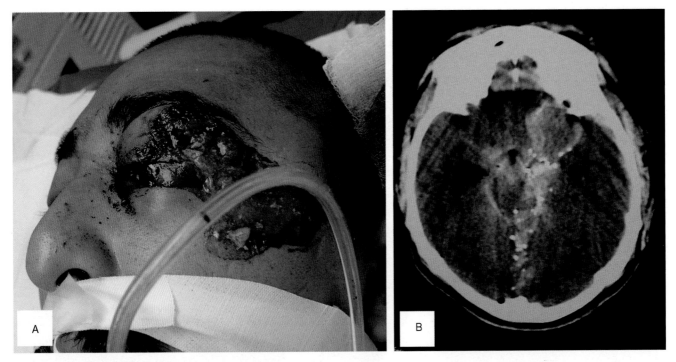

Figure 1.26 Gunshot wounds to the brain. (A) Patient with fatal gunshot with entry in the left orbit. (B) CT scan showing a massive nonsurvivable brain injury. The patient became an organ donor.

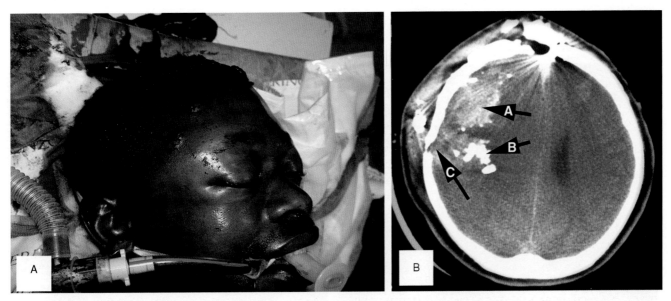

Figure 1.27 Gunshot wounds to the brain. (A) Patient with multiple gunshot wounds to the head. Note the cephalohematoma and periorbital ecchymosis. (B) CT scan of a gunshot wound showing a SDH, intraparenchymal hemorrhage (arrow A) and intraparenchymal bullet fragments (arrow B), and an open frontotemporal skull fracture (arrow C).

multiple wounds of the chest, neck, or abdomen that may take priority in terms of restoring hemodynamic stability to the patient. As with open skull fractures, bleeding from a gunshot wound of the head may be profuse, but hemorrhagic shock is uncommon with isolated head injuries, and other associated injuries

should be sought to explain the shock. Because there is open communication with the environment, an epidural hematoma associated with a penetrating injury may decompress spontaneously. Surgical debridement and control of cerebral hemorrhage may be life-saving. The incidence of post-traumatic

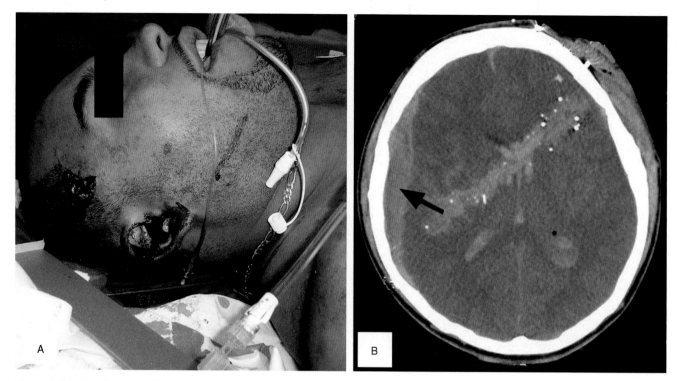

Figure 1.28 Gunshot wounds to the brain. (A) Fatal gunshot wound to the right frontotemporal area. (B) CT scan showing a nonsurvivable transaxial bullet tract, a right acute subdural hemorrhage (arrow), blood in the ventricles and metallic fragments.

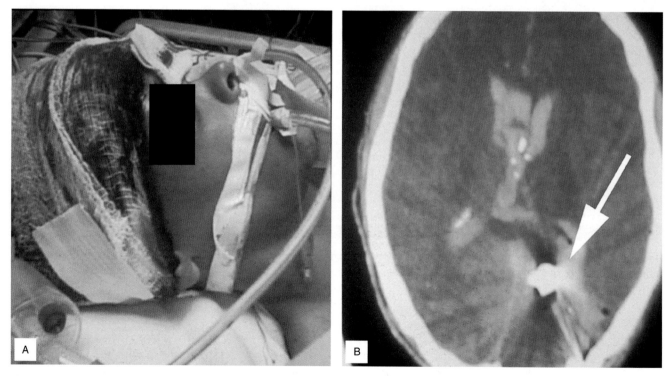

Figure 1.29 Gunshot wounds to the brain. (A) Pediatric victim with a fatal gunshot wound to the head. (B) The CT scan shows intraventricular and intracerebral hemorrhages and a bullet in the occipital area (arrow).

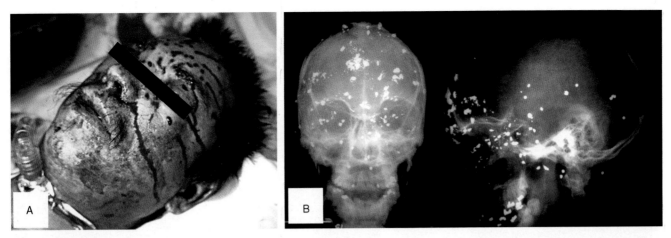

Figure 1.30 Shotgun wounds to the brain. (A) Victim of a fatal shotgun injury to the head, with multiple pellet wounds to the face and head. (B) Radiographs in the same patient showing multiple shotgun pellets of the face and skull.

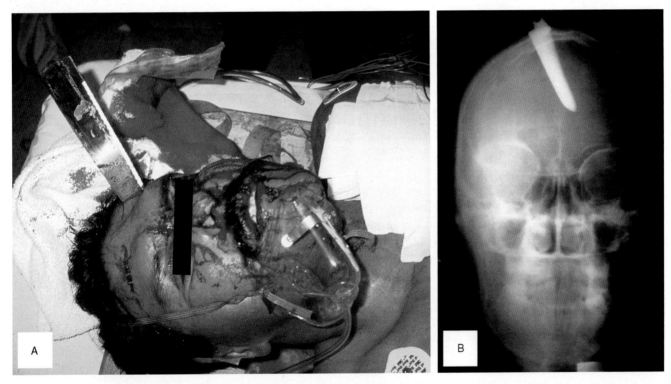

Figure 1.31 Knife injuries to the head. Foreign bodies should be removed only after an angiogram or in the operating room. (A) Stab wound to the head with an embedded knife in the frontal area. The patient was awake and alert. (B) Anteroposterior radiograph revealing the knife blade within the cranium. The knife was pulled out in the operating room without any complication.

seizures is more than 50%, and use of anticonvulsant medication is routine in these cases.

Injuries that result in exposed brain matter, especially gunshot wounds, are associated with a high incidence of coagulopathy (massive release of tissue thromboplastin from the injured brain), diabetes insipidus, hemodynamic instability, arrhythmias, hyperglycemia, and neurogenic pulmonary edema.

The prognosis after gunshot wounds to the head is poor and the mortality is higher than 90%. However, these cases should be treated aggressively because they often become organ donors.

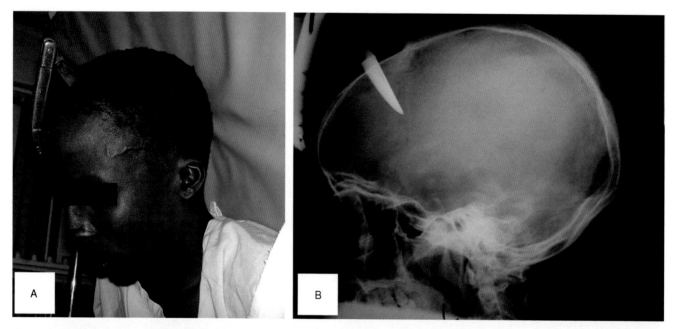

Figure 1.32 Knife injuries to the head. (A) Stab wound to the head with a switchblade impaled in the cranium. The patient is awake and alert. (B) Lateral skull radiograph revealing the knife penetrating the skull and impaled in the brain parenchyma. The knife was pulled out in the operating room without any complication.

1.5 Transtentorial Herniation

Herniation is the result of progressive expansion of one segment of the brain under the pressure of hemorrhage or edema formation, with the resultant compression and dysfunction of adjacent brain structures. If compression of the brainstem occurs, loss of vital functions such as respiration and vasomotor control result in rapid demise. There are four main types of herniation described:

1. Uncal herniation: The most common form of herniation results from edema or hematoma in one cerebral hemisphere that causes a shift of that hemisphere across the midline, under the falx, and downward across the tentorium, resulting in compression of the midbrain. The patient becomes somnolent or comatose. Compression of the ipsilateral cranial nerve III produces ipsilateral ptosis, a fixed and dilated pupil, and loss of extraocular movements. Compression of the ipsilateral cerebral peduncle results in weakness or abnormal posturing (decorticate, then decerebrate) of the contralateral limbs. In up to 30% of cases the opposite cerebral peduncle is compressed, resulting in a false localizing sign (Kernohan's notch phenomenon). Respiratory abnormalities progress from central neurogenic hyperventilation to Cheyne–Stokes breathing, to ataxic breathing, and finally to apneustic respiration.

2. Central herniation: Compression of the brainstem by a frontal or apical mass lesion that expands downward produces pinpoint pupils, downward gaze preference, and other brainstem dysfunction described previously. Bilateral motor findings (posturing, paralysis) may occur.

3. Cingulate gyrus herniation: Pressure in one cerebral hemisphere may result in herniation of the ipsilateral medial cingulate gyrus under the falx.

4. Cerebellar tonsillar herniation: Mass lesions or edema of the cerebellum can result in expansion of the cerebellar tonsils into the foramen magnum, compressing the posterior brainstem. This presents as sudden loss of consciousness and loss of brainstem function with consequent apnea and hypotension. This condition has extremely high mortality, so cerebellar lesions must be recognized before the onset of herniation to salvage the patient.

Patients who achieve hemodynamic stability should be treated with a cerebral resuscitation protocol

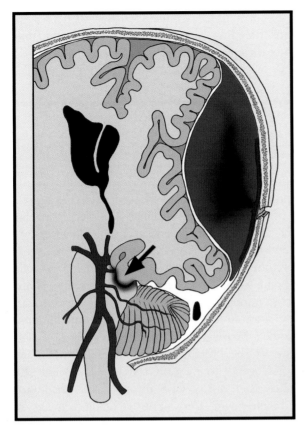

Figure 1.33 Brain stem herniation. Illustration of an epidural hematoma with acute mass effect and compression of the ipsilateral cerebral peduncle resulting in uncal herniation and compression of the brain stem (arrow).

including rapid sequence intubation (RSI), moderate hyperventilation to a pCO_2 of 35 mm Hg, osmotic and loop diuresis, sedation with cerebrally protective agents (e.g., propofol, etomidate, pentobarbital), and mild elevation of the head once the cervical spine is "cleared." Early placement of a ventriculostomy is indicated for monitoring and control of intracranial pressure by removal of CSF. Cerebral perfusion pressure is maintained by infusion of fluids and pressors if needed.

Cerebral blood flow (CBF) is governed by the relationship of mean arterial pressure (MAP) and intracranial pressure (ICP) as follows:

$$CBF = MAP - ICP.$$

Consequently, as ICP increases, every effort must be made to maintain or elevate MAP. Once ICP exceeds MAP no blood flow to the brain can occur and this is one definition of "brain death."

Complications of herniation affect all organ systems. Neurologic manifestations occur as described above, but also include derangements of the neurohormonal axis which can result in hemodynamic instability, diabetes insipidus, and dysregulation of temperature and metabolic control. Cardiac complications include tachyarrhythmias, hemodynamic lability, and electrocardiographic abnormalities. Pulmonary complications include neurogenic

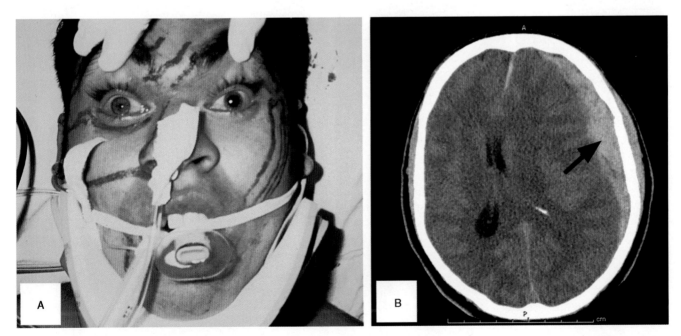

Figure 1.34 Brain stem herniation. (A) Patient with transtentorial herniation from blunt head trauma. The right pupil is constricted normally; the left pupil is fixed and dilated. (B) CT scan shows a large left subdural hematoma (arrow) with midline shift. This compression resulted in brainstem herniation.

pulmonary edema which occurs in response to the excessive catecholamine release. As mentioned earlier, release of tissue thromboplastin can result in a consumptive coagulopathy with resultant severe bleeding from minor injuries and mucus membranes.

1.6 Diffuse Cerebral Edema

Occasionally blunt head trauma results in diffuse hyperemia or edema formation rather than mass lesions (epidural or subdural hematoma, cerebral contusion). In most cases the edema is primarily vasogenic in nature, resulting from the loss of autoregulation and subsequent exposure of cerebral arterioles to the full force of arterial pressure. Transudation of plasma fluid into the extracellular compartment results in an increase in cerebral water content and swelling of the affected part of the brain. Elevated venous pressure contributes to the process of edema formation by decreasing the resorption of brain water. Progression of edema can result in herniation with brainstem compression and death.

Diffuse cerebral edema may be associated with mass lesions or may occur in isolation. It is more common in children and infants than in adults. Cerebral contusions are prone to develop severe focal edema in the surrounding tissues. Treatment is directed at decreasing brain water content with osmotic and loop diuretics, while preserving cerebral blood flow and perfusion pressure. Hypertonic saline may also be considered to reduce cerebral edema, it can be given as intermittent boluses over 20 minutes. A meta-analysis of hypertonic saline resuscitation in trauma patients demonstrated improved outcomes; however, this remains a subject of active debate in the literature. It is important when using osmotic agents to monitor sodium levels and serum osmoles. Removal of CSF through a ventriculostomy may be life-saving. Decompressive craniectomy or even brain lobectomy may also be considered in refractory cases with some hope of survival.

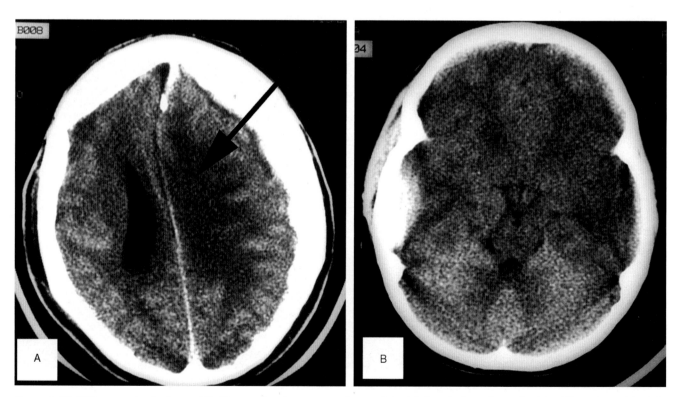

Figure 1.35 Diffuse cerebral edema. (A) CT scan showing severe edema of the left hemisphere (arrow) with obliteration of the left ventricle and midline shift. (B) CT scan with diffuse brain edema and obliteration of both ventricles.

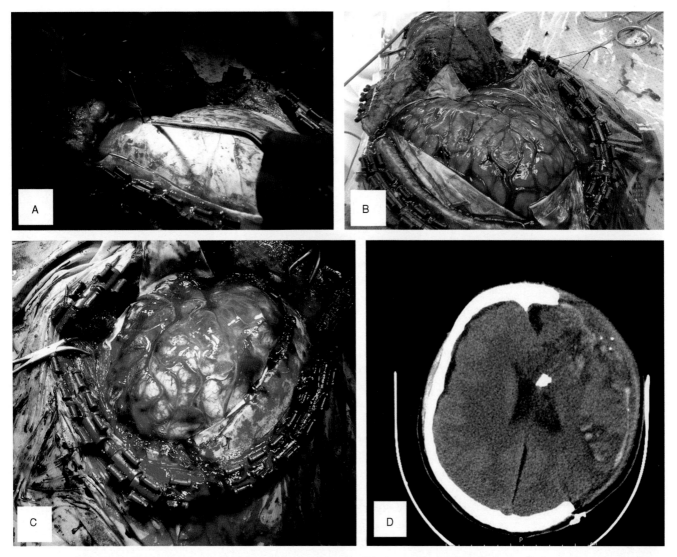

Figure 1.36 Diffuse cerebral edema. (A) Intraoperative photograph after removal of the skull shows cerebral edema with tense and bulging dura. (B) Edematous brain bulging from the cranium after release of the dura with engorged cerebral vasculature. (C) Brain material bulging beyond the cranial vault with herniation through the craniectomy site. (D) CT scan of the same patient with herniation of the brain beyond the edges of the craniectomy site.

1.7 Pediatric Head Injury

Children commonly sustain injury to the head for several reasons. First, young children in the course of exploring their environment are often oblivious to the dangers of certain situations (e.g., fall from a window or down a flight of stairs, wandering into traffic). Second, they are often less agile in escaping a dangerous situation than older children or adults. Third, the size and mass of a child's head relative to the body is much greater than in adults. Consequently, children are commonly thrust forward or fall headfirst, and the major impact is often onto the head. Finally, children are at the mercy of their caregivers and may be physically abused. Abuse in infants often takes the form of violent shaking of the baby and can result in characteristic patterns of injury known as the shaken baby syndrome or shaken impact syndrome.

Physiologically, the child's skull is more compliant than that of adults because it is less densely calcified and has unfused sutures that allow movement of one section of the skull on another. In spite of this, skull

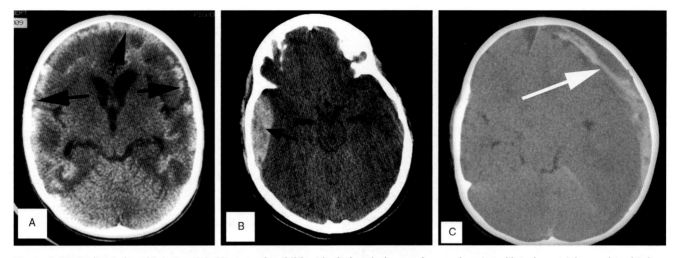

Figure 1.37 Pediatric head injuries. (A) CT scan of a child with shaken baby syndrome showing dilated ventricles and multiple cortical calcifications (arrows) suggestive of multiple previous SDHs. (B) Large epidural hematoma (arrow) in a 10-year-old patient. (C) CT scan of the head of a child with shaken baby syndrome showing a chronic SDH with acute rebleeding on the left (arrow), as well as diffuse cerebral edema and compressed ventricles.

fractures are still relatively common in children. Because of the greater compliance of the skull, more kinetic energy can be transmitted directly to the brain during trauma. Cerebral contusion and subdural hematomas are common injuries. EDHs are relatively more common in young children because of the loose adherence of the dura to the inner table of the skull.

Children are less susceptible to mass lesions than adults and more frequently develop diffuse cerebral hyperemia or diffuse edema as their principal injury pattern. Because of this propensity for diffuse hyperemia, mannitol is used with caution in young children with evidence of elevated ICP following head trauma. Mannitol causes a transient increase in cerebral perfusion and expands the vascular compartment temporarily before exerting its diuretic effect. Many authors recommend using loop diuretics and mild hyperventilation rather than mannitol when managing elevated ICP in a young child.

Another injury that occurs almost exclusively in children with head trauma is transient cortical blindness. The actual incidence of this complication is unknown but is thought to be secondary to vasospasm induced by trauma. Children also manifest cerebral concussion differently from adults. The "infant concussion syndrome" consists of the transient appearance of pallor, diaphoresis, vomiting, tachycardia, somnolence, and weakness, often occurring in an infant after relatively minor head trauma (e.g., falling off a changing table). CT scan is invariably normal, and the child often will make an equally dramatic recovery while still in the emergency department. Small infants may bleed sufficiently into the head to develop hemorrhagic shock, although this is rare. Separation of cranial sutures, a bulging fontanelle, or increasing head circumference may rarely be the initial clues to head injury in infants, but the diagnosis of serious head injury is generally made by CT scan.

The principal concern in evaluating children with head trauma is to consider the possibility of nonaccidental trauma. A history incompatible with the severity of injury or that involves activities that the child would be developmentally incapable of performing can be an initial clue that the injuries may be due to abuse.

1.8 Diffuse Axonal Injury

Diffuse axonal injury results from disruption of neurons at the interface of gray matter and white matter in the brain due to sudden deceleration or acceleration injuries of the head. Gray matter has greater mass than white matter because of higher water content and, as a result of greater momentum during sudden deceleration, continues farther than white matter, producing shear forces at the gray–white interface. The resultant

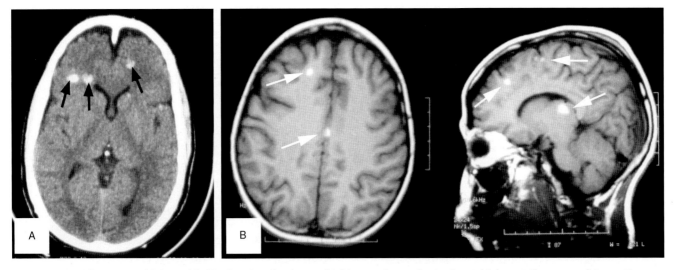

Figure 1.38 Diffuse axonal injury. (A) CT showing focal petechial hemorrhages in the frontal lobes at the gray–white matter junction (arrows) in a patient with diffuse axonal injury. (B) MRI showing multiple high-intensity focal hemorrhages (arrows) including those at the gray–white matter interface in a patient with diffuse axonal injury.

tearing of neurons produces neurologic dysfunction. Patients with extensive axonal shear injury present in profound coma that sometimes continues as a persistent vegetative state. Initial diagnosis is difficult as many other causes of coma must also be considered, including intoxication, encephalopathy, hypoglycemia, hypovolemic shock, and brainstem injury. Patients with less extensive areas of axonal shear injury may regain consciousness fairly rapidly (within 24 hours). More severe injuries may also heal over long periods of time, and occasionally a patient with this type of injury will awake after months of coma.

The CT scan in patients with diffuse axonal shear injury is often misleadingly normal or near normal. Findings include petechial hemorrhages seen mainly in the central part of the brain (corpus callosum, basal ganglia, and other medial structures). There may be additional, more evident injuries as well, such as EDH or SDH. MRI is more sensitive in delineating the extent of axonal disruption.

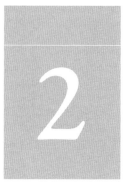

Facial Injury

Edward J. Newton

Introduction

Soft tissue injuries of the face are common in modern society. The majority of serious injuries occur in the context of vehicular trauma or assaults. Use of seatbelts and airbags has decreased the frequency but not eliminated facial trauma produced by motor vehicle accidents. In addition to direct impact of the face against the windshield, steering wheel, or dashboard, broken glass fragments frequently produce lacerations and eye injuries.

The lower face and neck contain structures that define and maintain the integrity of the airway. Consequently, facial injuries at times assume the highest priority in trauma management until airway patency and adequate ventilation can be established. Because facial tissues are highly vascularized, severe bleeding into the oral cavity can occlude the airway, especially when patients are obtunded from head injury or intoxication. In the presence of massive bleeding, airway compromise may be produced by placing the patient supine for spinal immobilization. Blood, secretions, fragments of teeth, and foreign bodies must be removed to avoid aspiration and airway occlusion. Although severe facial injuries are dramatic and often distract the inexperienced clinician from more critical tasks, treatment of most facial injuries can safely be deferred until life-threatening problems have been addressed.

The face and scalp also contain many structures that are essential for the special senses of sight, smell, taste, and hearing. Human communication is dependent not only on facial structures required for speech and hearing but also those involved in facial expression. In addition, many facial landmarks define human appearance, and their preservation is important cosmetically and psychologically. Injury to those structures can result in devastating disability which often can be avoided with early detection and repair.

Special attention is indicated in repairing facial injuries. Debridement of wound margins should be minimized, cartilaginous structures should be preserved, and fine sutures with minimal inflammatory properties should be used in closing the wounds. Complex lacerations involving delicate and essential facial structures such as the eyelid should be referred to a specialist.

Clinical Examination

1. Examination of the face

After completion of the primary survey, the face is examined for areas of swelling and tenderness that can indicate underlying fractures. Palpation of the facial bones for crepitus or abnormal motion can locate a fracture. Grasping the teeth and pulling forward can demonstrate Le Fort fractures with abnormal motion of the alveolar ridge, midface, or whole face. Lacerations are noted, and massive bleeding is tamponaded by direct pressure. Blind clamping of bleeding sites is dangerous in that it can injure nerves and other structures that run in proximity to vessels. Lacerations crossing the path of the parotid duct mandate examination of Stensen's duct in the mouth. Facial asymmetry can be due to direct trauma but also to facial nerve injury, and an assessment of the muscles of facial expression and facial sensation is made. In comatose patients corneal reflexes should be tested to assess these functions.

2. Examination of the eye

Anatomically, the orbit sits relatively protected by the orbital ridge, the malar prominence, and nose. The ciliary and corneal reflexes rapidly close the eyelid adding further protection to direct contact with the globe. Injuries to the eye range from minor (e.g., corneal abrasion) to critical (e.g., ruptured globe).

Examination of the eye and its adnexa is an important part of the secondary survey. Victims of motor vehicle crashes often have fragments of glass that can become embedded in the eye causing lacerations or corneal abrasions. Occasionally a patient's refractory agitation can be cured by treatment of corneal abrasion or removal of glass fragments in the eye that were initially unsuspected. Often patients have massive soft tissue swelling around the eye that makes examination difficult. In these cases devices to hold the eyelid open must be used and can be improvised by bending paperclips into blunt retractors and gently retracting the lids. Formal measurement of visual acuity may not be possible in the early phases of resuscitation but an initial estimate of vision can be made by having the patient count fingers or report light perception. Complete loss of vision in a previously normal eye requires immediate consultation with an ophthalmologist. The pupils are examined for symmetry and equality as well as reaction to light. The conjunctivae are assessed for foreign bodies and chemosis that can indicate rupture of the globe. A "peaked" pupil is highly suspicious for rupture of the globe, and the "peak" often points to the site of rupture. Visible scleral or corneal lacerations may indicate penetration of the globe by a foreign object and require radiographs or CT of the orbits to detect intraocular foreign bodies. The position of the globe in the orbit is noted for enophthalmos (blowout fracture) or exophthalmos (retro-orbital hematoma). Inability to perform all extraocular movements may indicate a brain lesion, cranial nerve injury, or entrapment of extraocular muscles. Lacerations involving the lacrimal duct and lid margins should be noted and referred to an ophthalmologist for repair. A brief fundoscopic exam is performed to assess the position of the lens and the presence of blood in the anterior chamber (hyphema) or retina.

3. Examination of the ear

The ear is inspected for the presence of lacerations or hematoma. Cartilaginous lacerations or avulsion require particular attention. The ear canal is examined with an otoscope for bleeding or CSF otorrhea indicating a ruptured tympanic membrane and basilar skull fracture. The tympanic membrane is examined for perforations or accumulation of blood in the middle ear that is seen as hemotympanum. Although it may take many hours to appear, inspection of the mastoid area for Battle's sign is important in detecting basilar skull fracture.

4. Examination of the nose

The nose is inspected for lacerations of overlying skin and of the cartilage. The presence of nasal fracture is often obvious clinically with deformity, crepitus, epistaxis, and tenderness to palpation. The nares are inspected for the presence of epistaxis and hematoma and for CSF drainage.

5. Examination of the mouth

The mouth is inspected for lacerations, avulsion or fracture of teeth, swelling of the tongue and oral mucosa, and misalignment of the teeth (indicating a mandible or maxilla fracture). Blood, loose teeth, and foreign bodies are removed manually or by suction. Simultaneously, an evaluation of the airway is made examining for stridor, dysphonia, gagging or drooling, and inability to handle oral secretions. The presence or absence of a gag reflex in obtunded patients often influences the decision to intubate the patient to protect against aspiration.

Investigations

After physical examination has indicated areas of suspected injury, specific radiographs or CT scans may be indicated to delineate injuries. Plain radiographs are useful in detecting most facial fractures and in locating radiopaque foreign bodies, but CT scan can more accurately identify these if the patient is sufficiently stable to undergo this examination. Certain radiographic views are indicated to clarify specific clinical findings such as a submentovertex view to detect zygomatic arch fracture or Panorex views for suspected mandible fractures. Leakage of CSF from the nose or ear can be assessed by examining the drainage for the presence of glucose (indicating CSF) or for a double ring sign when the drainage is applied to filter paper. Suspicion of injury to the lacrimal duct is best confirmed by an ophthalmologist using fine probes. Installation of fluorescein into the conjunctival sac and examination with a UV light source can demonstrate corneal abrasion, and Seidel's test can demonstrate leakage of aqueous humor from a ruptured globe. A detailed evaluation of the anterior chamber can be performed on stable patients using a slit lamp examination. Patients with suspected post-traumatic glaucoma or retro-orbital hematoma should undergo tonometry to measure the intraocular pressure, but this test should never be done if there is a possibility of a ruptured globe. Parotid duct laceration can be demonstrated by probing the duct or by performing a sialogram.

General Management

Airway management is of prime importance when facial injuries threaten the ability to ventilate the patient. Suction of secretions and manual removal of foreign bodies may establish airway patency, but often endotracheal intubation is indicated. Nasotracheal intubation should not be attempted with nasal, basilar skull, or Le Fort fractures or in apneic patients. Patients with massive facial injuries present a special problem, and the management of the airway in these cases is controversial. Use of paralytic agents to facilitate intubation may cause loss of airway patency, as the patient's voluntary effort to maintain an airway is lost. Consequently, some advocate the use of awake orotracheal intubation in these cases. This is a difficult and often unsuccessful task in an agitated, possibly hypoxic patient with severe bleeding in the oropharynx. Others have demonstrated the safety and efficacy of using rapid sequence intubation with paralytic drugs in this setting. The decision on the method of intubation should be based on the experience of the physician and the facilities of the emergency room. In selected cases in no need of immediate airway establishment, awake fiberoptic intubation by an experienced anesthesiologist or otolaryngologist is an excellent alternative. In all cases a physician should be immediately available to perform a cricothyroidotomy, if conventional intubation fails. Massive facial injuries that distort anatomic landmarks and produce severe bleeding may make orotracheal intubation impossible. Prolonged attempts at intubation are detrimental to the patient, and early use of cricothyroidotomy is essential and often life-saving. All physicians managing trauma should be familiar with this technique.

Facial injuries that do not threaten the airway can safely be deferred to the secondary survey and definitive care phases of trauma management. Active bleeding can usually be controlled by direct pressure or packing of wounds. However, prolonged bleeding from facial or scalp wounds can result in hemorrhagic shock and should not be ignored. Treatment of facial fractures can be deferred until the patient is hemodynamically stable.

Minor eye injuries (e.g., corneal abrasion, rust ring, eyelid laceration) can be deferred, but sight-threatening injuries should be dealt with immediately and consultation with an ophthalmologist is essential. Once the possibility of a ruptured globe has been established, the eye should be protected by use of a Fox shield or similar device to prevent further pressure on the globe. Retro-orbital accumulation of blood or air with deteriorating vision or massive elevation of intraocular pressure requires decompression by lateral canthotomy or creation of a communication from the retro-orbital space into the maxillary sinus. Entrapment of extraocular muscles by fractures should be relieved urgently.

Penetrating trauma of the ear is relatively uncommon and is managed by minimal debridement, irrigation, and primary closure. Blunt trauma is more common and often results in perichondrial hematoma formation. Because ear cartilage is dependent on its skin covering for blood supply, an interposed hematoma can result in ischemic necrosis of the cartilage. Consequently, the ear must be examined for this condition, and a hematoma should be aspirated. A pressure dressing is applied to prevent reaccumulation of the hematoma or abscess formation.

Avulsed cartilage from the ear or nose should be preserved in saline, as it is difficult to recreate the shape of these organs with other tissues.

Most facial fractures can be repaired electively with operative fixation and bone grafting if necessary. Intraoral lacerations are repaired with absorbable sutures. Antibiotics are unnecessary for most facial lacerations, although open fractures require prophylactic coverage.

Common Mistakes and Pitfalls

1. Severe oromaxillofacial trauma can produce delayed airway occlusion from swelling or bleeding. These patients should be intubated early or observed carefully in a monitored environment.
2. Attempts to perform endotracheal intubation in the presence of extensive facial trauma, without being prepared to perform a cricothyroidotomy, if intubation fails. The results can be catastrophic!
3. Failure to account for missing teeth. The missing teeth might be in the bronchial tree and cause a lung abscess.
4. Blind clamping of bleeding sites is rarely successful and it can injure nerves and other structures that run in proximity to vessels.
5. Injury to the cranial nerves is difficult to detect in severely injured patients, especially if they are comatose, intoxicated, or otherwise unable to cooperate with physical examination. Reassess again during the tertiary survey.

2.1 Eye Injuries

Corneal Abrasion

In spite of brisk protective reflexes, corneal abrasion is common. The usual cause is the patient's own finger as the eye is rubbed to relieve itching or remove a foreign body. Other causes are scraping by branches or twigs, broken glass, industrial injuries involving power grinders and saws, or welding without adequate eye protection. Clinically, the patient presents with a history of sudden onset of pain in the affected eye and the sensation of having a foreign body in the eye, with increased tearing and resultant blurred vision. Physical examination is often normal unless the eye is examined using a UV light source with magnification after fluorescein dye is instilled onto the conjunctival sac. If the patient is capable of sitting, ideally the examination should be with a slit lamp. Otherwise the examination can be made using a portable source of UV light such as a Wood's lamp. Areas of abrasion on the corneal surface show increased dye uptake and appear intensely fluorescent under UV light. The patient will experience complete relief of the pain after instillation of anesthetic drops onto the affected cornea. Treatment is supportive as most corneal abrasions heal within 48 hours.

Antibiotic drops are prescribed, oral analgesia with nonsteroidal anti-inflammatory drugs (NSAIDs) is appropriate, and tetanus vaccination should be updated if necessary. The use of eye patches is controversial but generally considered unnecessary for small abrasions.

Ocular Foreign Bodies

There are certain situations that merit special caution in dealing with apparent corneal abrasions. Patients who present with symptoms of corneal abrasion after high-speed grinding or hammering on metal should be suspected of having a perforated globe. Small fragments of metal can enter the eye at high speed, leaving only minimal evidence of their entry into the globe. CT scan of the orbit is indicated to locate these foreign bodies, as plain films are less sensitive. A metal foreign body that impacts the cornea at lower speed may become embedded in the cornea and produce a rust ring that can impair vision if it occurs in the visual axis. These should be removed electively after 1–2 days, when they are less adherent to the cornea. A retained wood foreign body is also important to detect, as fungal enophthalmitis can result.

Hyphema

Hyphema is the accumulation of blood in the anterior chamber of the eye. With the patient lying supine, the blood is less visible than in an upright position, when it forms a clearly visible layer of blood in the dependent portion of the anterior chamber. The initial bleeding usually resorbs without complication. However, in up to one-third of cases rebleeding will occur 2–5 days after the initial injury. Complications from hyphema include hemosiderin staining of the inner surface of the cornea with resulting loss of vision, as well as post-traumatic glaucoma due to fibrotic occlusion of the canals of Schlemm. Treatment is conservative and consists of bed rest with head elevated, sedation, and monitoring of intraocular pressure. Surgery is required occasionally for evacuation of blood or to decompress the anterior chamber.

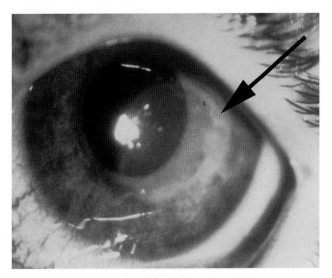

Figure 2.1 Photograph of corneal abrasion, after instillation of fluorescein dye showing bright yellow–green uptake of dye lateral to the pupil (arrow).

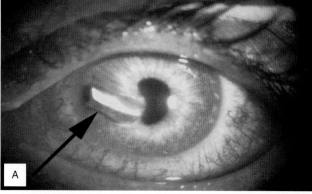

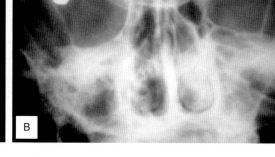

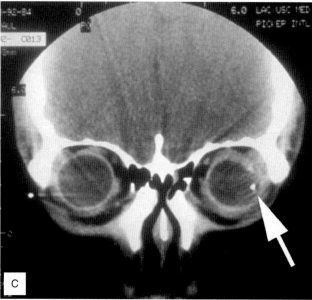

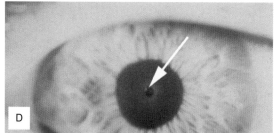

Figure 2.2 (A) Photograph of the eye showing a metallic foreign body on the cornea deforming the iris and the pupil (arrow). (B) Plain radiograph showing an intraocular bullet (arrow). (C) CT scan of the orbit showing one small intraocular foreign body of the left eye (arrow), and another lateral to the right orbit. (D) Photograph of the eye showing a central rust ring in the cornea (arrow). This rust ring is in the visual axis and will seriously impair vision if not removed.

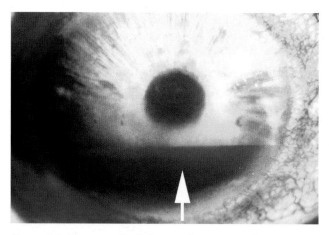

Figure 2.3 Photograph of the eye showing a collection of blood pooled (hyphema) in the inferior aspect of the anterior chamber (arrow).

Ruptured Globe

Rupture of the globe usually occurs after penetrating injury but can be caused by blunt trauma as well. Penetration of the sclera results in herniation of orbital contents through the wound and exposure of the choroid membrane, visible as a dark layer of tissue in the wound. Penetration of the cornea allows leakage of vitreous humor through the wound. In either case, distortion of the globe results in loss of functional vision at the time of injury although light perception may be preserved. Patients report pain and often resist eye examination.

Signs of globe rupture include enophthalmos, loss of eyeball turgor, a peaked pupil that points

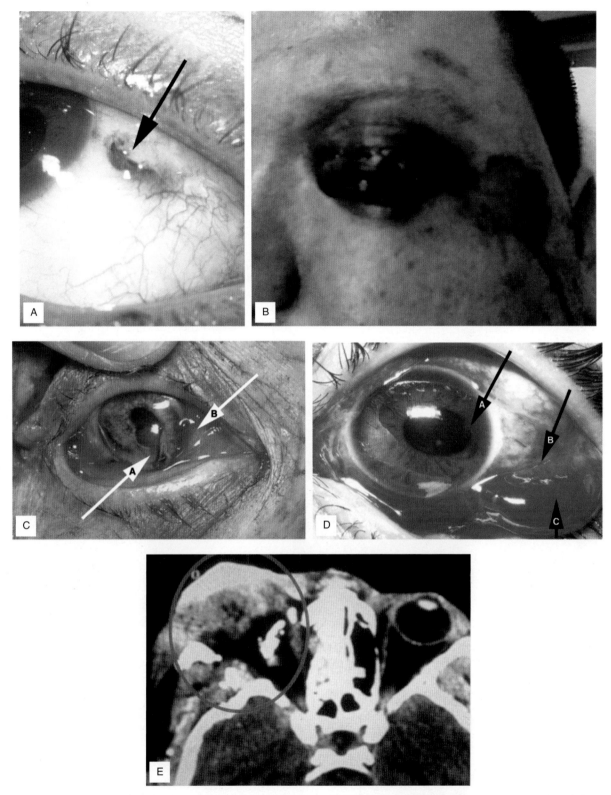

Figure 2.4 (A) Photograph of the eye showing a scleral laceration with exposure of the choroid (arrow). This is highly suggestive of rupture of the globe. (B) Photograph of a patient with a ruptured globe from blunt trauma. (Courtesy Manon Kwon, MD.) (C) Photograph of an irregular peaked pupil (arrow A), bulging chemosis (arrow B), and laceration of the iris due to a ruptured globe. (D) Photograph of a ruptured globe with a peaked pupil (arrow A), laceration of the inferior/lateral sclera (arrow B), and bulging chemosis (arrow C). The peak in the pupil points toward the laceration. (E) Gunshot wound of the right orbit with extensive destruction of the bone structures and the eye globe.

toward the site of injury, loss of pupillary reactivity, and a positive Siedel's test. The latter is performed by instilling fluorescein dye into the conjunctiva and observing the dye clearing from the cornea or sclera in the area of rupture because of the flow of aqueous humor from the anterior chamber. Although intraocular pressure is reduced in the presence of a ruptured globe, tonometry or any other maneuver that increases pressure on the globe is contraindicated. The conjunctiva is very distensible and often becomes edematous after trauma, resulting in bulging chemosis which frequently limits complete examination. Because of its common association with rupture of the globe, bulging chemosis itself should be considered a sign of possible ruptured globe. The ruptured globe is commonly enucleated if sight cannot be restored to avoid development of a sympathetic ophthalmoplegia in the normal eye.

Retrobulbar Hematoma

Trauma to the globe can result in bleeding from retro-orbital vessels including the ophthalmic artery and vein. In addition, fractures of the orbit that communicate with paranasal sinuses can result in the accumulation of air in the retro-orbital space. If air or blood accumulates under sufficient pressure, ischemic necrosis of the optic nerve can occur. Clinical evidence of this condition includes proptosis, impaired extraocular movements, and progressive loss of vision. Tonometry will indicate elevated intraocular pressure.

Treatment of a symptomatic retrobulbar hematoma is by lateral canthotomy or by surgically perforating the floor of the orbit to allow decompression of the retrobulbar space. In a lateral canthotomy, the lateral canthal ligaments are grasped with a forceps and crushed. Iris scissors are then used to divide the ligament, allowing the globe to protrude forward. If this is done in a timely

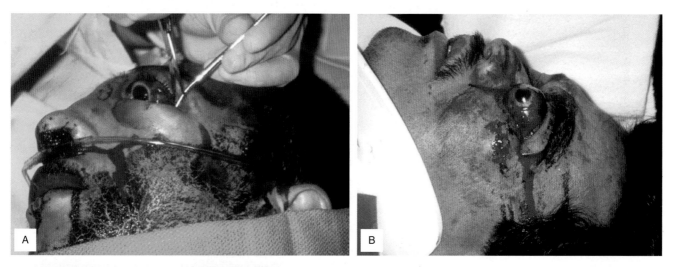

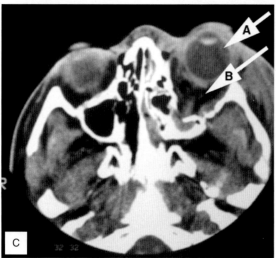

Figure 2.5 (A) Photograph of a lateral canthotomy in progress. (B) Photograph showing increased proptosis of the eye after lateral canthotomy. Allowing the eye to protrude further decreases the retrobulbar pressure on the optic nerve. (C) CT scan of the orbit showing proptosis (arrow A), retro-orbital blood and air (arrow B), and a fracture of the posterior orbital wall.

manner, normal vision can be restored once the globe is repositioned and the canthal ligament is repaired. Patients experience diplopia after repair of a lateral canthotomy but the brain gradually adapts and restores normal binocular vision over a period of months. Alternatively, a forceps can be introduced beneath the globe and the floor of the orbit fractured to allow drainage of the retro-orbital space into the maxillary sinus.

2.2 Periorbital Lacerations

In addition to the globe itself, there are numerous structures in the adnexa of the eye that merit special consideration. The lacrimal system ensures that a constant flow of tears stream across the surface of the eye, maintaining lubrication to facilitate ocular motion, preventing desiccation, and clearing debris, including potential infectious agents. Lacerations involving the lacrimal apparatus, lid margins, and lacrimal duct must all be sought out and referred to an ophthalmologist for repair. Lacerations of the lid margins are reapproximated exactly under microscopic vision to avoid a step-off that can result in constant dripping of tears onto the face. Injury to the lacrimal duct at the medial canthus of the eye is important to detect and repair as scarring and stenosis of the duct can result in a similar problem. Delayed repair of a stenotic lacrimal duct is very difficult and yields suboptimal results in most cases.

Laceration of the eyebrow is common and can be repaired in the ED. Exact alignment is essential to preserve facial expression. Consequently, the eyebrows should never be shaved in preparation for suturing as the alignment landmarks will be lost. Repair of each layer of tissue is done independently in a layered closure to preserve the mobility of the brow.

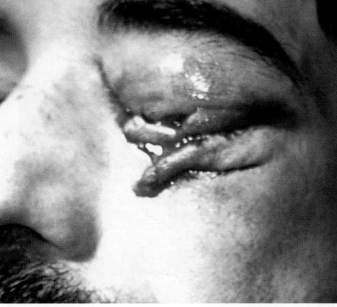

Figure 2.6 Photograph of a complex laceration of the eyelid that involves the lid margin.

2.3 Facial Fractures

Orbital Blowout Fracture

Blunt impact to the orbital area is common. The globe itself is usually spared when large objects strike the face because of protection afforded by the malar prominence, nose, and superior orbital ridge. However, smaller objects can strike the globe directly, resulting in a massive rise in intraocular pressure.

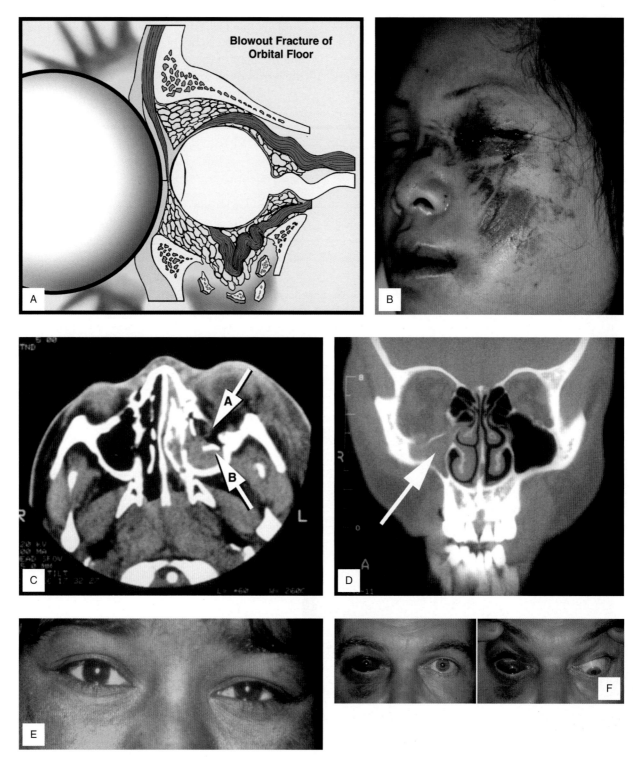

Figure 2.7 (A) Illustration showing typical mechanism of injury that produces an orbital blowout fracture. (B) Photograph of a patient with blunt trauma to the orbital area from an airbag deployment, who proved to have an orbital blowout fracture. (C) CT scan of the orbits showing fracture of the posterior/inferior orbital wall (arrow A) with herniation of orbital contents into the maxillary sinus on the left (arrow B). (D) CT scan showing fracture of the inferior orbital wall with opacification of the right maxillary sinus (arrow). (E) Photograph of a patient with blowout fracture showing enophthalmos of the left eye. (F) Photographs of a patient with blowout fracture of the right eye and subconjunctival hemorrhage. There is no evidence of divergent gaze with the eyes in neutral position. Downward gaze reveals entrapment of the extraocular muscles of the right eye, resulting in a subtle divergent gaze.

This pressure is transmitted to the bony orbit, often resulting in fracture at its weakest points, the orbital floor and the medial wall of the orbit (lamina papyracea). Fracture of the orbital floor by this means is called a "blowout fracture." This injury typically occurs in certain sports activities such as racquetball, lacrosse, boxing, and baseball but may also be seen in blunt eye trauma of any type. The patient presents with enophthalmos and pain in the orbital area. A common complication of this injury is that the inferior rectus muscle becomes entrapped in the fracture fragments, resulting in restricted upward gaze and diplopia when the patient attempts to look upward. Consequently, it is essential that physical examination should verify that extraocular movements are intact. Finding an entrapped inferior rectus muscle mandates surgical repair.

Plain radiographs of the face seldom reveal the actual orbital floor fracture. The characteristic finding is opacification of the maxillary sinus caused by herniation of periorbital fat and blood into the sinus. CT scan reveals the herniation as well, and special reconstructions of the orbit may reveal the fracture in detail.

Mandible Fracture

Fractures of the mandible are common after blunt facial trauma. The most common etiologies are vehicular-related trauma and assaults. Fractures are distributed almost equally between the condyles, angle, and body of the mandible. Clinically, patients present with swelling and tenderness over the fracture site. Dysarthria and drooling are common because any movement of the jaw is painful. Maximal incisor opening (normally 5 cm) is reduced, and the patient will note malocclusion of the teeth if the fracture fragments are displaced. Typically, the patient cannot hold a tongue blade with his teeth against the examiner's pull. At times bony crepitus can be elicited by examination or with voluntary movement of the mandible. Inspection of the mouth often reveals that the fracture is open, with gingival lacerations overlying the fracture site. Airway obstruction can occur in unconscious patients with bilateral mandibular rami fractures, as the tongue is unsupported and falls back into the posterior pharynx. Trauma to the temporomandibular joint is common and may result in dislocation of the joint or chronic pain with chewing.

Plain films are usually adequate to reveal a mandibular fracture, particularly if it is displaced. However, a Panorex view of the jaw is more accurate and should be used if available. CT scan is not indicted for a suspected isolated mandible fracture but these fractures are readily visible on facial CT scans obtained for complex facial injuries. Treatment is operative, with wiring or plating of the fracture fragments into anatomic position. Open fractures of the mandible should be treated with antibiotics that are active against mouth flora (e.g., penicillin or clindamycin) because osteomyelitis and abscess formation can occur.

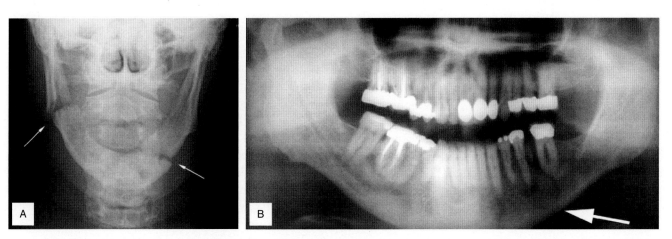

Figure 2.8 (A) Anteroposterior radiograph of the mandible showing bilateral displaced fractures of the angles of the mandible (arrows). (B) Panorex view of the mandible showing an undisplaced fracture of the left mandibular ramus (arrow).

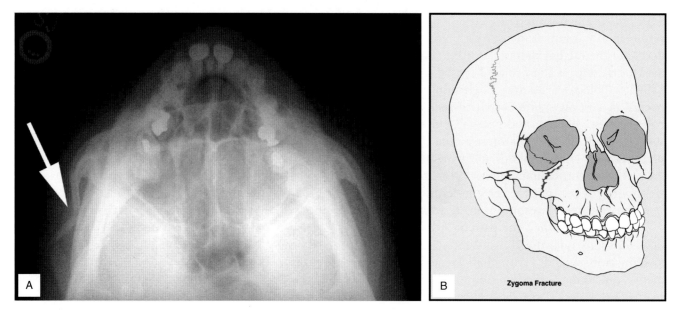

Figure 2.9 (A) Submentovertex plain radiograph showing a depressed right zygomatic arch fracture (arrow). (B) Illustration outlining a tripod fracture of the zygoma (see Figure 2.10E as well).

Zygoma Fractures

The zygoma provides the bony support to the cheek and thus is commonly implicated in blunt trauma to the face. Because of its arched structure, comminuted fractures are typically seen. Associated injury to the infraorbital nerve should be sought out. The patient typically presents with loss of the malar prominence on the affected side and this is best appreciated by looking at the patient's face from above. In the acute phase, however, swelling may mask this finding, so careful palpation of the facial bones to detect pain, a bony step-off, and crepitus of the zygoma should be routine. Injury to the infraorbital nerve may occur and results in anesthesia of the upper lip. Impingement of the zygoma onto the coronoid process of the mandible may result in limited excursion of the mandible and trismus. Diagnosis is made by plain radiographs. The submentovertex view (or "bucket handle" view) clearly demonstrates fractures of the zygoma and should be ordered if this fracture is suspected clinically. Treatment of displaced zygoma fractures is surgical elevation of the fragments to restore a normal facial contour.

A more complex zygoma fracture is the tripod fracture which involves fractures at the origins of the zygoma, resulting in a large triangular fragment. The fractures occur at the zygomaticofacial and zygomaticofrontal sutures and through the inferior orbital foramen. The result is a free-floating fragment of bone that often requires surgical repair. Because the fracture often involves the infraorbital foramen, hypesthesia of the ipsilateral midface down to the upper lip is often present.

Le Fort Fracture

Le Fort fractures result from high-energy facial trauma and are classified according to their location. Le Fort II and III fractures are potentially life-threatening in that they are commonly associated with airway compromise, massive bleeding, basilar skull fracture, and intracranial injury. Nasal intubation and nasogastric tubes must be avoided in these patients, as fatal intracranial insertion may result. Patients often have combinations of injuries such as Le Fort II on one side with Le Fort I on the other.

Le Fort I This fracture separates the upper alveolar ridge from the face and extends into the nasal fossa. Clinically, the patient will have mobility of the upper teeth when they are grasped and pulled forward. Airway compromise is rarely associated with this fracture.

Le Fort II The Le Fort II fracture separates the midface from the skull, resulting in a pyramid-shaped large fragment of the central maxilla and nasal bones. Pulling

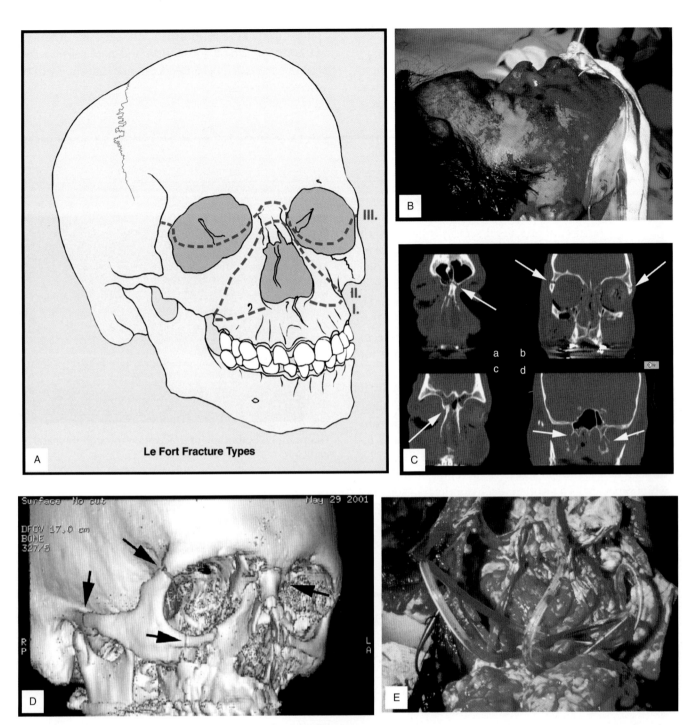

Figure 2.10 (A) Schematic showing three types of Le Fort fracture. (B) Photograph of a patient who had a garage door crush his face. The abnormal concavity of the face ("dish face") is characteristic of a Le Fort III fracture. (C) CT scan of the face showing Le Fort III fracture: (a) anterior ethmoid fracture (arrow); (b) mid ethmoid and lateral orbit fractures (arrows); (c) frontal sinus fracture (arrow); (d) pterygoid fractures (arrows). (D) CT scan 3-D reconstruction of a Le Fort III fracture showing multiple fractures, including a tripod fracture of the zygoma (arrows). (E) Photograph at autopsy of a nasogastric tube coiled intracranially.

on the upper teeth demonstrates mobility of the entire midface. Radiographs reveal fracture lines through both maxillae extending upward to include the nasal bones. Associated basilar skull fracture is common, and

CSF rhinorrhea can occur. Massive epistaxis may require nasal packing or surgery to control the bleeding.

Le Fort III The most severe form of Le Fort fracture results in complete craniofacial dissociation due to fractures of both maxillae, zygomas, nasal bones, ethmoids, and vomer, as well as bones at the base of the skull. Complications such as intracranial injury, airway compromise, basilar skull fracture, cervical spine injury, CSF rhinorrhea, and massive epistaxis are common. Nasal intubation and nasogastric tubes should be avoided because of the risk that they will be inserted intracranially.

2.4 Nasal Injuries

Superficial lacerations of the nose are common and easily repaired, but several serious injuries merit discussion. Laceration extending through nasal cartilage must be repaired in separate layers using absorbable sutures for the cartilage repair. Avulsed cartilage should be preserved in saline if repair can be done urgently or in a subcutaneous pocket if repair is delayed. Reconstruction of the nose can be done in delayed fashion, but finding appropriate cartilage for reconstruction is difficult.

Nasal fractures may be treated conservatively if undisplaced. Deviation of the septum or impairment of nasal breathing is an indication for repair within the first week after injury. Open fractures should be treated with antibiotics. The nasal septum should be inspected for the presence of a septal hematoma, which appears as a swollen, ecchymotic area separating the nasal mucosa from underlying cartilage. The septal hematoma must be drained and the nose packed to avoid reaccumulation of the hematoma.

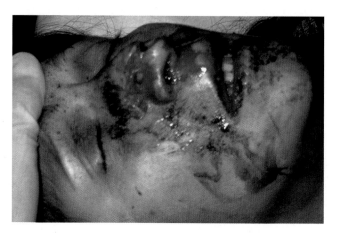

Figure 2.11 Photograph of a laceration through the nasal cartilage.

Because the blood supply to the cartilage depends on the nasal mucosa, increasing the distance for diffusion causes ischemic necrosis of the cartilage, and eventually a saddle-nose deformity results.

2.5 Penetrating Facial Trauma

While the vast majority of facial trauma is blunt in nature, penetrating wounds of the face due to gunshots, stab wounds, and impalement injuries are not uncommon.

The face is divided into three zones, each with structures at particular risk from penetrating injury. Zone I extends from the hairline to the superior orbital ridge and includes the ears. Injuries in this area are at risk for intracranial penetration and wounds of the frontal sinuses are at risk for serious infection. Zone II extends from the superior orbital ridge to the upper lip. Wounds in this zone are at risk for arterial injury, globe damage, and airway compromise. Zone III extends from the upper lip to the hyoid bone. Injuries in this area are at high risk for airway compromise and carotid artery injuries.

The first priority in examining patients with penetrating facial trauma is to establish the patency of the airway. If suction of blood and debris from the airway does not restore adequate air exchange, orotracheal intubation is indicated. Endotracheal intubation under these circumstances is difficult because of distorted anatomy and copious bleeding into the oropharynx. Surgical cricothyroidotomy may be required. Arterial bleeding may be readily apparent as pulsatile hemorrhage of bright red blood but more often is apparent indirectly. Arterial injury is often inaccessible to vascular clamping or even direct pressure if it occurs deep to the bony facial structures. For example, an injury within the maxillary sinus may present as massive oral bleeding or epistaxis. The presence of an expanding or pulsatile hematoma is another indication of potential vascular injury.

Diagnosis of penetrating injuries relies heavily on CT scanning. In addition to a head CT, specific views of the orbits and facial bones may be indicated. CT angiography is indicated for suspected vascular injuries. Location of missiles is important because the irregular angles of facial bones and the base of the skull can deflect bullet fragments away from their expected course.

Treatment of penetrating facial injuries ranges from simple wound care and suturing of superficial lacerations to operative repair of more extensive injuries. Early debridement and operative fixation of fractures can be undertaken if the patient is sufficiently stable. Examination of the parotid duct, branches of the facial nerve, and major vessels is best done in the operating room. In rare cases, uncontrollable hemorrhage may require ligation of the ipsilateral external carotid artery.

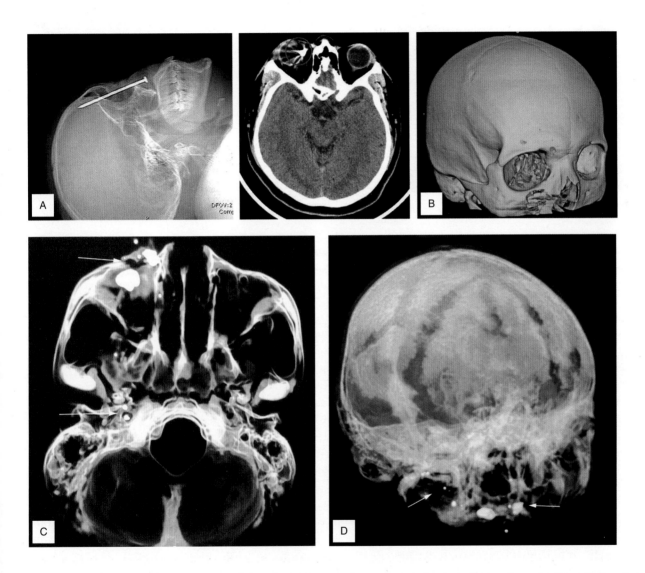

Figure 2.12 (A) CT scout film of the head showing a large nail penetrating through the face into the frontal lobe of the brain (left). The patient complained of diplopia and a 5 mm infraorbital entrance wound. He stated he had fallen off his bicycle 2 days earlier. CT scan of the same patient showing the metal foreign body medial to the globe. There was a small laceration of the globe but the patient's sight was preserved and there were no apparent neurological deficits (right). (B–E) CT scan reconstructions showing a gunshot wound of the face with a complex fracture of the zygoma and a bullet path through the orbit (B); CT reconstruction showing bullet fragments impacted at the anterior maxillary wall and extending posteriorly to the base of the skull (arrows) (C); CT reconstruction highlighting the bullet fragments (D); CT scan 3-D reconstruction showing extensive facial and cranial fractures (E).

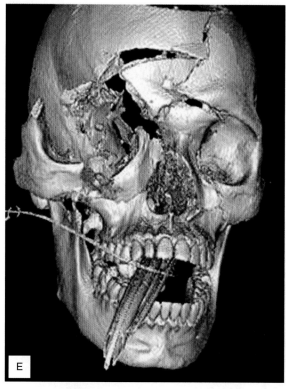

E

Figure 2.12 (*cont.*)

2.6 Complex Oromaxillofacial Trauma

Massive facial injury can result from blunt force trauma or penetrating injury from gunshot or shotgun wounds. The primary challenge in these cases is to secure an airway. Massive facial injury can result in airway obstruction either by loss of the supporting bony framework of the face or by accumulation of blood, debris such as fractured teeth, edema, or tissue flaps that occlude the larynx. Immediate restoration of a patent airway is the highest priority in trauma management. Initially, simple airway maneuvers such as chin lift, suctioning blood and secretions, and placement of an oral airway should be attempted. If these are unsuccessful in restoring air flow, a definitive airway must be obtained rapidly. Orotracheal intubation is difficult because of massive bleeding and edema, distorted anatomic landmarks, and debris, including avulsed teeth, fragments of bone, and bullet fragments. Use of paralytic agents for orotracheal intubation may cause loss of voluntary muscle maintenance of a patent airway, but on the other hand, will facilitate intubation in a struggling, hypoxic patient. Attempted awake orotracheal intubation, although often recommended in these cases, is similarly extremely difficult and usually unsuccessful. Consequently, use of a cricothyrotomy is often the only viable choice to establish a patent airway and should be employed early in the management.

Once the airway is secured, the spine is immobilized and the remainder of the primary survey and resuscitative interventions are completed. Massive facial injuries are dramatic and often distract clinicians from a systematic primary survey. Unless there is massive bleeding present, repair of the vast majority of facial injuries can be deferred until the patient is stable. Repair of facial lacerations can produce surprisingly good results, providing that tissue has not been avulsed and the arterial supply is intact. Debridement of tissue should be kept to a minimum, and tissues should be closed in layers, with individual muscle layers, subcutaneous tissues, and skin closed separately. Fine sutures with minimal inflammatory properties are used to close the skin. Revision of wounds should attempt to orient wounds parallel to the natural wrinkle lines

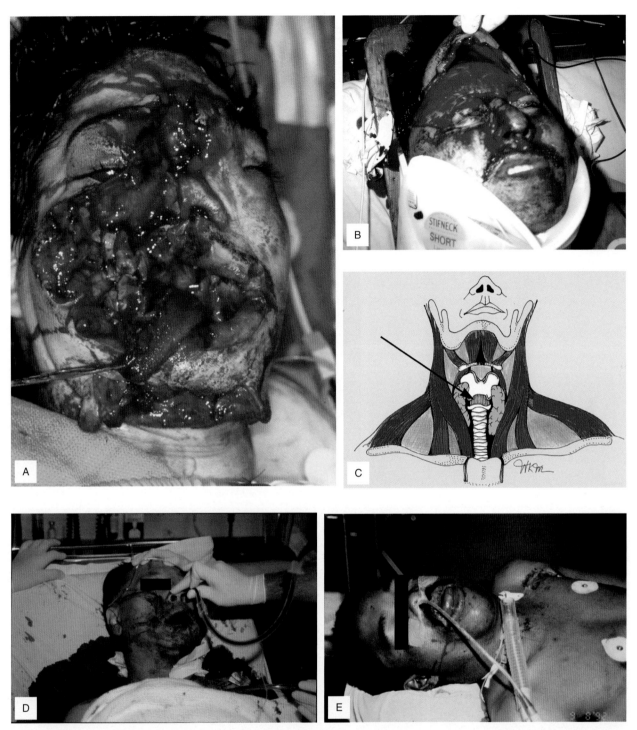

Figure 2.13 (A) Photograph of a patient with a shotgun wound of the face. Airway management is extremely difficult in these cases, as anatomic landmarks are severely distorted. (B) Photograph of a patient with avulsion of the scalp. Primary suturing is usually highly successful because of the excellent blood supply of the scalp. (C) Emergency cricothyroidotomy: schematic showing the cricothyroid membrane (arrow) and its relationship to the thyroid cartilage (above) and the cricoid cartilage (left). The cricothyroidotomy incision may be transverse or vertical, about four fingers above the suprasternal notch (right). Tracheostomy tube secured in place (right). (D) Fiberoptic endotracheal intubation in a patient with gunshot wound of the face and extensive hematoma and bleeding. (E) Gunshot wound to face with a large hematoma causing airway obstruction. The patient required an emergency cricothyroidotomy.

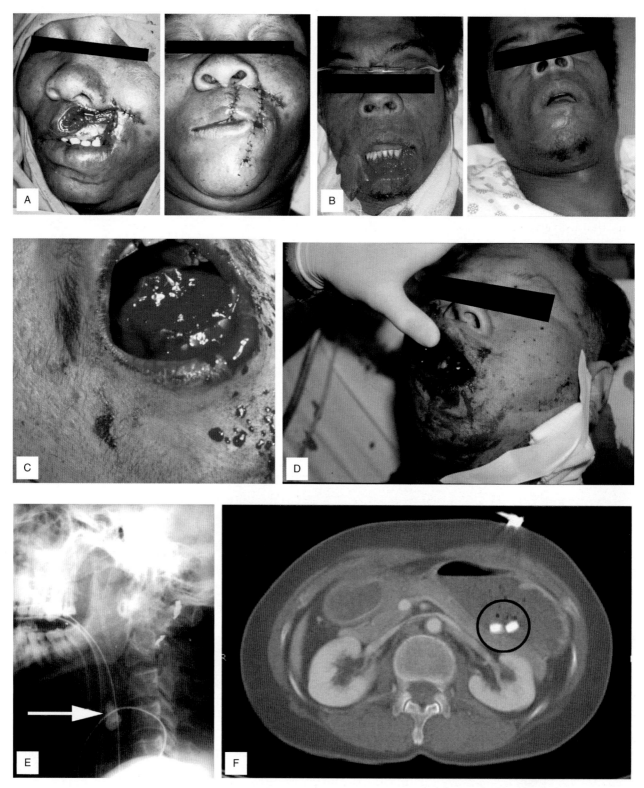

Figure 2.14 (A) Photographs of a patient with a complex facial laceration involving loss of tissue from the upper lip with avulsion of almost half the upper lip (left). After careful alignment of the vermilion border and restoration of the "cupid's bow," an acceptable cosmetic result is obtained (right). (B) Photographs before (left) and after (right) repair of a complex laceration of the lower lip caused by a human bite. An acceptable cosmetic result is obtained. (C) Amputation of the distal tongue caused by a human bite from the patient's girlfriend. (D) Patient with gunshot wound to the mouth and missing teeth. This patient should undergo radiological evaluation of the neck, chest, and abdomen to locate the missing teeth. (E) Lateral radiograph of the soft tissues of the neck showing an aspirated tooth anterior to C-4. (F) CT scan showing two avulsed teeth in the stomach.

of the face, as these scars will be less noticeable. Scars that are perpendicular to the natural wrinkle lines are much more apparent.

Oral Trauma

Lacerations of the lips occur commonly as the lip is crushed between a striking object and the underlying teeth. Because the blood supply to the lips is excellent, uncomplicated healing is the rule. However, care must be taken to properly align lacerations that traverse the vermilion border because even minor misalignment in this area is noticeable and disfiguring.

Intraoral lacerations should be repaired using soft, absorbable sutures. With through-and-through lacerations involving the skin and mucosal surfaces of the mouth, the mucosal laceration is repaired first, followed by skin closure. Lacerations of the tongue should be repaired using absorbable sutures after removal of clots and irrigation of the wound. Because of its rich vascularity, the tongue is capable of massive swelling, and delayed airway compromise is possible.

Missing teeth should be accounted for and x-rays of the neck, chest, and abdomen should be obtained in the appropriate cases. In cases of aspiration in the trachebronchial tree endocopy and removal of the tooth should be performed in order to avoid serious infectious complications in the lung.

2.7 Facial Nerve Injury

Penetrating facial trauma can occasionally result in transection of the facial nerve as it courses through the face. The facial nerve exits the base of the skull, enters the face just anterior to the tragus of the ear, and continues as a large trunk for approximately 1 cm before it subdivides

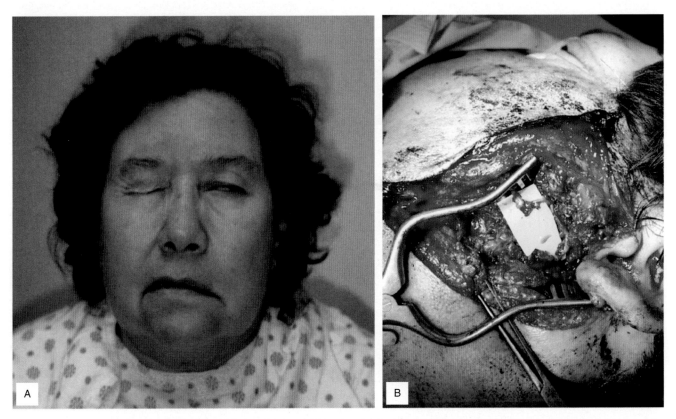

Figure 2.15 (A) Photograph of a patient with facial nerve injury on the left side showing loss of the left nasolabial fold, incomplete eyelid closure, and facial droop. (B) Intraoperative photograph showing a transected facial nerve.

extensively into smaller branches. Lacerations in the vicinity of the tragus should prompt careful examination of the muscles of facial expression because facial nerve injury is frequently missed during the initial examination of patients with multiple trauma. Injury of the smaller branches of the facial nerve may also merit exploration and surgical repair depending on the severity of the deficit. Care should be taken to moisten the conjunctivae with artificial tears to avoid desiccation and ulceration of the cornea due to incomplete closure of the eyelid.

2.8 Parotid Gland Injury

The parotid gland lies anterior to the tragus of the ear and extends to the midpupillary line external to the maxilla. Lacerations of the parotid gland may result in delayed sialocele or salivary cutaneous fistula. Laceration of the parotid duct, however, commonly results in persistent fistula. The parotid duct courses through

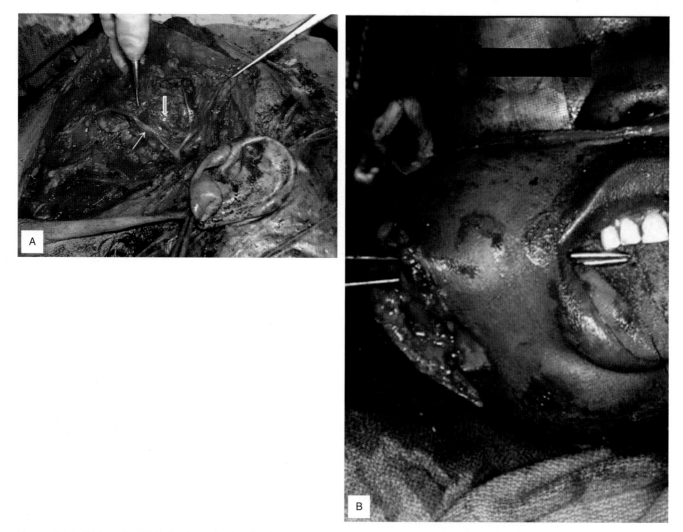

Figure 2.16 (A) Repair of inferior branch of right facial nerve (white arrow) and right parotid duct (wide arrow) following transection from facial laceration (courtesy Dr. U. Sinha). (B) Patient with extensive right facial nerve and parotid gland injuries. Neither structure could be repaired due to the extensive damage to the parotid gland (courtesy Dr. U. Sinha).

the parotid gland along a line drawn from the tragus to the upper lip and enters the mouth as Stensen's duct at the level of the second upper molar. Lacerations that cross this line proximal to the entry of the parotid duct into the mouth should be suspected of transecting the duct. Examination of the duct is performed by milking the parotid gland while examining Stensen's duct intraorally. Expression of saliva suggests that the duct is intact. Expression of blood or failure to express saliva suggests transection of the duct. If injury is suspected, Stensen's duct is probed retrograde, and the wound is examined for the probe. Careful surgical repair of the duct will prevent formation of a salivary-cutaneous fistula.

3 Neck Injury

Demetrios Demetriades and Lydia Lam

Introduction

Neck injuries, especially penetrating ones, are difficult to evaluate and manage because of the dense concentration of so many vital structures in a small anatomical area and the difficult surgical access to many of these structures. However, very few patients with blunt trauma and only 15–20% of cases with penetrating trauma require operative treatment. The combination of a meticulous clinical examination and appropriate investigations can safely identify those patients requiring operative treatment. Advanced trauma life support (ATLS) principles should always be followed.

During the primary survey, the following life-threatening conditions in the neck should be identified and treated:

1. Airway obstruction due to laryngotracheal trauma or compression by external hematoma.
2. Tension pneumothorax.
3. Severe active bleeding, externally or in the thoracic cavity.
4. Spinal cord injury or ischemic brain damage due to carotid artery occlusion.

During the secondary survey, the following neck pathologies should be identified and managed:

1. Occult vascular injuries.
2. Occult laryngotracheal injuries.
3. Occult pharyngoesophageal injuries.
4. Cranial or peripheral nerve injuries.
5. Small hemopneumothoraces.

Clinical Examination

Clinical examination according to a carefully written protocol is the cornerstone of the diagnosis and management. The examination should be systematic and evaluate the vessels, the aerodigestive tract, the spinal cord, the nerves, and the lungs:

1. Vascular structures: "Hard" signs and symptoms highly diagnostic of vascular trauma include active bleeding, shock not explained by other injuries, expanding or pulsatile hematoma, absent or significantly diminished peripheral pulses, and a bruit. "Soft" signs and symptoms suggestive but not diagnostic of vascular trauma include mild shock, stable hematoma, slow bleeding. The presence of a seatbelt mark in the neck is a suspicious sign of associated vascular trauma. Unexplained neurological findings (coma, hemiplegia) may be due to a vascular injury. This group of patients requires specialized vascular investigations.
2. Aerodigestive tract: Hard signs or symptoms highly diagnostic of significant laryngotracheal trauma include respiratory distress, air bubbling through a neck wound, and massive hemoptysis. There are no hard signs diagnostic of esophageal trauma. Soft signs and symptoms suspicious of aerodigestive trauma include subcutaneous emphysema, hoarseness, odynophagia, and minor hemoptysis.
3. Nervous system: The examination should include Glasgow Coma Score, localizing signs, pupils, cranial nerves (VII, IX–XII), spinal cord, brachial plexus (median, ulnar, radial, axillary, musculocutaneous nerves), the phrenic nerve, and the sympathetic chain (Horner's syndrome). Many patients with neck trauma have associated head injuries and abnormal neurological examination. Also, in injuries to the carotid or vertebral arteries the patient may present with neurological signs, such as low GCS or hemiplegia.

Investigations in Neck Trauma

History and clinical examination will determine the need and type of investigations in the evaluation of neck trauma. Patients with hard signs of major vascular or laryngotracheal injuries should be operated on without any delay for ancillary investigations. Specific investigations should be considered only in stable patients.

1. Plain chest and neck films: They can diagnose foreign bodies, fractures, pneumothorax, subcutaneous emphysema, and hematomas.
2. CT scan of the neck is the most valuable investigation in both blunt and penetrating trauma.
3. CT angiogram: It is the investigation of choice in suspected vascular or laryngotracheal injuries. In addition, it can reliably identify the bullet tract, i.e., near or away from vital structures, and help decide about the need for more specific investigations.
4. Angiography: Diagnostic angiography should be reserved only for cases with shotgun injuries and multiple pellets, or when the CT angiography is not conclusive. However, it has a definitive therapeutic role for embolization of a bleeding vessel or endovascular stenting of a false aneurysm or an arteriovenous fistula.
5. Color flow Doppler (CFD): CFD is noninvasive, accurate, and cost-effective. In addition, it does not require additional intravenous contrast if the patient has already received contrast for other investigations. The combination of a good physical examination and CFD can detect or highly suspect all vascular injuries, including minor ones. It has some limitations in the visualization of the proximal left subclavian artery in obese patients, the internal carotid artery near the base of the skull, and parts of the vertebral artery under the bony part of the vertebral canal. It is a good option for blunt trauma, especially in patients with a seatbelt sign on the neck, to rule out carotid or vertebral artery injuries.
6. Esophagogram: This should be considered in patients sustaining penetrating trauma with subcutaneous emphysema, odynophagia, or hematemesis, especially if the CT shows a wound tract near the esophagus. Very often it is supplemented by esophagoscopy.
7. Endoscopy: Esophagoscopy and laryngoscopy/tracheoscopy are indicated in patients with suspicious findings, such as subcutaneous emphysema, or a wound tract near the esophagus or trachea.

General Management

In an urban environment, the "scoop and run" principle should be applied in penetrating neck injuries. Any external bleeding should be controlled by direct pressure. Protective C-spine collars should be applied loosely and with caution because of the risk of airway obstruction in patients with large neck hematomas. Neck collars are not necessary in knife injuries, and though gunshot wounds to the spine can cause fractures, in neurologically intact patients they rarely are unstable.

Airway compromise may occur because of an external compressing hematoma, a laryngotracheal hematoma, or a major transection of the larynx or trachea. Orotracheal intubation can be a difficult and potentially dangerous task in the prehospital environment and should not be undertaken lightly.

The initial assessment in the emergency department should always follow ATLS guidelines. Approximately 10% of penetrating neck injuries present with airway compromise. Endotracheal intubation should be attempted only in the presence of a surgeon who can perform a cricothyroidotomy, in case of intubation failure. In fairly stable patients with airway compromise, fiberoptic nasotracheal intubation should be attempted first. For attempted orotracheal intubation, muscle relaxants should be used only in selected cases and by experienced intubators, because of the risk of airway loss. On the other hand, intubation without pharmacological paralysis may aggravate bleeding and airway obstruction due to patient coughing and straining, and thus the optimal method of airway establishment should be individualized.

Any external bleeding is controlled by direct pressure or by balloon tamponade using a Foley catheter. In order to avoid air embolism, all patients with suspected venous injuries should be put in the Trendelenburg position. Intravenous lines should be avoided on the same side as the injury because of the possibility of a proximal venous injury.

Patients arriving in the emergency department with imminent or established cardiac arrest should have an emergency department thoracotomy performed. As part of the resuscitation efforts, the right ventricle of the heart should be aspirated for air embolism.

Following a careful initial physical examination and appropriate investigations, a decision should be made about operation or observation. Overall, only about 15–20% of penetrating neck injuries require surgical intervention. The selection of the type of management can safely be made on the basis of a good clinical examination and appropriate investigations.

Common Mistakes and Pitfalls

1. Pharmacological paralysis for emergency endotracheal intubation in the presence of a large neck hematoma without being ready or not having the skills for a cricothyroidotomy. The loss of airway may be lethal.

2. Attempts to insert a nasogastric tube in an awake patient in the presence of a large neck hematoma or suspected vascular injury. Straining and coughing may precipitate bleeding. If a nasogastric tube is needed, wait until the patient is anesthetized.

3. Insertion of an intravenous line in the arm on the same side as the neck injury. Any infused fluids may be extravasated from an injury to the axillary or subclavian vein. Always use the opposite side.

4. Failure to perform a clinical examination according to a written protocol (see Table 3.1 below). The inexperienced physician can easily miss important signs and symptoms.

5. Failure to evaluate for vascular injuries in patients with unexplained neurological findings.

Penetrating Neck Injuries

3.1 Anatomical Zones of the Neck

The description of penetrating neck injuries according to zones is useful in the evaluation and management of the patient. The incidence of significant injuries with zone I wounds is about 15%, in zone II 25%, and in zone III 25%. About 12% of patients with zone I injuries, 14% with zone II, and 5% with zone III injuries require surgical intervention. Also, vascular evaluation in zones I and III is more difficult than in zone II. The vessels in these areas are not easily accessible to CFD studies, and CT angiographic evaluation may be more appropriate.

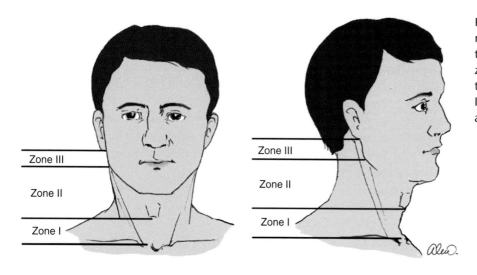

Figure 3.1 Anatomical zones of the neck. Zone I is confined between the clavicle and the cricoid cartilage, zone II between the cricoid and the angle of the mandible, and zone III between the angle of the mandible and the base of the skull.

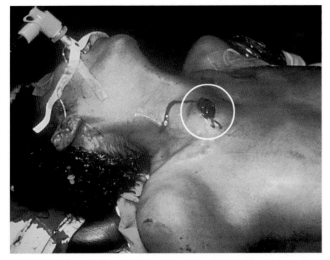

Figure 3.2 Zone I penetrating injury.

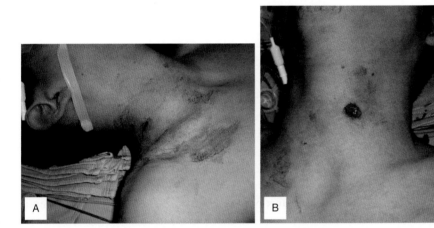

Figure 3.3 Zone II penetrating injuries. (A) Knife wound. (B) Gunshot wound.

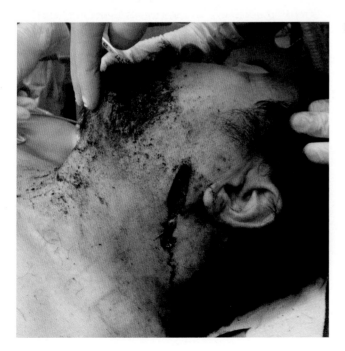

Figure 3.4 Zone III stab wound to the neck.

3.2 Epidemiology of Penetrating Neck Trauma

Overall, about 35% of all gunshot wounds and 20% of stab wounds to the neck result in significant injuries to vital structures. Transcervical gunshot wounds are associated with the highest incidence (75%) of significant injuries. The most commonly injured structures are the vessels (22% of patients), followed by the spinal cord, aerodigestive tract, and nerves (about 7% each).

Overall, only about 20% of gunshot wounds and 10% of stab wounds require operation. The remaining patients can be managed nonoperatively. The selection of patients for operation or observation can safely be made by physical examination and special investigations such as radiography, CT angiography, CFD studies, angiography, endoscopy, and contrast swallow studies.

3.3 Physical Examination of Penetrating Injuries of the Neck

Physical examination is very reliable in diagnosing or highly suspecting significant injuries requiring surgical repair. In order to avoid missing significant signs or symptoms, it is strongly recommended to perform the examination according to a written protocol. A careful examination in penetrating neck trauma is more important than in any other anatomical region.

Hard signs diagnostic of vascular trauma include severe bleeding, unexplained severe shock, absent or diminished peripheral pulses, bruits, and large, expanding hematomas. Soft signs suggestive but not diagnostic of vascular trauma include stable hematomas, mild hypotension responsive to small amounts of fluid resuscitation, abnormal brachial–brachial index (BBI), proximity injuries, and unexplained neurological findings. Only about 22% of patients with soft signs have significant vascular injuries.

These patients need further investigation by means of CFD or CT angiogram.

Hard signs diagnostic of aerodigestive tract trauma include respiratory distress, air bubbling through the wound, and major hemoptysis. These patients need an operation without any special investigations. Soft signs suggestive but not diagnostic of aerodigestive injuries include subcutaneous emphysema, minor hemoptysis, hoarseness, and odynophagia. Only about 15% of these patients have significant aerodigestive injuries. These patients require CT evaluation and possibly further investigation by means of endoscopy and/or contrast swallow studies.

Asymptomatic patients are highly unlikely to have any significant trauma requiring surgical treatment.

Depending on the findings of clinical examination, a CT angiogram or CFD may be indicated.

Table 3.1 Physical examination protocol for penetrating injuries of the neck

A. URGENT PRIORITIES
1. Control any active bleeding (pressure, packing, Foley's catheter).
2. If active bleeding: Trendelenburg position to prevent air embolism.
3. Secure airway.
4. IV fluids (no IV line on the side of the injury).

B. SYSTEMIC EXAMINATION
1. Dyspnea: ☐ yes   ☐ no
2. Blood pressure:
3. Pulse:
4. Color: ☐ pale   ☐ normal

C. LOCAL EXAMINATION
Vascular structures
1. Active bleeding: ☐ minor   ☐ severe   ☐ nil
2. Expanding hematoma: ☐ small   ☐ large   ☐ nil
3. Pulsatile hematoma: ☐ yes   ☐ no
4. Peripheral pulses (compare with
    normal side, Doppler?):   ☐ normal   ☐ diminished   ☐ absent
5. Bruit: ☐ yes   ☐ no

D. LARYNX–TRACHEA–ESOPHAGUS
1. Hemoptysis: ☐ yes   ☐ no
2. Air bubbling through wound
    (ask patient to cough):   ☐ yes   ☐ no
3. Subcutaneous emphysema: ☐ yes   ☐ no
4. Pain on swallowing sputum: ☐ yes   ☐ no

E. NERVOUS SYSTEM
1. Glasgow Coma Scale (GCS):
2. Localizing signs:
3. Cranial nerves:
    • Facial nerve: ☐ yes   ☐ no
    • Glossopharyngeal nerve: ☐ yes   ☐ no
    • Recurrent laryngeal nerve: ☐ yes   ☐ no
    • Accessory nerve: ☐ yes   ☐ no
4. Spinal cord: ☐ normal   ☐ abnormal
5. Brachial plexus injury:
    • Median nerve: ☐ yes   ☐ no
    • Ulnar nerve: ☐ yes   ☐ no
    • Radial nerve: ☐ yes   ☐ no
    • Musculocutaneous nerve: ☐ yes   ☐ no
    • Axillary nerve: ☐ yes   ☐ no
    • Horner's syndrome: ☐ yes   ☐ no

F. INVESTIGATIONS (only in fairly stable patients): Chest x-ray (erect), neck x-ray:
    ☐ hemopneumothorax
    ☐ subcutaneous emphysema
    ☐ widened upper mediastinum
    ☐ retained knife blade or missile

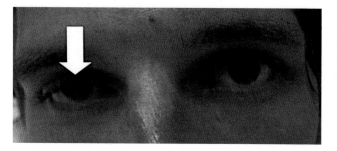

Figure 3.5 Horner's syndrome after penetrating trauma in zone I. It consists of ptosis of the upper eyelid (arrow), miosis of the ipsilateral eye, and anhidrosis of the ipsilateral side of the face. It is the result of injury of the stellate ganglion (on the neck of the first rib) of the sympathetic chain.

3.4 Protocol for Initial Evaluation and Management of Penetrating Injuries to the Neck

Clinical examination according to a written protocol remains the cornerstone for the selection of the appropriate treatment and investigation of a patient with penetrating neck trauma.

The selection of investigation (e.g., CT angiogram versus CFD) should also take into consideration the experience and facilities of the particular trauma center.

Table 3.2 Algorithm for the Management of Penetrating Injuries of the Neck

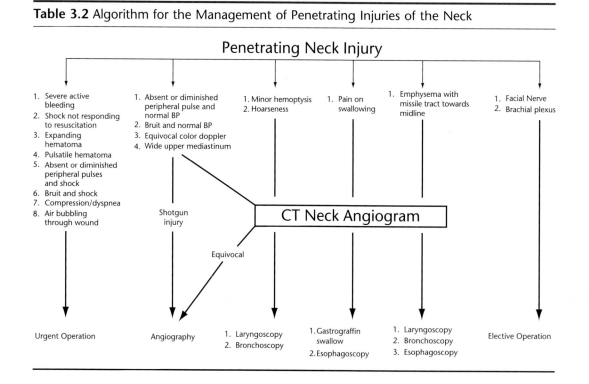

3.5 Radiological Investigations for Penetrating Neck Trauma

Plain Radiography

Anteroposterior and lateral films of the neck should be obtained in all patients with penetrating neck trauma who are hemodynamically stable. Important radiological findings include hematoma, subcutaneous emphysema, fractures, and foreign bodies. A chest film is also recommended in all stable patients. In about 15% of patients with penetrating neck trauma, there is an associated pneumothorax or hemothorax. A widened upper mediastinum is suggestive of a hematoma secondary to a vascular injury, and an elevated diaphragm may be due to a phrenic nerve injury.

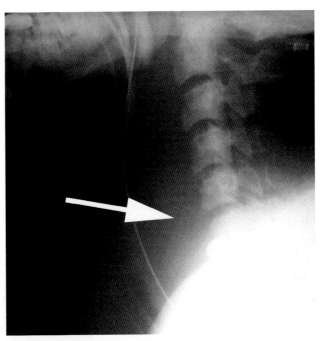

Figure 3.7 Lateral neck x-ray, in a patient with a gunshot wound, shows a large prevertebral hematoma (arrow).

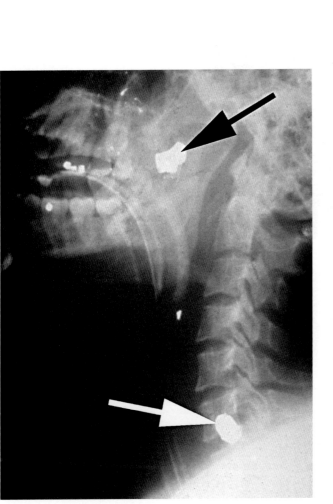

Figure 3.6 Plain film of the neck shows two bullets, one in zone I and another in zone III.

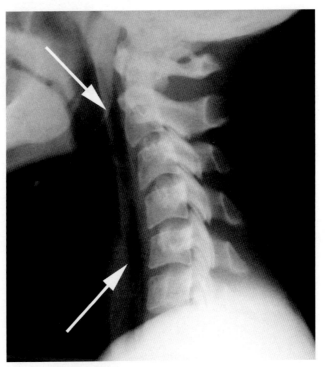

Figure 3.8 Lateral neck x-ray in a patient with a knife wound to neck shows prevertebral air (arrows). This finding is highly suspicious of aerodigestive trauma.

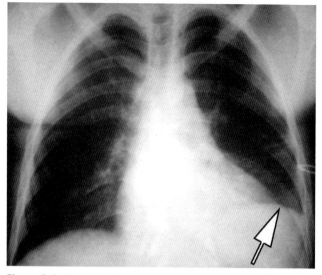

Figure 3.9 Patient with a stab wound to the neck. Chest x-ray showing elevated left hemidiaphragm (arrow) secondary to phrenic nerve injury.

CT Angiogram in Penetrating Neck Trauma

A CT angiogram should be a routine investigation in all hemodynamically stable patients with penetrating neck trauma. The CT may provide information about the site and nature of any fracture, involvement of the spinal cord, the presence of fragments in the spinal canal, the presence of any hematomas compressing the cord, vascular injuries including pseudoaneurysms, dissections, thrombosis, or extravasation, and/or subcutaneous emphysema indicating aerodigestive injury. In addition, the direction of the bullet tract may help the physician determine the need for further diagnostic studies including esophagogram or endoscopy.

A brain CT scan may be helpful in patients with penetrating neck trauma and unexplained neurological deficits. It may identify an anemic infarction or brain edema secondary to a carotid artery injury or an associated direct brain injury due to a missile.

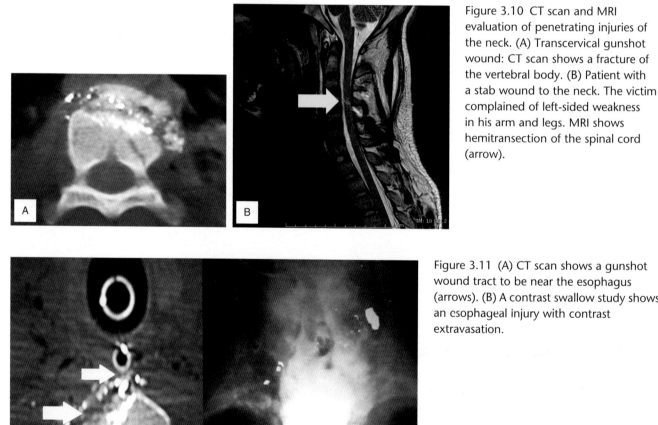

Figure 3.10 CT scan and MRI evaluation of penetrating injuries of the neck. (A) Transcervical gunshot wound: CT scan shows a fracture of the vertebral body. (B) Patient with a stab wound to the neck. The victim complained of left-sided weakness in his arm and legs. MRI shows hemitransection of the spinal cord (arrow).

Figure 3.11 (A) CT scan shows a gunshot wound tract to be near the esophagus (arrows). (B) A contrast swallow study shows an esophageal injury with contrast extravasation.

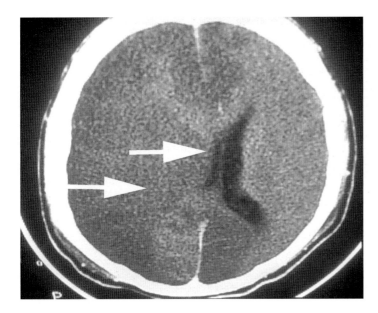

Figure 3.12 CT scan of the head on a patient in coma following a gunshot wound to the right internal carotid artery. The CT scan shows an anemic infarction of the right hemisphere, brain edema, and midline shift (arrows).

3.6 Evaluation of the Vascular Structures in the Neck

Asymptomatic patients are highly unlikely to have significant vascular injuries requiring surgical intervention or angiographic embolization. However, in about 8% of asymptomatic patients investigated by angiography, there is a vascular injury not requiring any type of treatment.

Patients with soft signs of vascular trauma need evaluation either by CT angiogram or CFD. The combination of physical examination and either of these diagnostic studies will detect almost all vascular injuries.

In zone I injuries, the presence of a peripheral pulse does not preclude a significant subclavian or axillary arterial injury. It is essential that the pulse is compared with the contralateral one. An objective measurement is the brachial–brachial index (BBI). The BBI is measured by taking the systolic pressure of the arm on the injured side and comparing it to the systolic pressure of the arm on the uninjured side. An index >0.90 is unlikely to be associated with significant arterial injury. It is recommended that all asymptomatic zone I penetrating injuries be evaluated routinely by BBI and either CT angio or CFD.

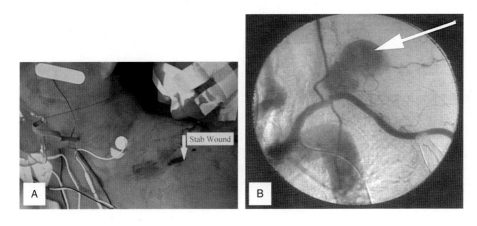

Figure 3.13 Zone I injury with vascular trauma. (A) Stab wound to zone I of the neck (arrow). The patient has peripheral pulse present in his left arm. (B) Angiogram showing pseudoaneurysm (arrow) of the left subclavian artery. The presence of peripheral pulses does reliably rule out a vascular injury.

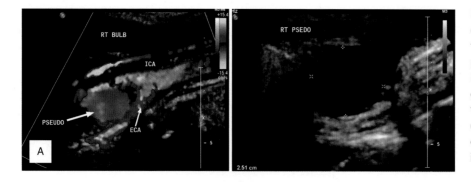

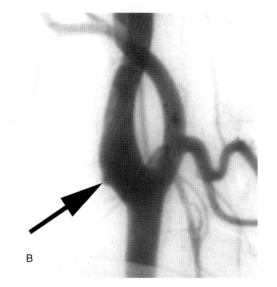

Figure 3.14 (A) Color flow Doppler (CFD) showing pseudoaneurysm of the internal carotid, following penetrating trauma. Color flow Doppler evaluates the flow and the gray scale duplex demonstrates the pseudoaneurysm (within stars). (B) Angiogram confirms the presence of a carotid pseudoaneurysm (arrow) in same patient.

Color Flow Doppler

Color flow Doppler (CFD) is an excellent investigation for suspected vascular trauma in most patients who are hemodynamically stable. The combination of physical examination and CFD imaging is a safe and cost-effective alternative to intravenous contrast angiography. It is noninvasive, can be performed at the bedside, has a high sensitivity and specificity, and is relatively inexpensive. However, it is operator-dependent and has some limitations in the visualization of the internal carotid artery near the base of the skull, sections of the vertebral artery directly underneath the bony part of the vertebral canal, and the proximal subclavian vessels, especially on the left side and in obese patients. In patients where the CFD is inconclusive, a CT neck angiogram should be considered.

Angiography for Penetrating Injuries of the Neck

Angiography may be used for diagnostic or therapeutic purposes in penetrating neck trauma. Its diagnostic advantage compared to the CT scan is the ability to digitally subtract any interfering objects, especially in cases with shotgun injuries. However, with the high sensitivity and specificity of the CT scan and the ease to obtain it, angiography is now used mostly for therapeutic interventions after diagnosis of vascular injuries.

Diagnostic indications: (a) shotgun injuries; (b) foreign bodies obscuring CT scan; and (c) embedded knife blade before removal.

Therapeutic indications for stenting or embolization: (a) bruit; (b) ongoing, slow, continuous bleeding from suspected vertebral artery injury; (c) continuous bleeding following a gunshot wound to the face; and (d) CT angio diagnosis of false aneurysms or arteriovenous fistula.

Failure to perform a meticulous physical examination and the appropriate investigations may result in missing significant injuries and serious complications. Auscultation is an important part of physical examination in penetrating neck trauma.

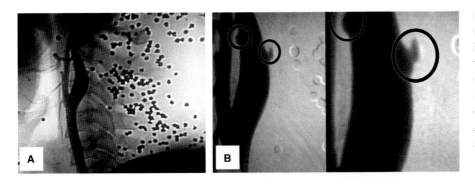

Figure 3.15 In the presence of multiple pellets following shotgun injuries, a formal angiogram remains the gold standard for evaluating the neck vessels. (A) The presence of multiple pellets makes a CT scan evaluation problematic. (B) Angiography in the depicted case shows two pseudoaneurysms (circles).

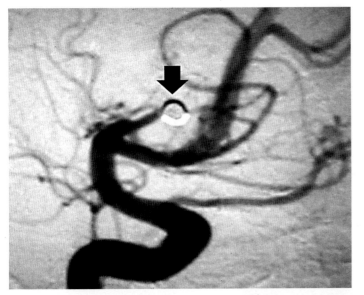

Figure 3.16 Shotgun wound to the neck. Angiography identifies a pellet embolization (arrow) to the middle cerebral artery.

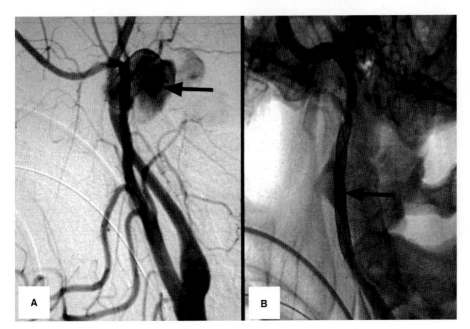

Figure 3.17 Penetrating injury to zone III of the neck resulted in this pseudoaneurysm of the internal carotid artery (A). The patient underwent endovascular repair using a stent-graft (B).

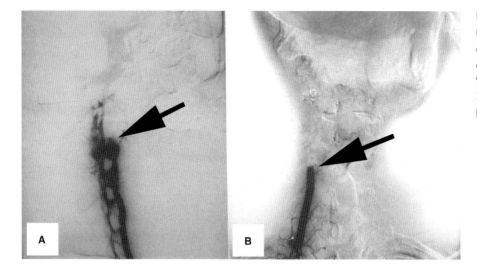

Figure 3.18 Gunshot wound to the neck with a hematoma and bruit on auscultation. Angiogram shows an arteriovenous fistula between the vertebral artery and veins (A). Successful angioembolization was performed (B).

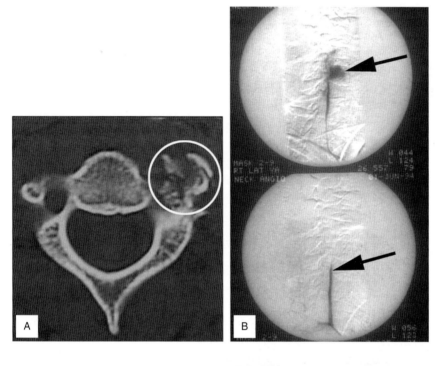

Figure 3.19 (A) Gunshot wound of the cervical spine with fracture of the transverse foramen (circle). In these cases the vertebral artery should always be evaluated by CT angio or a formal angiogram. (B) Angiography shows a false aneurysm of the vertebral artery (top), successfully managed with embolization (bottom).

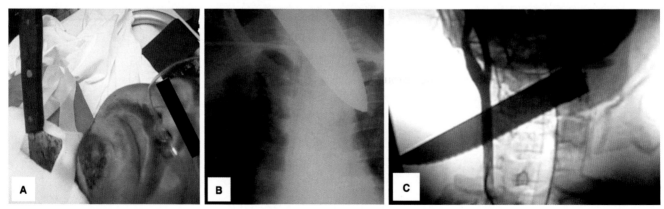

Figure 3.20 Knife embedded in the neck. It should be removed only in the operating room or after angiography. (A) Patient with a knife embedded in zone I of the neck. (B) X-ray showing the knife blade embedded deep in the tissues. (C) Angiography revealed no vascular injury and the knife was removed.

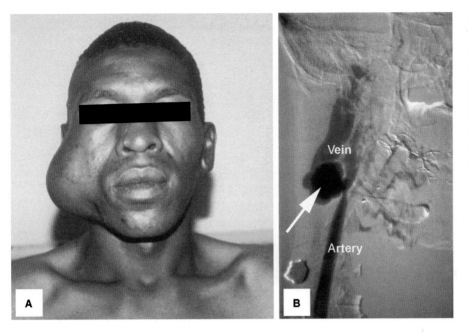

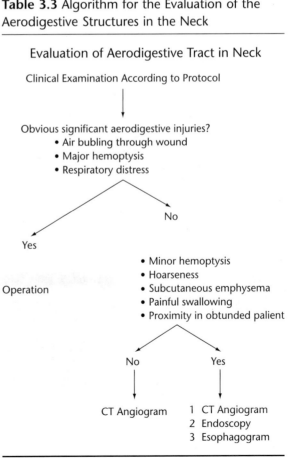

Figure 3.21 Photograph of a patient with penetrating trauma to zone III (A), who presented a few weeks after the injury. Physical exam found a pulsatile mass with a bruit. Angiogram (B) shows a pseudoaneurysm (arrow) of the internal carotid artery and communication with the internal jugular vein. The patient was successfully managed with an endovascular stent-graft.

3.7 Evaluation of the Aerodigestive Tract in the Neck

Asymptomatic patients are highly unlikely to have a significant injury requiring surgical management. Unevaluable patients or patients with soft symptoms of aerodigestive injuries need investigation by CT scan of the neck and in the appropriate cases, by endoscopy and/or contrast swallow studies.

The esophagus is evaluated by means of esophagography or endoscopy. The combination of the two investigations has a sensitivity of 100%. Rigid esophagoscopy is superior to flexible esophagoscopy in evaluating the upper esophagus; however, rigid endoscopy can be performed only under general anesthesia. Thus, this investigation is best reserved for patients undergoing anesthesia for another reason.

Patients with hard signs diagnostic of laryngotracheal injuries (respiratory distress, air bubbling through the wound, and major hemoptysis) need an emergency operation without any special investigations. However, patients with soft signs (subcutaneous emphysema, minor hemoptysis, hoarseness) require evaluation by means of endoscopy.

Table 3.3 Algorithm for the Evaluation of the Aerodigestive Structures in the Neck

Evaluation of Aerodigestive Tract in Neck

Clinical Examination According to Protocol

Obvious significant aerodigestive injuries?
- Air bubling through wound
- Major hemoptysis
- Respiratory distress

No

Yes

Operation

- Minor hemoptysis
- Hoarseness
- Subcutaneous emphysema
- Painful swallowing
- Proximity in obtunded palient

No

Yes

CT Angiogram

1 CT Angiogram
2 Endoscopy
3 Esophagogram

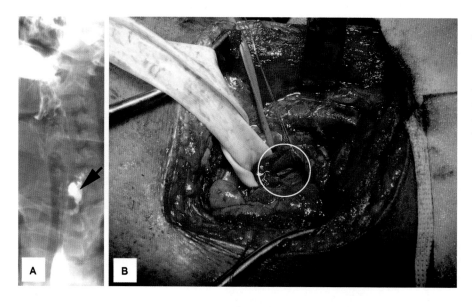

Figure 3.22 Esophageal injury following a gunshot wound to the neck. (A) Contrast extravasation on gastrografin swallow study (arrow) shows a perforation of the cervical esophagus. (B) Intraoperative appearance of esophageal injury with the nasogastric tube in view (circle).

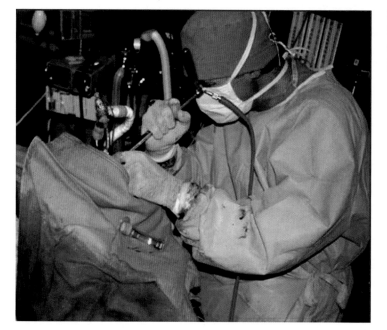

Figure 3.23 Rigid esophagoscopy is a reliable investigation in the evaluation of the cervical esophagus, but it can be performed only under general anesthesia in the operating room.

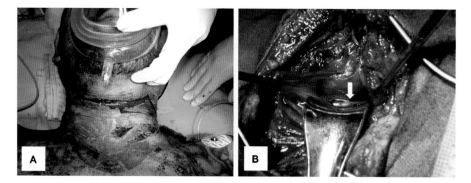

Figure 3.24 A patient with a stab wound to the neck in zone II, presenting with hematemesis (A). Operative exploration showing a large laceration in the pharynx exposing the nasogastric tube (B, arrow).

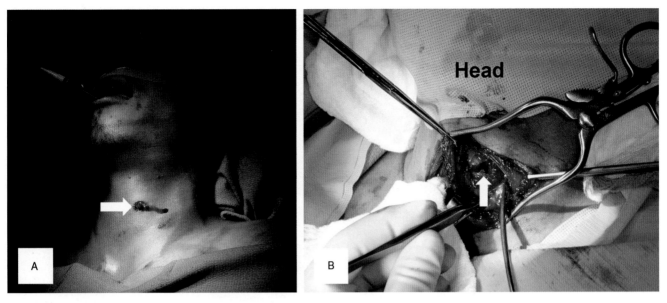

Figure 3.25 Patient with a zone II gunshot wound, presenting with hemoptysis and air bubbling through the wound (A). He was taken to the operating room without any diagnostic tests. Exploration shows an injury to his trachea (B, arrow).

3.8 Airway Establishment in the Presence of a Neck Hematoma

About 10% of patients with penetrating neck trauma present with airway compromise due to direct trauma to the larynx or trachea or due to external compression by a large hematoma. Airway establishment in the emergency department or the operating room in the presence of a large neck hematoma can be a difficult and potentially dangerous procedure. Pharmacological paralysis for endotracheal intubation should always be performed in the presence of an experienced physician ready to perform a cricothyroidotomy, if the intubator cannot visualize the cords. Orotracheal intubation without pharmacological paralysis should be avoided, if possible, because patient straining may precipitate massive hemorrhage. For the same reason, insertion of a nasogastric tube should be avoided in the awake patient. In addition, in the presence of a neck hematoma due to penetrating trauma, a cervical collar should be applied loosely because it may precipitate or aggravate an airway obstruction. The best approach is fiberoptic nasotracheal intubation under light sedation. It must be remembered that in the presence of a large neck hematoma a cricothyroidotomy may be a difficult and bloody procedure.

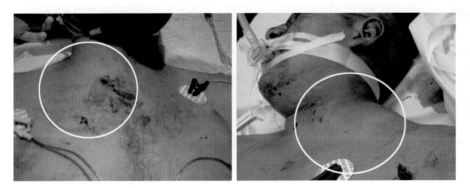

Figure 3.26 Patients with large neck hematomas may pose significant airway challenges and require early intubation. The decision on the technique of airway establishment should be based on the condition of the patient and the experience of the physicians.

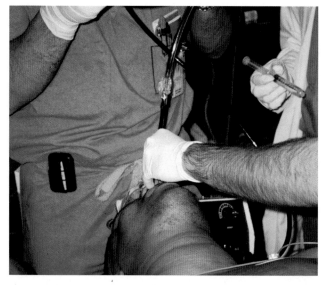

Figure 3.27 Awake, fiberoptic intubation of a patient with a large neck hematoma from a gunshot wound. This approach should be considered in fairly stable patients without severe respiratory distress.

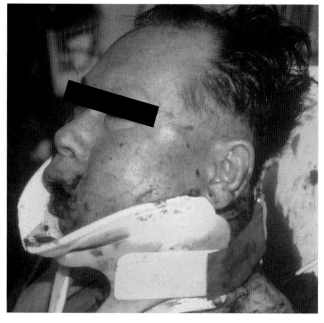

Figure 3.28 Patient with a large neck hematoma following penetrating trauma. Application of a firm cervical collar may aggravate the airway obstruction.

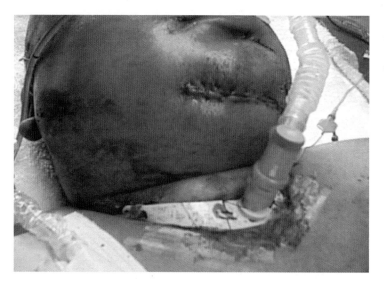

Figure 3.29 Patient who required an emergency cricothyroidotomy following failed endotracheal intubation, due to a large neck hematoma and airway compromise.

3.9 Bleeding Control in the Emergency Department

In most cases, the bleeding may be controlled by direct digital pressure in the wound. However, in some cases, especially in zones I and III, direct pressure is not effective. In these situations, insertion of the tip of a Foley catheter into the wound and inflation of the balloon with sterile water may control the bleeding.

Some patients with neck vascular injuries arrive in the emergency room with no vital signs or suffer a cardiac arrest soon after admission, due to massive blood loss. In these cases a resuscitative thoracotomy should be performed. The subclavian vessels can be accessed and the bleeding controlled through the thoracotomy, at the apex of the pleural cavity.

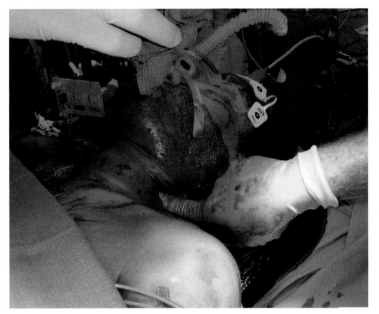

Figure 3.30 Digital compression and hemorrhage control can be a life-saving maneuver.

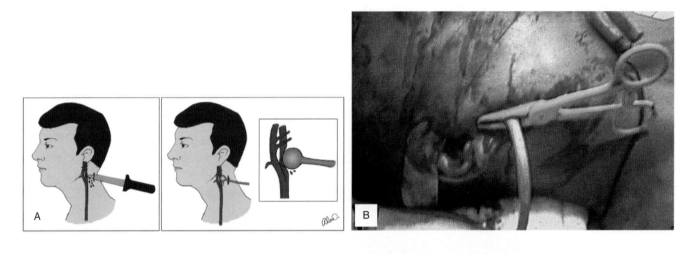

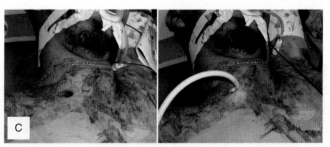

Figure 3.31 Balloon tamponade of difficult bleeding from the neck. (A) Illustration of balloon tamponade of severe bleeding from a zone III internal carotid injury. (B) Balloon tamponade with a Foley catheter and bleeding control in a patient with a zone III gunshot injury. Digital compression was not possible because of the small bullet entry. (C) This patient with a gunshot wound to zone I of the neck was admitted with severe hypotension but no active bleeding (left). However, after fluid resuscitation there was severe bleeding, successfully controlled with Foley catheter tamponade (right). At operation he was found to have an injury to the proximal common carotid artery.

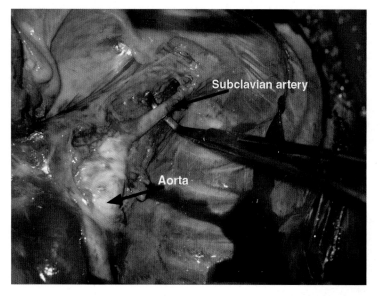

Figure 3.32 Emergency Room resuscitative thoracotomy following cardiac arrest due to severe blood loss from a left subclavian artery injury. Subclavian vessel control can be achieved through the chest, at the apex of the pleural cavity.

3.10 Penetrating Trauma to the Carotid Artery

Carotid artery trauma is diagnosed in about 8% of all penetrating injuries to the neck and the overall mortality is about 60%. Due to close anatomical proximity, there is often associated injury to the internal jugular vein. The victim should always be placed in the Trendelenburg position to prevent air embolism in cases with venous injuries. Bleeding control can temporarily be achieved by digital exploration or balloon tamponade, as described above. Timely operative intervention in cases with active bleeding remains the cornerstone of survival. Patients with pseudoaneurysms, especially in the distal internal carotid artery which is difficult to access surgically,

should be considered for angiointervention and stent-graft placement.

Traumatic thrombosis of the common or internal carotid artery may result in ipsilateral anemic infarction and brain edema, although in some cases this may be well tolerated due to an intact circle of Willis. Early revascularization, ideally within the first 4 hours, is associated with good results. Delayed revascularization after the establishment of an anemic infarction may worsen the brain edema or lead to a hemorrhagic infarction. Early surgical reconstruction remains the mainstay of management of penetrating carotid injuries.

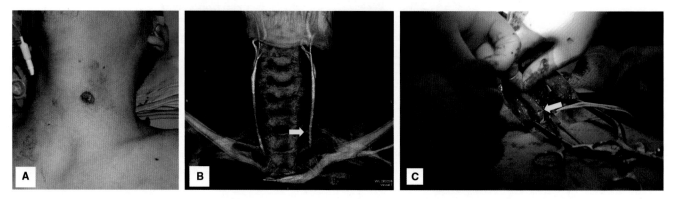

Figure 3.33 Zone II injury with carotid artery trauma. (A) Patient with a stab wound in zone II. (B) CT angiogram, with 3-D reconstruction, shows a common carotid pseudoaneurysm (arrow). (C) Intraoperative appearance of the carotid injury (arrow).

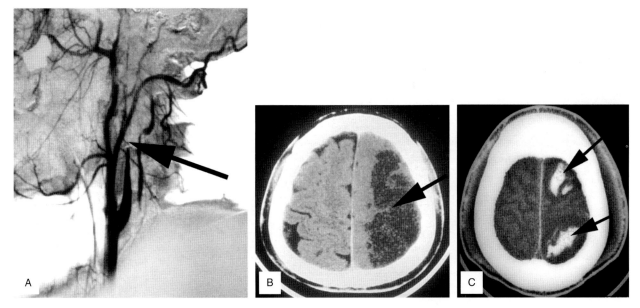

Figure 3.34 Carotid injury with brain infarction. (A) Angiogram of patient admitted to the hospital 4 hours after a gunshot wound to the neck shows injury with thrombosis of the internal carotid artery (arrow). (B) CT scan of the brain shows an ischemic infarct (arrow). The patient underwent revascularization about 6 hours after the injury. (C) CT scan of the brain 1 day after revascularization shows conversion of the anemic infarction to a hemorrhagic one (arrows).

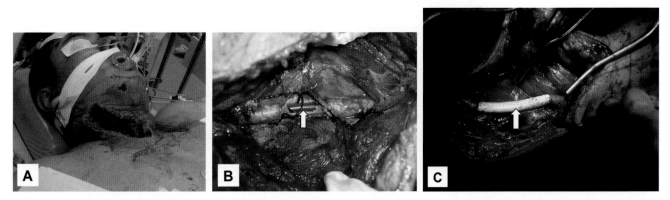

Figure 3.35 Penetrating carotid trauma. Patient with a gunshot wound to the neck. He arrived in severe shock and was taken emergently to the operating room. Operative exploration through an incision along the anterior border of the sternomastoid muscle (A) shows an injury to the right carotid artery (B). The artery was temporarily shunted (arrow) to establish flow to the brain and avoid infarction. (C) Definitive repair of the carotid artery with a PTFE interposition graft (arrow).

3.11 Penetrating Trauma to the Vertebral Artery

Vertebral artery trauma is diagnosed in about 3% of all penetrating injuries to the neck and the mortality in patients reaching hospital is about 5%.

Occlusion of a vertebral artery is usually tolerated well, and there is no need to attempt revascularization. In rare occasions with insufficient collateral circulation, occlusion of a vertebral artery may cause neurological deficits. The majority of vertebral artery injuries can be managed by observation or angiographic embolization. Surgical intervention is indicated only in the presence of severe active bleeding or in cases where angiographic embolization has failed.

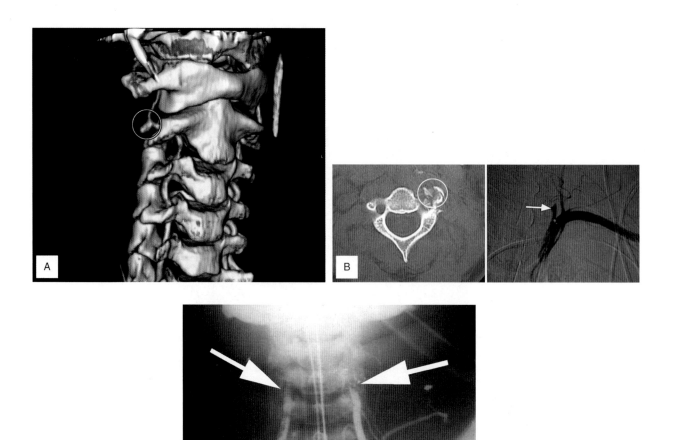

Figure 3.36 Penetrating injuries to the vertebral artery. (A) Patient with gunshot wound in zone III of the neck. CT angiogram with 3-D reconstruction shows a pseudoaneurysm of the distal vertebral artery (circle). (B) Patient with a gunshot wound to the neck. The CT scan shows fracture of the vertebral foramen (left, circle). In such cases there is concern of injury to the vertebral artery that travels through the foramen. Angiography confirms injury and thrombosis of the vertebral artery (right, arrow). (C) Patient with a transcervical gunshot wound to the neck and fracture of the cervical spine. Angiography showing thrombosis of both vertebral arteries (arrows). The patient had no neurological deficits from this injury.

3.12 Penetrating Trauma to the Subclavian Vessels

Subclavian vascular injuries are diagnosed in about 3% of hospital admissions with penetrating neck trauma, and the overall mortality is about 60%. More than 20% of these patients have no vital signs on admission and may benefit from an emergency room resuscitative thoracotomy. The deaths are the result of massive bleeding or air embolism in cases of venous injury. The bleeding can temporarily be controlled by digital exploration or balloon tamponade, as described above. The victim should always be placed in the

Trendelenburg position to prevent air embolism. Timely operative intervention in cases with active bleeding remains the cornerstone of survival. Patients with no active bleeding (pseudoaneurysm, thrombosis, or arteriovenous fistula) should be considered for angiointervention and stent-graft placement.

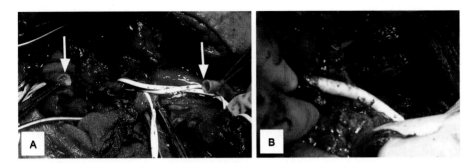

Figure 3.37 Subclavian vascular injuries. (A) Intraoperative appearance of severe injury to the subclavian artery following a gunshot wound to the neck. There is significant tissue loss (arrows) and reconstruction with a prosthetic graft is necessary. (B) Reconstruction of the arterial defect with a synthetic vascular graft.

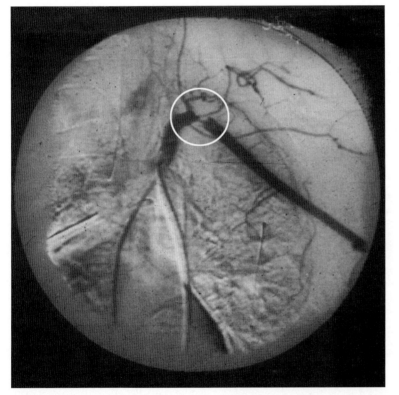

Figure 3.38 Angiogram of a patient with a stab wound in zone I of the neck. The patient had diminished radial pulse. The angiogram shows stenosis (circle) of the proximal subclavian artery. This patient can be managed with an endovascularly placed stent-graft.

Blunt Neck Trauma

Blunt trauma to the neck usually involves the musculoskeletal structures. However, in some cases it may involve the vessels or the laryngotracheal tract.

3.13 Vascular Injuries

Cervical cerebrovascular injuries occur in less than 1% of all blunt trauma admissions and may involve the carotids or the vertebral arteries. These injuries are often asymptomatic initially and because of the low index of suspicion they are often missed. Failure to treat them early can result in delayed neurological deficits due to thrombosis. This complication may occur many days or even weeks after the initial injury. It is essential that patients at risk for this injury should be screened. Criteria for screening for cerebrovascular injuries include: seatbelt mark signs or any bruising or hematoma to the neck after blunt trauma, unexplained neurological deficits, severe maxillofacial injuries, cervical spine fractures with subluxation, especially if there is involvement of the transverse foramen, and skull fracture of the base of the skull with carotid canal involvement.

The usual mechanism is overextension of the neck, although overflexion of the head or direct trauma to the neck may result in such injuries as well. The most common site of blunt carotid trauma is the proximal internal carotid artery, near the bifurcation. Another site of injury is the internal carotid at the C2 level, due to stretching of the vessel over the transverse process of the C2, after neck overextension. The clinical picture may vary from an asymptomatic seatbelt mark sign or neck hematoma to severe neurological deficits such as hemiparesis or hemiplegia or coma.

Multislice CT angiography (CTA), especially with 3-D reconstruction, is the best screening tool. In addition, it provides information about any skeletal or laryngotracheal injuries. CFD study may be useful but it is not always available, and can miss injuries near the base of the skull or in the vertebral artery canal. Formal angiogram is the diagnostic gold standard, but its routine use for screening purposes is limited because of its invasiveness. It has a significant role in the endovascular management of selected cases with dissection or pseudoaneurysm.

The treatment depends on the site of carotid injury and the experience of the surgeon. In low lesions that are surgically accessible, an operation with reestablishment of the blood flow by means of a homologous venous graft is recommended, provided that the diagnosis is made early.

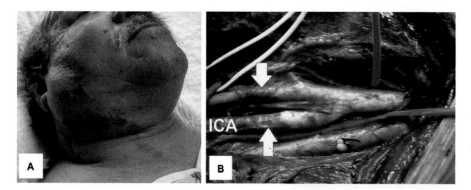

Figure 3.39 Patient with seatbelt sign on the right side of the neck and unexplained hemiplegia. (A) A "seatbelt" sign on the neck should increase suspicion for vascular injury. (B) The intraoperative findings show the carotid contusion and underlying thrombosis of the internal and external carotid arteries (arrows).

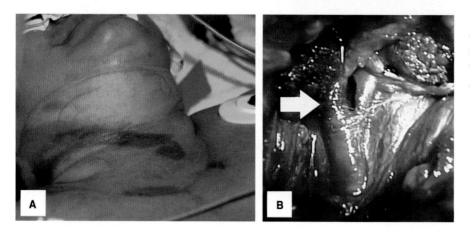

Figure 3.40 Patient with seatbelt sign on the neck (A). Surgical exploration shows bruising and underlying thrombosis of the internal carotid artery (arrow) (B).

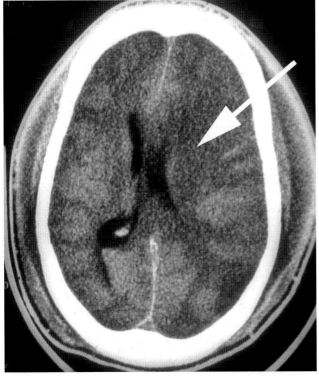

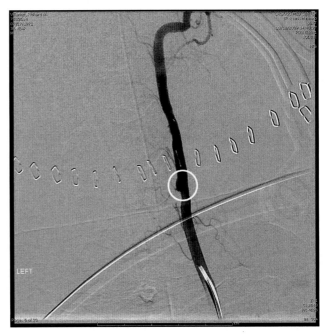

Figure 3.41 Patient who was involved in a motor vehicle accident. On initial evaluation, besides a small seatbelt mark sign on the left side of the neck, he was asymptomatic and was discharged home. He returned 4 days later with hemiplegia. CT scan shows anemic infarction and brain edema of the left hemisphere due to thrombosis of the left internal carotid artery.

Figure 3.42 Angiography showing a pseudoaneurysm of the distal internal carotid artery (circle), following a motor vehicle injury. This patient was managed with endovascularly placed stent-graft combined with antiplatelet therapy.

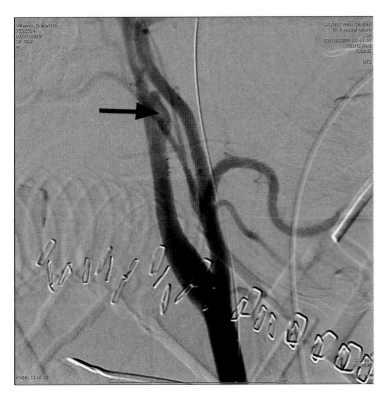

Figure 3.43 Angiogram after blunt trauma shows a pseudoaneurysm in the right vertebral artery (arrow). These injuries should be managed with anticoagulation and antiplatelet therapy.

Most of the cases with blunt cerebrovascular trauma are managed with anticoagulation, initially with heparin and later on with antiplatelet agents. The treatment should be continued for 3–6 months. Early anticoagulation has been shown to reduce the risk of progression of the thrombus and stroke. Angiographically placed stents should be considered in selected cases with internal carotid trauma. The recommended management of blunt vertebral artery trauma is antiplatelet therapy for a few months.

3.14 Blunt Laryngotracheal Trauma

Blunt trauma to the larynx or trachea may occur as a result of direct trauma to the neck, hanging injuries, or anteroposterior crush trauma to the chest, which causes intratracheal high pressures while the glottis is closed. Also, deceleration injuries may cause shearing injuries at fixed points, such as the cricoid or the carina. These injuries may vary from submucosal hematomas to complete transection.

The patient often complains of pain in the neck, dyspnea, hemoptysis, or hoarseness. Physical examination usually reveals subcutaneous emphysema. The diagnosis is confirmed by CT scan of the larynx and endoscopy.

About 28% of patients with blunt laryngotracheal trauma require emergency airway control. Depending on the severity of the injury and the condition of the patient, the airway can be established by orotracheal intubation, fiberoptic intubation, or surgical airway. Many patients with no airway problem and with no major disruption of the laryngotracheal structures may be managed nonoperatively. Perforation of the larynx or trachea or major fractures of the thyroid or arytenoid cartilages or the hyoid bone often need surgical intervention.

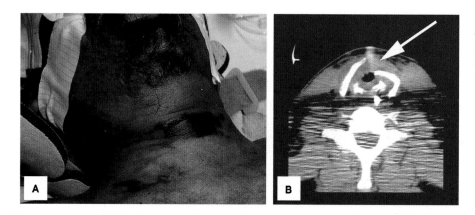

Figure 3.44 (A) Patient with blunt force trauma to the anterior neck. (B) CT scan showing fracture of the larynx.

4 Thoracic Injury

Demetrios Demetriades and Peep Talving

Introduction

Chest trauma is estimated to be the primary cause of death in 25% of traumatic mortalities and a contributing factor in another 25% of deaths. Good understanding of the pathophysiology of chest trauma and timely selection of the appropriate investigations and treatment are all critical components for optimal outcome.

Clinical Examination

Advanced trauma life support (ATLS) principles are particularly important in the initial evaluation and management of the chest trauma patient.

During the primary survey, there are six life-threatening conditions that need to be identified and treated:

1. Airway obstruction
2. Tension pneumothorax
3. Open pneumothorax with a "sucking wound"
4. Flail chest
5. Massive hemothorax
6. Cardiac tamponade.

During the secondary survey, there are another six potentially lethal chest injuries that should be identified and treated. The diagnosis of these conditions may need more complex and time-consuming investigations.

1. Lung contusion
2. Myocardial contusion
3. Aortic rupture
4. Diaphragmatic rupture
5. Tracheobronchial rupture
6. Esophageal injury.

Investigations

History and clinical examination will determine the type and timing of investigations necessary for the safe and efficient evaluation of the chest trauma patient. Very often, in unstable patients, therapeutic interventions such as thoracostomy tube insertion or thoracotomy may be initiated without any investigations.

Investigations are necessary in fairly stable patients when the diagnosis is uncertain. The following investigations may be useful in chest trauma:

1. Chest x-ray: Ideally it should be taken during deep expiration and erect position for more accurate detection of small pneumothoraces, small hemothoraces, and mediastinal abnormalities. In many cases this is not possible because of associated hemodynamic instability, depressed level of consciousness, or concern about spinal injury. The following radiological findings should be sought: pneumothorax, hemothorax, lung contusion, subcutaneous or mediastinal emphysema, fractures, mediastinal widening, enlarged cardiac shadow, pneumopericardium, elevated diaphragm or suspicious shadows suggestive of diaphragmatic hernia, free air under the diaphragm, and foreign bodies.
2. Electrocardiogram (ECG): It should be performed in all patients with severe blunt chest trauma and suspected cardiac trauma. In addition, it might be useful in some stable patients with suspected penetrating cardiac injuries.
3. Focused assessment with sonography for trauma (FAST) is an important investigation and should be available in the emergency department. Emergency physicians and trauma surgeons should be trained in its use, as it allows early diagnosis of cardiac tamponade or hemoperitoneum at the bedside with high accuracy. Emergency room

ultrasound is also a useful tool in the diagnosis for pneumothoraces and in placement of central venous catheters.

4. Pericardiocentesis: This diagnostic procedure has little or no value in the evaluation of suspected cardiac trauma in a modern trauma center as it is associated with an unacceptably high incidence of false-negative results because of clot formation in the pericardium. In addition, it is a potentially dangerous procedure because of the risk of myocardial or coronary vessel perforation, especially if performed in the absence of hemopericardium. It might have a role for temporary decompression of a tense hemopericard in selected cases where a surgeon is not available.

5. Subxiphoid pericardial window: This major invasive procedure has been used by many surgeons to diagnose cardiac tamponade. With FAST to evaluate the pericardium, it has little or no place in a modern trauma center. Intraoperative transdiaphragmatic window during an exploratory laparotomy has a definitive place in thoracoabdominal injuries with suspected cardiac involvement.

6. Chest computed tomography (CT) including CT angiography (CTA): CT is very valuable in blunt trauma in the evaluation of the mediastinum, the thoracic spine, and suspected lung contusions. All stable blunt trauma patients with a suspicious mechanism of injury (high-speed accidents, falls from height) or those with an abnormal mediastinum on chest films should be evaluated by CTA for aortic rupture. CTA is highly sensitive and specific in detecting aortic rupture and has replaced aortography to a great extent. CT scan is also useful in the evaluation of suspected lung contusions or persistent opacifications on chest x-ray following insertion of a thoracostomy tube. In these cases, the differential diagnosis between atelectasis, contusion, and residual hemothorax may be difficult or impossible on the basis of clinical examination and chest x-ray.

CTA also has a definitive role in the evaluation of selected patients with penetrating chest trauma. In patients with transmediastinal gunshot wounds who are hemodynamically stable, a multi-slice CT scan may be useful in identifying the bullet track and in determining the need for further investigations such as endoscopy or esophageal contrast swallow studies. If the direction of the bullet track is away from the major vessels, esophagus, and other important mediastinal structures, no further investigations are necessary.

7. Angiography: In recent years, most trauma centers have replaced diagnostic angiography with CTA. Formal angiography still has an important role in the evaluation of patients with shotgun injuries with multiple pellets. However, therapeutic angiography and placement of stent-grafts play a major role in the management of traumatic thoracic aortic injuries, false aneurysms, and arteriovenous fistulas of the major thoracic inlet arteries.

8. Color flow Doppler: Color flow Doppler (CFD) ultrasound is a very good noninvasive vascular study that can reliably evaluate the subclavian and neck vessels and is recommended for hemodynamically stable patients with thoracic inlet penetrating injuries. Its major weaknesses are its operator-dependent accuracy and inability to visualize the left proximal subclavian vessels, especially in obese patients.

9. Endoscopy: Esophagoscopy and bronchoscopy may be necessary for suspected aerodigestive tract injuries, usually as a result of mediastinal penetrating trauma.

10. Laparoscopy: Laparoscopy has a definitive role in the evaluation of the diaphragm in asymptomatic patients with left thoracoabdominal or right anterior thoracoabdominal penetrating injuries. Failure to recognize and repair a diaphragmatic injury may result in a diaphragmatic hernia at a later stage. Right posterior thoracoabdominal injuries do not need evaluation and repair of any diaphragmatic laceration because the presence of the liver protects against herniation of intra-abdominal organs.

11. Thoracoscopy: Thoracoscopy is used in the evaluation of diaphragmatic injuries, especially in the posterior region. It is particularly useful in cases with residual hemothorax that can be evacuated through the port. It has the disadvantage of needing double lumen intubation and lung collapse, which may be technically demanding and sometimes not well tolerated by the patient.

12. Troponin levels: Serial troponin measurements have replaced cardiac enzymes (e.g., CPK-MB) for monitoring in suspected myocardial contusion. Though routinely used, troponin levels do not correlate with the severity of the myocardial trauma. In addition, many patients with severe extrathoracic injuries, such as head trauma, may have elevated troponin levels.

13. Arterial blood gas: Arterial blood gases are indicated in all severe chest trauma cases in order to assess severity, plan treatment, and monitor progress of treatment.

General Management

In an urban environment, there is no place for prehospital attempts to stabilize patients with severe chest trauma, and the principle of "scoop and run" should be applied. The patient should be placed on a spinal board, receive oxygen by mask, and be transferred without any delay to the nearest trauma hospital. Intravenous access should be attempted in the ambulance en route. In patients with severe respiratory distress and clinical suspicion of tension pneumothorax, a needle thoracostomy may be attempted. Open sucking wounds should be covered with a clean square gauze taped only on three sides to avoid a tension pneumothorax. Patients with respiratory failure will need prehospital intubation or bag-valve mask ventilation en route. In the emergency department, the primary survey will determine the need and type of immediate treatment. Patients with imminent or established cardiac arrest should be managed with an emergency department resuscitative thoracotomy. Any bleeding is controlled by sutures or clamping. Aortic cross-clamping is performed, and cardiac massage is initiated. Transfusions with O-negative blood, cardiac drugs, calcium, and sodium bicarbonate and defibrillation are administered as necessary. If cardiac activity returns, the operation is completed in the operating room.

Patients with severe hypotension and suspicion of cardiovascular trauma should be taken directly to the operating room with minimal investigations. A FAST is very valuable in determining the source of hypotension in patients with multiple injuries as it can evaluate the pericardial, pleural, and peritoneal spaces.

Hemodynamically stable patients are examined carefully, and further investigations are performed as indicated. Thoracostomy tubes, analgesia, intubation, and mechanical ventilation may be necessary.

Elderly patients with multiple rib fractures or significant lung contusions, despite a normal respiratory status on initial examination, should be admitted to the intensive care unit (ICU) for close monitoring. Early, liberal endotracheal intubation and mechanical ventilation should be considered because elderly patients often deteriorate rapidly and with little warning. Adequate analgesia by means of epidural or patient-controlled analgesia (PCA) is a critical component of the management of these cases as these patients often deteriorate a few hours after admission.

Indications for Thoracotomy

Fewer than 5% of blunt chest traumas, about 15% of stab wounds, and about 20% of gunshot wounds require thoracotomy. The majority of patients with chest trauma can safely be managed with a thoracostomy tube and other supportive treatment. The indications for emergency thoracotomy are generally the following:

- Cardiac arrest or imminent cardiac arrest
- Evidence of cardiovascular injury, such as severe hypotension or severe active external or internal bleeding
- Immediate blood loss in the thoracostomy tube more than 1,000–1,200 ml
- Diagnosis of esophageal or tracheobronchial injury.

Semielective thoracotomies are indicated for large residual hemothoraces or persistent major air leaks.

Common Mistakes and Pitfalls

1. Elderly patients with multiple rib fractures or lung contusions may seem stable on admission, but rapid respiratory deterioration may occur a few hours later. Consider admission to the intensive care unit for close monitoring and early endotracheal intubation and mechanical ventilation.
2. Patients with flail chest may seem stable on admission. Decompensation with severe respiratory failure may occur during prolonged radiological investigation with potentially catastrophic consequences. Liberal early intubation is recommended before these patients are transferred to the radiology suite.
3. A widened mediastinum following a traffic accident or a fall from height may be due to rupture of the thoracic aorta or to fractures of the thoracic spine.
4. Traumatic rupture of the thoracic aorta may not be associated with an abnormal mediastinum on chest x-ray. In high-speed deceleration trauma all patients should be evaluated by chest CT scan to rule out aortic injuries.
5. In left thoracoabdominal or anterior right thoracoabdominal penetrating injuries, routine laparoscopy should be performed on all asymptomatic patients. Diaphragmatic injuries are common and radiology is usually not reliable.

4.1 Chest Wall, Soft Tissues

Seatbelt marks on the thoracic wall are indicators of severe trauma, and 20% of these patients have significant intrathoracic injuries. These patients should have routine evaluation for lung contusion, myocardial contusion, aortic rupture, and hemopneumothorax.

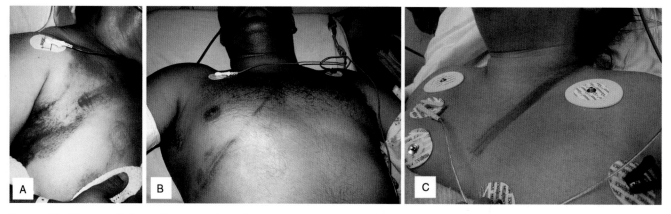

Figure 4.1 Chest seatbelt marks are markers of significant internal injuries and should be evaluated by CT scan, ECG and troponin levels.

4.2 Rib Fractures

Fractures of the Upper (First or Second) Ribs

Fractures of the upper ribs, especially the first rib, are associated with a high incidence of subclavian and other major vascular injuries. A CTA or CFD evaluation of the vessels will help exclude this injury. The force required to fracture an upper rib is severe, and thus mediastinal structures, including the aorta, are also at high risk with this mechanism. Children have a much more compliant chest wall, and thus any rib fractures are significant.

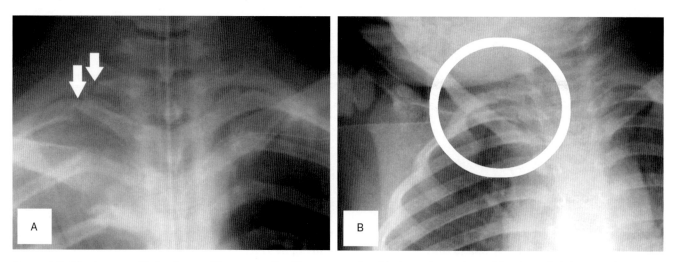

Figure 4.2 Chest x-ray with fractures of the upper ribs. These cases should always be evaluated for thoracic inlet vascular injuries, especially the subclavian vessels.

Fractures of Middle (Third to Eighth) Ribs

Rib fractures are diagnosed clinically (pain aggravated by breathing or coughing, pain on anteroposterior chest compression) or radiologically. Fractures at the costochondral junction may not show on x-rays. Associated injuries include hemopneumothorax, lung contusion, cardiac trauma, and diaphragmatic tear. Pain relief is extremely important, especially in elderly patients with multiple rib fractures, in order to prevent atelectasis and pneumonia. PCA or epidural analgesia should be considered in multiple fractures.

Rib fractures in children are uncommon and signify severe impact to the chest wall, and there is a high incidence of underlying lung contusion.

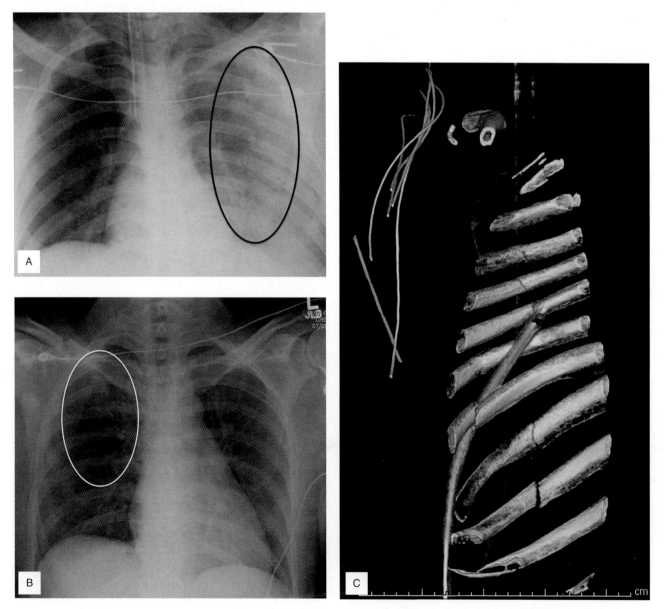

Figure 4.3 (A–B) Plain radiographs of multiple mid rib fractures, with underlying lung contusion (A). Adequate analgesia with epidural or patient-controlled analgesia should be considered early, especially in elderly patients. (C) 3-D reconstruction of multiple mid rib fractures and a thoracostomy tube in place.

Fractures of the Lower (Ninth to Twelfth) Ribs

Fractures of the lower ribs are often associated with injuries to the kidneys, liver, or spleen. Liberal use of abdominal CT scan should be considered.

Flail Chest

Flail chest is the result of anterior or lateral double fractures of at least three adjacent ribs. In most cases there is an underlying lung contusion. Clinically the flail segment moves paradoxically to

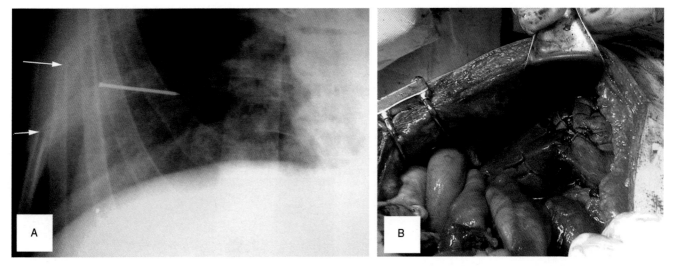

Figure 4.4 (A) Radiograph showing fractures of the right lower ribs (arrows) (left). Injuries to intra-abdominal solid organs are common and CT scan evaluation should be considered. (B) Intraoperative photograph of the associated liver injury in the same patient.

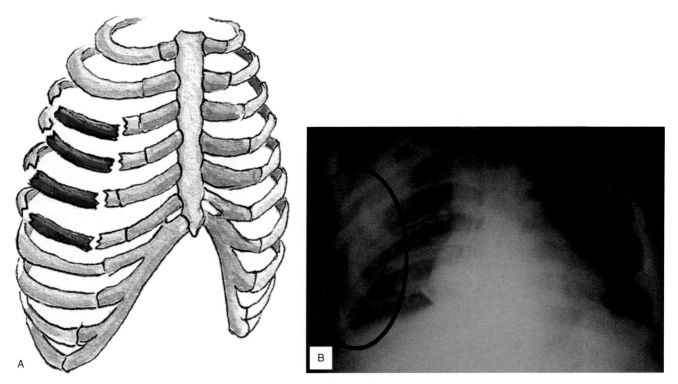

Figure 4.5 Flail chest. (A) Double fractures of at least three adjacent ribs are required in order to produce a flail chest. (B) Chest x-ray showing a left flail chest with underlying lung contusion. (C) Patient with a flail sternal segment; Note the midsternal depression (right).

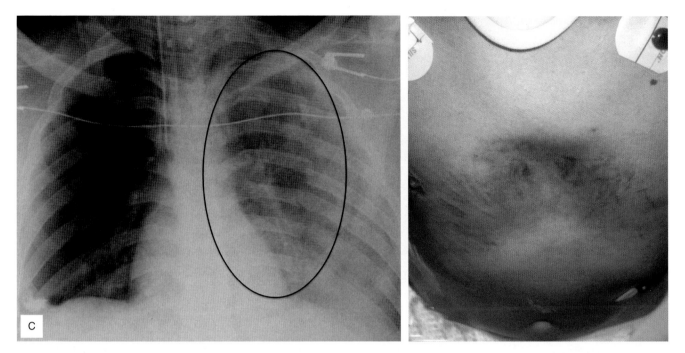

Figure 4.5 (*cont.*)

normal chest wall motion, and the patient may be in respiratory distress. All patients with flail chest should have a thoracostomy tube inserted and be monitored in an ICU setting with serial blood gases and continuous pulse oximetry. Analgesia by means of PCA or epidural anesthesia should always be used. Mechanical ventilation is necessary for respiratory failure or imminent failure. Internal, operative fracture fixation may be useful in selected cases without underlying lung contusion and in patients having difficulty weaning off mechanical ventilation.

4.3 Hemo-Pneumothorax

Pneumothorax

A pneumothorax may be due to blunt or penetrating trauma. Small pneumothoraces are usually asymptomatic and can safely be managed without a chest drain, provided the patient does not need mechanical ventilation or air transportation. In these cases, any size pneumothorax should be treated with a thoracostomy tube to avoid the creation of tension pneumothorax. Large pneumothoraces may cause respiratory distress, and tension pneumothoraces can cause cardiorespiratory failure. The diagnosis of simple pneumothorax is usually made by plain chest film or CT scan. An erect chest x-ray in deep expiration is the most suitable film to identify small pneumothoraces.

Tension Pneumothorax

In tension pneumothorax, air leaks into the pleural cavity with no escape route on account of a one-way valve effect. It is a life-threatening condition because of the severe cardiorespiratory failure that ensues. The patient is panicky and has dyspnea, cyanosis, shock, and distended neck veins. The trachea is shifted to the opposite side, there are

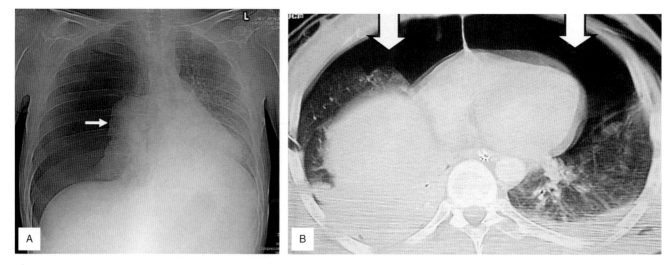

Figure 4.6 Pneumothorax. (A) Large right pneumothorax on chest x-ray. Arrow points to collapsed lung. (B) Bilateral pneumothoraces on CT scan (arrows).

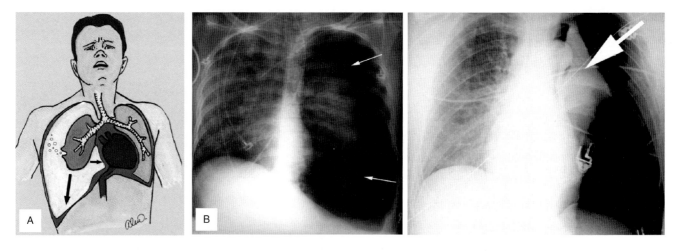

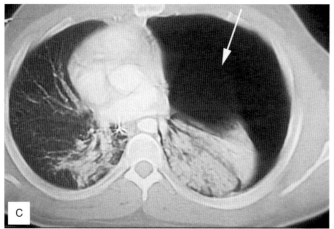

Figure 4.7 Tension pneumothorax. (A) Illustration showing mechanism of tension pneumothorax. Extrapulmonary air under tension collapses the lung, depresses the diaphragm, and pushes the heart toward the opposite side. The normal lung is compressed in the contralateral pleural cavity. These changes cause cardiorespiratory failure. (B) Chest x-rays showing a large tension pneumothorax on the left side, mediastinal shift to the opposite side, and downward displacement of the left hemidiaphragm. Arrows point to tension pneumothorax. (C) Tension pneumothorax on the CT scan (arrow). Note the deviation of the heart to the right.

no breath sounds and there is hyperresonance on percussion in the affected hemithorax. Immediate life-saving therapy is needle decompression of the chest, followed by formal thoracostomy tube insertion. The mere suspicion of a tension pneumothorax is an absolute indication for a needle decompression whenever a thoracostomy tube cannot be inserted immediately (prehospital stage,

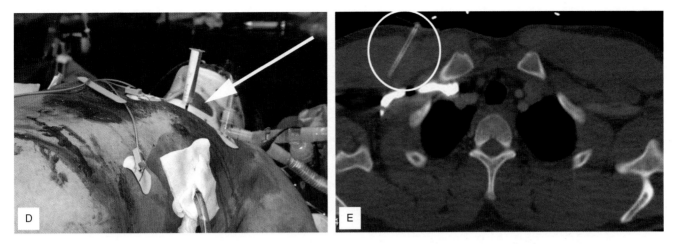

Figure 4.7 (*cont.*) (D) Photograph showing a thoracostomy needle in place, below the middle of the clavicle. (E) CT scan shows that the thoracostomy needle is located into the subcutaneous tissues, outside the pleural cavity. This is a common technical problem.

areas outside the emergency department or operative room). A thoracostomy tube should be subsequently inserted as soon as possible.

Hemothorax

A hemothorax can be due to blunt or penetrating trauma. Large hemothoraces may present with hypovolemia or dyspnea, but small hemothoraces can be asymptomatic. On physical examination, the breath sounds are diminished, there is dullness on percussion, and the affected hemithorax moves poorly. A chest x-ray, preferably in the erect position, confirms the diagnosis, although many times it cannot distinguish between a hemothorax and intrapulmonary hematoma, contusion, or atelectasis. A supine chest film may miss small hemothoraces.

The treatment of significant hemothoraces is thoracostomy tube insertion through the fourth or fifth intercostal space, in the midaxillary line. A thoracotomy should be considered if the initial thoracostomy tube output exceeds 1,000–1,500 ml of blood, or if the patient is hemodynamically unstable.

Significant residual hemothorax following thoracostomy tube insertion should be evaluated by means of CT scan and evacuated within 3–5 days. Barring contraindications, thrombolytic agents such as tissue plasminogen activator (tPA) or urokinase delivered through the chest tube have resulted in high success rates as a first line of treatment. In cases selected for operative approach, a thoracoscopy within 7 days of diagnosis or a small anterolateral thoracotomy as a last resort should be performed. Delayed evacuation is difficult because of clot organization and inflammation, and it requires a thoracotomy with decortication.

An undrained significant hemothorax is associated with increased risk of empyema and may cause respiratory compromise due to fibrosis.

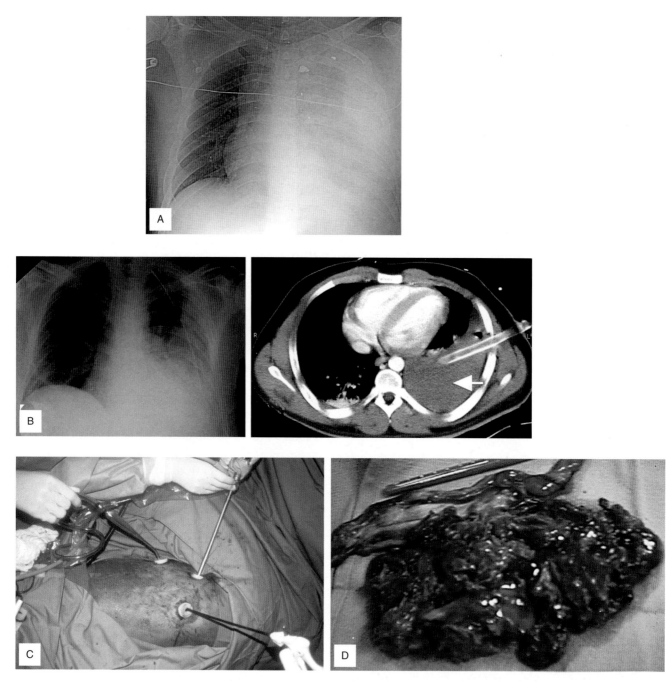

Figure 4.8 Hemothorax. (A) Chest radiograph with extensive opacification of the left hemithorax due to massive hemothorax with mediastinal shift to the opposite side and retained fragments of a missile. (B) Gunshot wound to the left chest with suspected "residual hemothorax" on chest x-ray (left) 2 days after injury. Residual hemothorax is confirmed by CT scan (right). (C) Thoracoscopic evacuation of the residual hemothorax. The procedure should be performed within the first 5 days of injury, before organization of the clot and fibrin encapsulation of the lung. (D) Photograph of material removed during decortication for persistent residual hemothorax and lung entrapment, a few weeks after injury. Delayed evacuation of a clotted hemothorax is difficult and requires thoracotomy and decortication.

Thoracostomy Tube Insertion

Chest tube can be inserted with an open or a percutaneous dilational technique. The site and technique of the insertion of the thoracostomy tube are the same for both hemothorax and pneumothorax. The patient is placed in the supine position and the arm abducted at 90 degrees. The insertion site is the fourth or fifth intercostal space, mid-axillary line.

With the open technique, a 1.5–2 cm incision is made through the skin and subcutaneous fat. A Kelly forceps is inserted into the pleural cavity. Finger exploration should be performed in all patients with previous chest trauma or infection in order to evaluate for adhesions and avoid the risk of intrapulmonary placement of the tube. The drain is inserted 8–10 cm into the pleural cavity, aiming posteriorly towards the apex. Standard thoracostomy tube sizes are adult male, 28–36; adult female, 28–34; newborn, 10; 4 years, 16–20; 8 years, 20–24; and 12 years, 24–28.

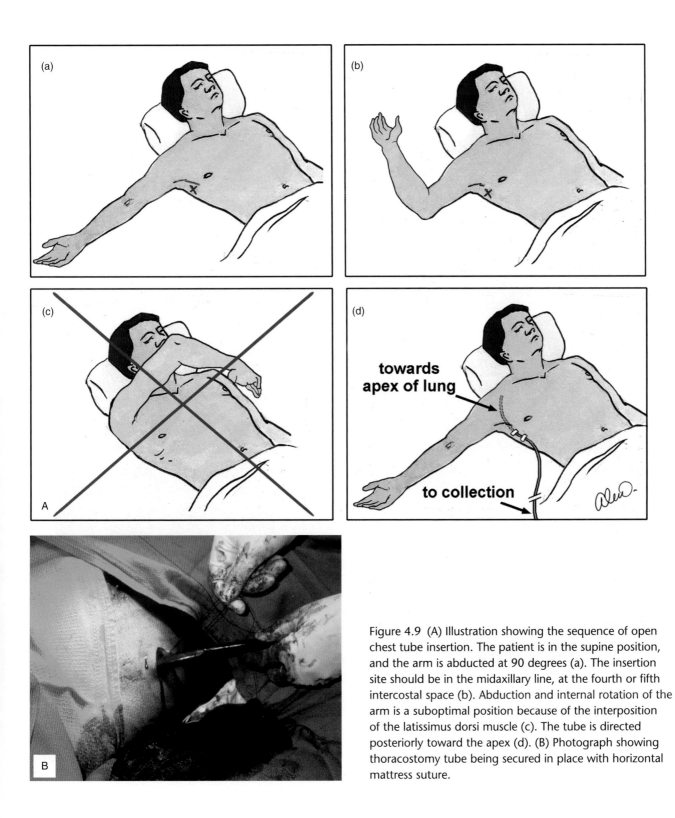

Figure 4.9 (A) Illustration showing the sequence of open chest tube insertion. The patient is in the supine position, and the arm is abducted at 90 degrees (a). The insertion site should be in the midaxillary line, at the fourth or fifth intercostal space (b). Abduction and internal rotation of the arm is a suboptimal position because of the interposition of the latissimus dorsi muscle (c). The tube is directed posteriorly toward the apex (d). (B) Photograph showing thoracostomy tube being secured in place with horizontal mattress suture.

The percutaneous insertion technique is less painful and less traumatic. The method employs the Seldinger guidewire concept which is extensively used for central venous catheter placement.

The trocar technique should be avoided because of the high incidence of serious iatrogenic injuries.

The most common complications associated with chest drain insertion include injury and bleeding from the intercostal vessels and injury to the lung parenchyma. Other serious complications include perforation of the heart, the diaphragm, liver, and spleen.

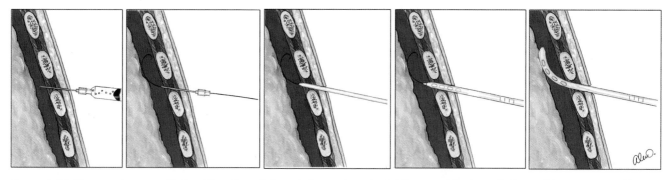

Figure 4.10 The percutaneous dilational insertion of chest drain employs the Seldinger guidewire technique with progressive dilation.

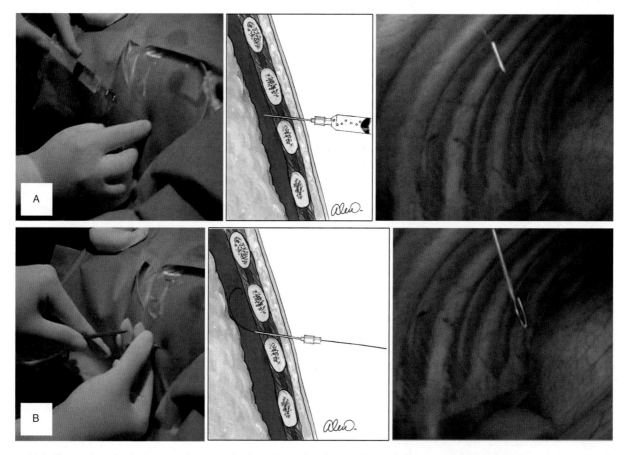

Figure 4.11 Illustration depicting step by step the insertion of a chest tube with the percutaneous dilational technique (illustration, photograph of procedure, thoracoscopic view): The needle, attached to a syringe containing sterile water, is inserted through the fourth to fifth intercostal space, close to the superior border of the rib, in order to avoid injury to the intercostal vessels. (A) Aspiration of air or blood confirms the intrathoracic position of the needle. (B) A guidewire is inserted though the needle into the thoracic cavity. Serial dilatation over the wire (C) is followed by insertion of the chest tube over the guidewire (D).

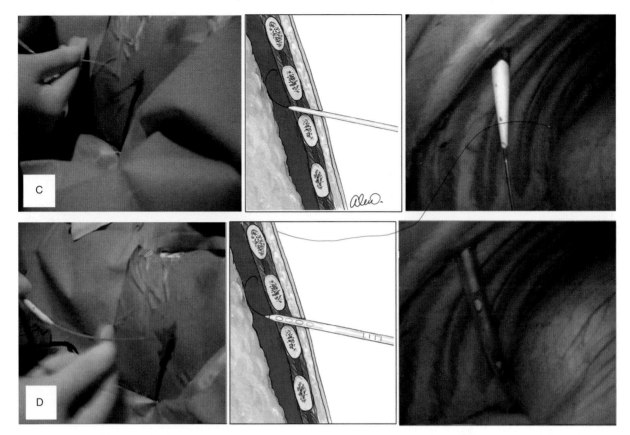

Figure 4.11 (*cont.*)

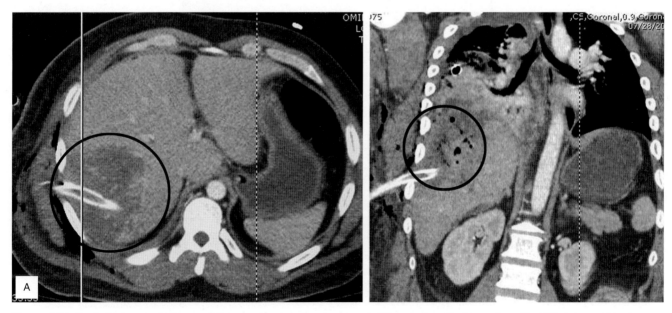

Figure 4.12 Technical complications of thoracostomy tube placement. (A) Insertion site lower than the fifth intercostal space may result in injury to the diaphragm or the intra-abdominal solid organ. The CT scans show the tube in the liver parenchyma. (B) CT scans show the chest drain in the subcutaneous tissues. (C) Chest x-ray showing insertion of the tube too far in the pleural cavity with kinking.

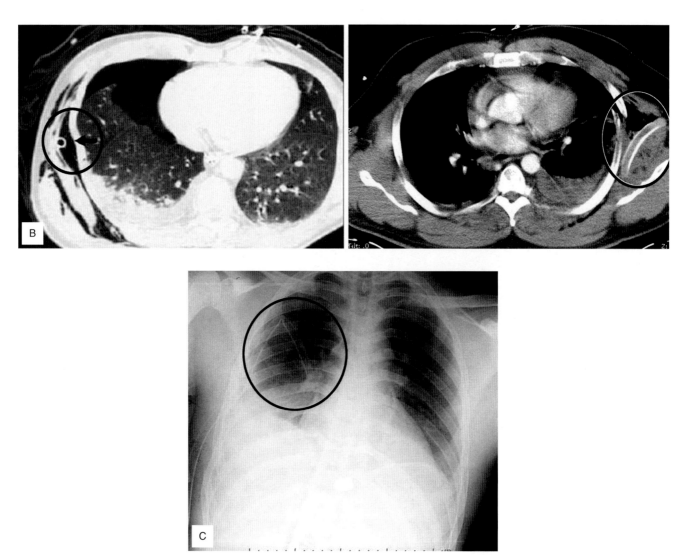

Figure 4.12 (*cont.*)

Autotransfusion of Blood in Chest Trauma

Blood autotransfusion following chest trauma is easy, safe, and cheap. The system is recommended for use in all patients with suspected large hemothoraces. Anticoagulant (1 ml citrate per 10 ml of blood) is advisable but not necessary.

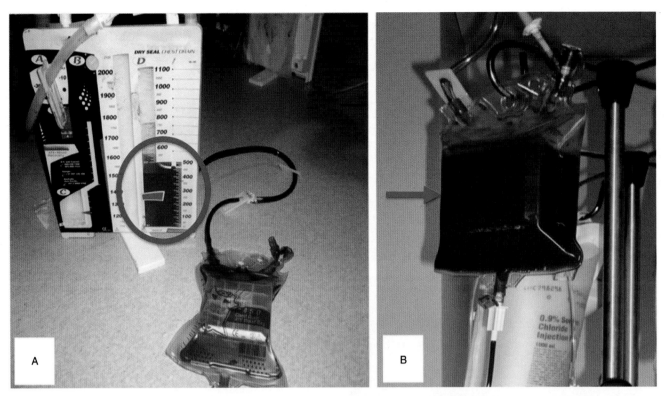

Figure 4.13 Autotransfusion system utilization in hemothorax. The collection chamber of the drainage system (circle) is connected to a negative pressure autotransfusion bag and the blood is actively sucked into the bag (A). (1 ml of citrate per 10 ml of blood is added to the collection system before drainage.) The collected blood is autotransfused using standard techniques (B).

4.4 Lung Contusion

Lung contusion may occur after blunt trauma to the chest, rapid deceleration injuries, or gunshot wounds to the lung. Associated rib fractures are a common finding in adults but not in children. The symptoms may vary from minor chest discomfort or hemoptysis to severe dyspnea, massive hemoptysis, and respiratory failure. The treatment is

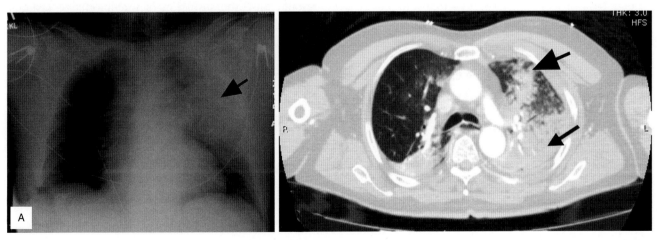

Figure 4.14 (A) Lung contusion: chest x-ray with large opacification in the left lung, highly suspicious for lung contusion (left). Chest CT scan confirms the presence of lung contusion (right).

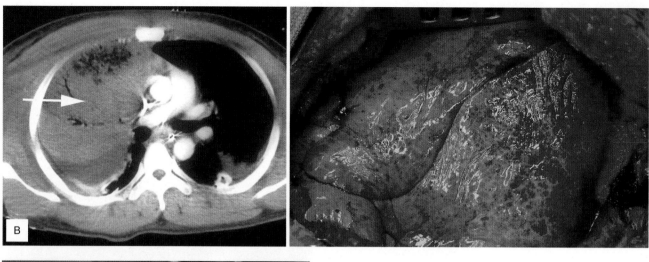

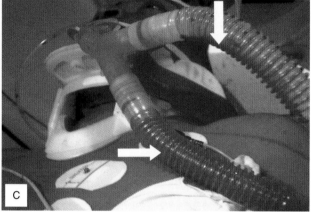

Figure 4.14 (*cont.*) (B) Lung contusion: CT scan appearance of a large contusion (arrow) (left). Intraoperative appearance of the lung contusion (right). (C) Bronchial bleeding in respiratory tubing is a common finding in severe lung contusions. Flooding of the normal lung may result in respiratory failure. Double-lumen endotracheal tube and independent lung ventilation should be considered.

symptomatic, and mechanical ventilation may be necessary. High-frequency percussive ventilation (HFPV), airway pressure release ventilation (APRV), or independent lung ventilation (ILV) may be necessary in patients who do not respond to conventional ventilation.

The radiological diagnosis of a lung contusion is not always easy with plain chest radiography because it has a similar appearance to hemothorax or atelectasis. CT scan delineates lung parenchyma well and provides an accurate diagnosis.

The contusion usually improves and resolves within a few days. Failure to improve radiologically should raise the suspicion of pneumonia or residual hemothorax.

4.5 Subcutaneous Emphysema

Subcutaneous emphysema may be secondary to a pneumothorax or aerodigestive tract perforation. A poorly placed thoracostomy tube, with a fenestration outside the pleural cavity, may also result in extensive emphysema. The first step in evaluating the cause of the emphysema is to check the position of any thoracostomy tube. For massive, unexplained emphysema, endoscopy should be performed to evaluate the aerodigestive tract. Subcutaneous emphysema rarely causes symptoms, and the treatment is directed toward the underlying cause.

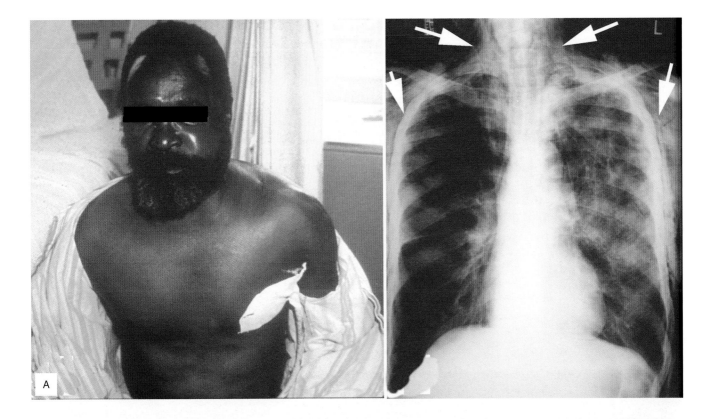

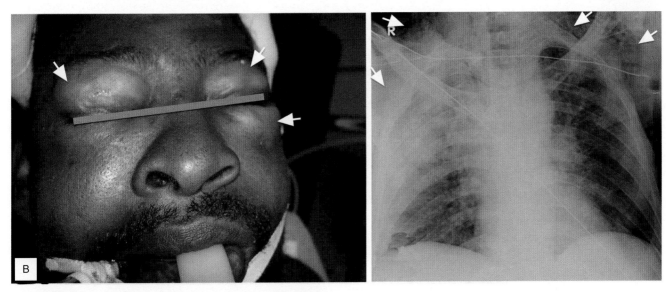

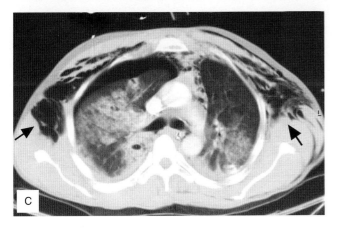

Figure 4.15 Subcutaneous emphysema. (A) Patient and chest x-ray with extensive subcutaneous emphysema in the face, neck, and chest wall. (B) Patient with extensive subcutaneous emphysema involving the face and neck. Chest x-ray and CT scan demonstrate extensive subcutaneous emphysema in the chest wall (arrows). (C) CT scan shows extensive bilateral subcutaneous emphysema and a right pneumothorax.

4.6 Penetrating Cardiac Injury

More than 80% of patients with penetrating cardiac injuries die at the scene. For those who reach the hospital alive, early diagnosis and operation are critical factors for survival.

Clinically the patient is restless, and the inexperienced physician often mistakes it for alcohol or drug intoxication. The victim is almost always in shock, although in cases with small cardiac wounds and short prehospital times, the initial blood pressure may be normal. Beck's triad (hypotension, distant cardiac sounds, distended neck veins) is found in about 90% of cases with tamponade. Pulsus paradoxus is rarely found in acute tamponade.

Stab wounds usually involve the right ventricle, and the prognosis is fairly good, with a hospital survival of about 65%. Bullet injuries usually involve multiple cardiac chambers and the prognosis is poor, with an overall hospital survival of about 15%. High-velocity bullets cause massive injury and are always fatal.

The outcome of penetrating cardiac trauma depends on many factors: Short prehospital times, an experienced trauma team, low-velocity injuries, right ventricular injuries, and the presence of cardiac tamponade are favorable factors for survival.

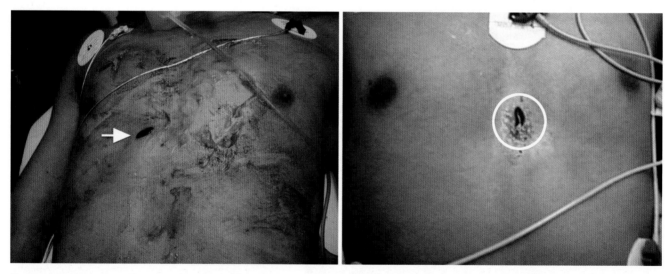

Figure 4.16 Patients with precordial penetrating wounds. Every penetrating injury to the chest, especially in the presence of hypotension, should be considered as a cardiac injury until proven otherwise.

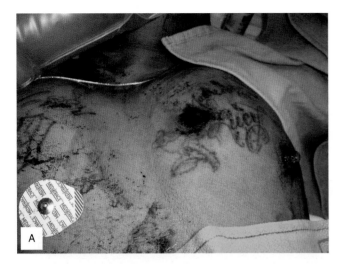

Figure 4.17 Cardiac wounds. (A) Patient with precordial gunshot wound. In these cases, especially in the presence of hypotension, a cardiac injury should be suspected. (B) Cardiac injury explored through sternotomy demonstrating a pericardial penetration (arrow) (left). Sutured injury to the right ventricle of the heart (arrow) (right).

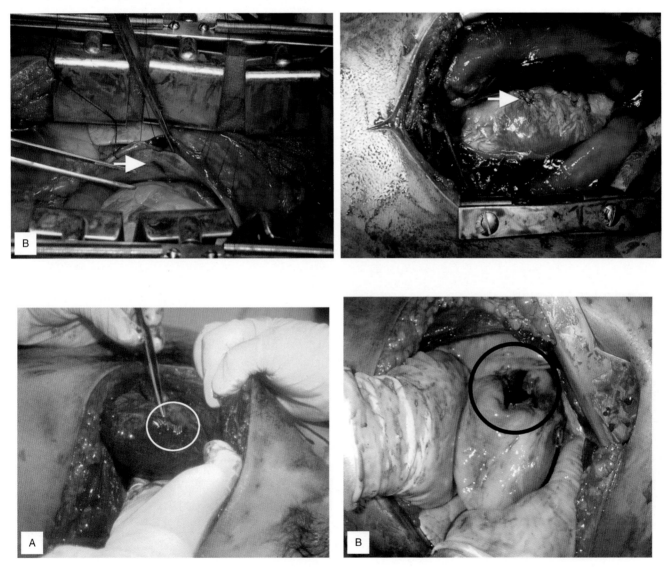

Figure 4.18 (A) Photograph of a stab wound to the heart (stapled during a resuscitative emergency room thoracotomy).

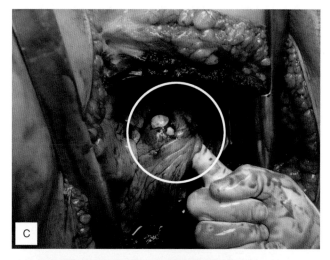

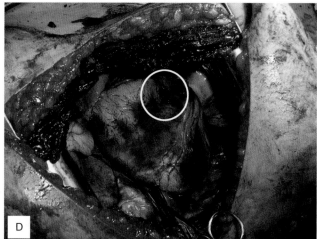

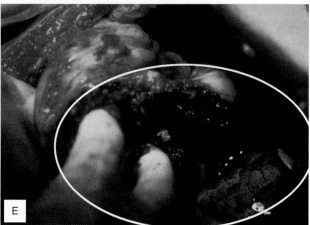

Figure 4.18 (*cont.*) (B–D) Photographs of low-velocity bullet injuries to the heart. (E) Photograph of a massive trauma to the heart from a high-velocity bullet injury.

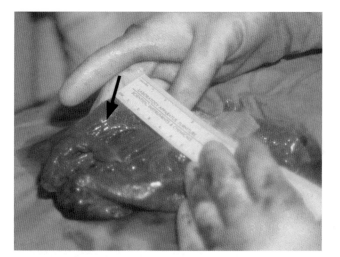

Figure 4.19 Autopsy photograph of the heart. The right ventricle has relatively thick wall (4 mm) and relatively low pressures. This is an optimal combination for survival. The left ventricle is thick (12 mm) but has high pressures, which result in a tense tamponade or rapid exsanguination, and thus the prognosis is poor.

Diagnosis of Cardiac Injury

The diagnosis of penetrating cardiac injury is usually clinical and can be confirmed by pericardial FAST performed in the emergency department by emergency physicians or surgeons, and thus it should be part of the standard primary survey. A chest film may be helpful in about half the cases with cardiac trauma. Radiological signs suggestive of cardiac trauma include an enlarged cardiac shadow, a widened upper mediastinum (due to a dilated superior vena cava), and pneumopericardium (a sign of pericardial violation).

An ECG may be diagnostic in about 30% of cases. It may show low-voltage QRS complexes, elevated ST segments, inverted T waves, electrical alternans, and other nonspecific findings.

Subxiphoid window is a major invasive procedure and has a very limited role in the diagnosis of cardiac tamponade. Similarly, pericardiocentesis has little or no place in a modern trauma center. The blood in the pericardial sac usually clots, and this results in high incidence of false-negative pericardiocentesis.

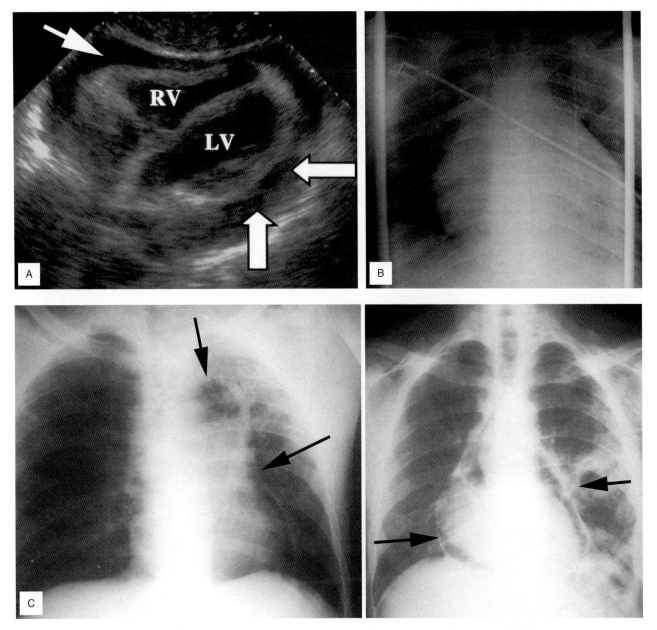

Figure 4.20 Investigations for cardiac injury. (A) Focused assessment with sonography for trauma (FAST) showing a circumferential pericardial effusion (arrows) diagnostic of cardiac tamponade. (B) Chest x-ray showing enlargement of the cardiac shadow suggestive of cardiac tamponade. (C) Chest x-rays depicting pneumopericardium suggestive of pericardial violation.

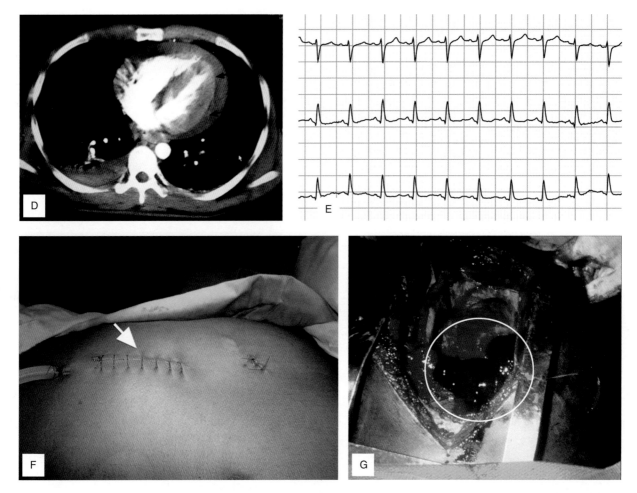

Figure 4.20 (*cont.*) (D) CT scan showing pericardial effusion following a superficial stab wound to the heart. The patient developed late cardiac tamponade symptoms. (E) ECG with sinus tachycardia and low-voltage QRS complexes in a patient with cardiac tamponade. (F) Subxiphoid window on a patient with a precordial stab wound. It is a major invasive diagnostic procedure and has a limited role in a modern trauma center. (G) Intraoperative photograph of a clot within the pericardial sac. A pericardiocentesis would have been falsely negative.

Retained Cardiac Missiles

The diagnosis of retained cardiac missile is suspected on the chest x-ray and confirmed by echocardiogram or CT scan. All missiles diagnosed at the acute stage should be removed because of the risk of delayed hemorrhage, embolization, false aneurysm, and endocarditis. Retained missiles that have been diagnosed long after the injury and are asymptomatic do not need routine removal.

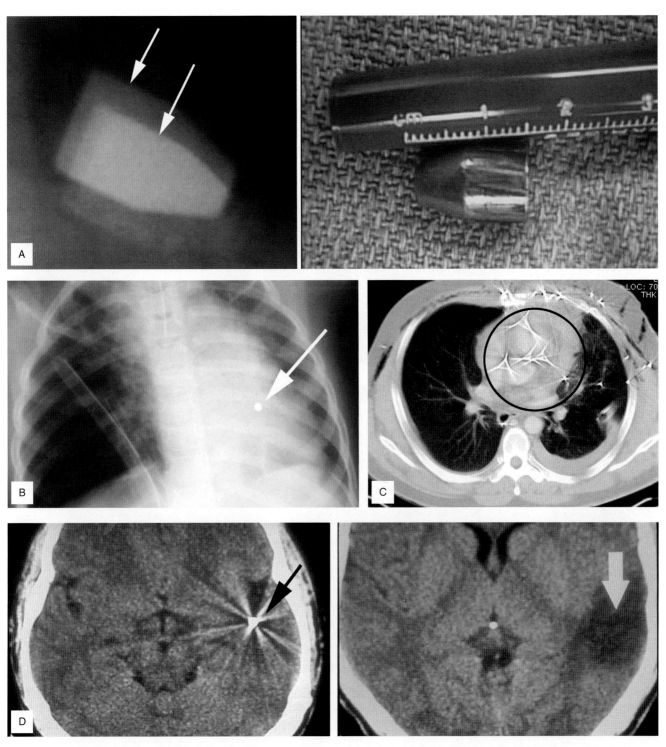

Figure 4.21 Retained foreign bodies in cardiac injuries. (A) Chest x-ray of a retained bullet. The double shadow of the bullet on chest x-ray is diagnostic of contact with the beating heart (left). Removed bullet postoperatively (right). (B) Chest radiograph showing a retained cardiac pellet following a shotgun injury (arrow). (C) Chest CT scan depicting multiple pellets in the myocardium. (D) Brain CT scan shows brain embolization of a pellet (black arrow) and anemic infarction (white arrow) following a shotgun injury to the heart.

Emergency Department Thoracotomy

Patients with cardiac arrest or imminent cardiac arrest in the emergency department should be managed with an immediate left anterolateral thoracotomy, through the fourth or fifth intercostal space (under the nipple in males or the inframammary crease in females). A lower incision may injure the diaphragm while a

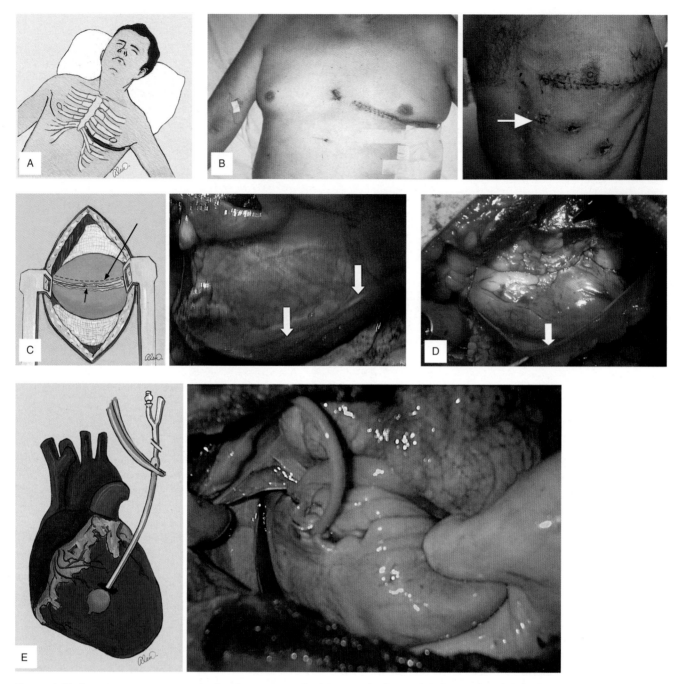

Figure 4.22 Emergency room resuscitative thoracotomy for injury to the heart. (A) Illustration of the incision for a resuscitative emergency department left anterolateral thoracotomy. (B) Photographs showing incisions for resuscitative thoracotomy, in a female and a male patient. (C–D) Illustration and photo of the pericardium at thoracotomy. The phrenic nerve is seen on the lateral aspect of the pericardium. The pericardium should be opened above the nerve (C). The pericardium is opened and the heart exposed (D). (E) Illustration and intraoperative photograph showing the use of a Foley catheter for temporary bleeding control from a cardiac wound.

higher incision does not provide a good exposure of the heart.

The pericardium is opened longitudinally to avoid injury to the phrenic nerve, and the clot is evacuated. The cardiac wound is repaired by suturing or stapling. A Foley catheter balloon may be useful in achieving temporary control of bleeding. In the presence of cardiac arrest, the aorta is cross-clamped just above the diaphragm, and direct cardiac massage is performed. Sodium bicarbonate and calcium should be administered intravenously, preferably through a central venous line. Adrenaline or

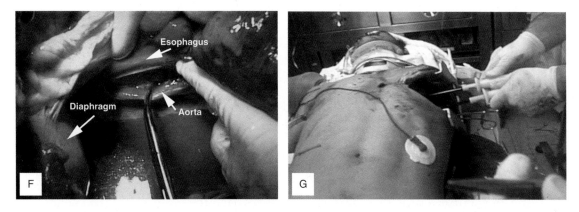

Figure 4.22 (*cont.*) (F) Photograph of a cross-clamping of the thoracic aorta. The clamp should be applied about 3–4 cm above the diaphragm. (G) Photograph of internal cardiac defibrillation during emergency room resuscitative thoracotomy.

defibrillation may be administered when the heart is full, and their use in an empty heart reduces the chances of successful resuscitation. Internal cardiac pacing may be useful in cases that do not respond to conventional treatment. If cardiac activity returns, the operation is completed in the operating room. The survival rate for emergency department thoracotomy is about 7%.

Indications of emergency department thoracotomy include cardiac arrest or imminent cardiac arrest due to both penetrating and blunt trauma, excluding fatal head injuries. Some of the survivors suffer brain death, but they may become organ donors.

Late Sequelae of Penetrating Cardiac Injuries

Late post-traumatic cardiac sequelae include anatomical defects (pericardial effusion, atrial or ventricular septal defects, valvular or papillary muscle lesions) and functional abnormalities (dyskinesia, hypokinesia). All survivors should be evaluated early and late postoperatively, clinically and by means of ECG and echocardiography. Many abnormalities may not manifest early, and a late cardiac evaluation performed about 1 month post injury is essential.

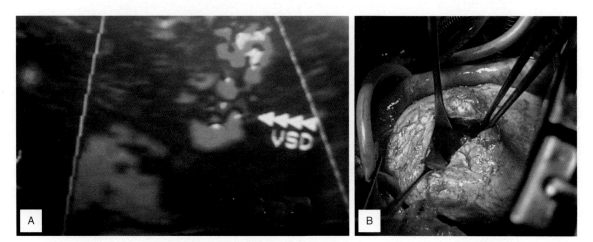

Figure 4.23 (A) Postoperative echocardiogram in a patient with penetrating cardiac injury demonstrates a ventricular septal defect (VSD). (B) Intraoperative photograph of a post-traumatic VSD.

4.7 Blunt Cardiac Trauma

There are no uniform criteria for the diagnosis of blunt cardiac trauma. Many patients are asymptomatic with only ECG changes or troponin elevations. Others may present with tachycardia, arrhythmia, or cardiogenic shock. All patients with a suspicious mechanism of injury or fractured sternum or anterior ribs should be evaluated by means of trauma ultrasound, ECG, and troponin levels. If these tests are normal, no further investigation is needed. If the ECG is abnormal or the troponin levels are elevated, the patient should be monitored closely and evaluated with formal echocardiogram. Symptomatic patients may need inotropes or antiarrhythmic treatment.

Cardiac rupture may result from major anteroposterior chest compression, rapid deceleration, perforation by fractured ribs or sternum, or massive sudden crushing forces on the abdomen. Blunt cardiac rupture is diagnosed at autopsy in about 30% of fatal blunt trauma. Patients with blunt cardiac rupture rarely reach the hospital alive. These patients are in severe shock, and the diagnosis can be confirmed by trauma ultrasound or during an emergency department thoracotomy. Most ruptures involve the right heart. In these cases, immediate thoracotomy with cardiac repair should be performed.

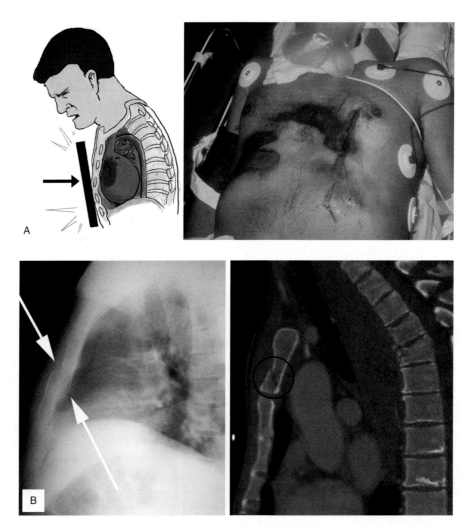

Figure 4.24 (A) Illustration of the mechanism of blunt cardiac injury from steering wheel (left). Photograph of blunt chest trauma to the anterior chest from a steering wheel injury (right). This patient arrived in ventricular tachycardia. (B) Lateral chest radiograph and CT scan showing sternal fractures. This injury is often associated with cardiac trauma. These patients should be evaluated by ECG and serial troponin levels.

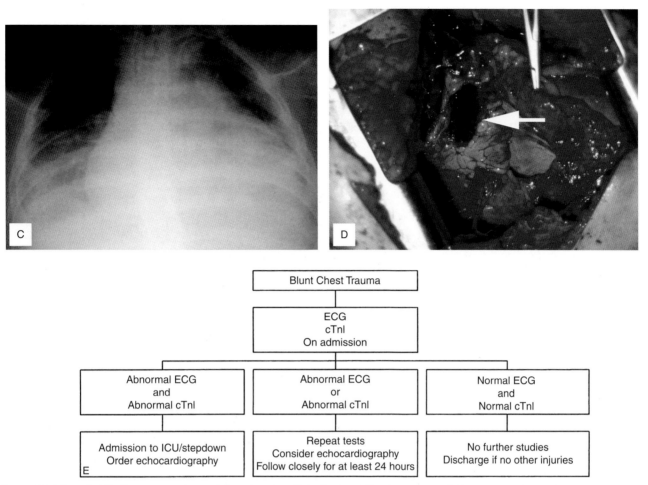

Figure 4.24 (*cont.*) (C) Chest x-ray shows delayed pericardial effusion following myocardial contusion due to blunt trauma. (D) Photograph of cardiac rupture (right atrium) following blunt trauma. (E) Algorithm for the evaluation of suspected cardiac trauma.

4.8 Blunt Thoracic Aortic Injury

Blunt thoracic aortic injury usually occurs after deceleration injuries, such as high-speed traffic accidents or falls from heights. In about 93% of cases, the rupture occurs just distal to the left subclavian artery and in about 7% the rupture occurs in the ascending aorta. About 34% of all fatalities due to blunt trauma have a rupture of the thoracic aorta at autopsy. Most of the victims die at the scene, with only about 20% of patients reaching hospital care. The diagnosis is based on the history of the injury and suspicious chest x-ray findings. Radiological findings suggestive of aortic rupture include a widened mediastinum, left apical pleural cap, obliteration of the aortic knob, and deviation of the nasogastric tube or the left main bronchus to the right. However, in many cases of aortic rupture, the chest x-ray may be normal. All patients with a suspicious mechanism of injury should be evaluated by means of CTA after stabilization. Diagnostic aortography should be reserved for patients requiring angiography for another reason (e.g., angioembolization for pelvic fracture) or cases when the CTA is not definitive. However, therapeutic aortography with endovascular stent-graft aortic repair has rapidly evolved and is becoming the standard of care treatment in aortic lesions distal to the left subclavian artery. The endovascular repair is associated with significantly lower in-hospital mortality, complications, and blood transfusions compared to the traditional open operative repair. While preparing for definitive aortic repair, judicious fluid management and the addition of beta-blockers or nitroprusside may be needed to maintain the systolic blood pressure 90–100 mm Hg in order to minimize the risk of free rupture. Other major associated injuries, such as intra-abdominal trauma or head injury, should be addressed before the definitive management of the aortic injury. The aortic repair can safely be delayed for a few days, as long as the blood pressure is controlled.

There is some evidence that multitrauma elderly patients with minor aortic injuries can safely be managed nonoperatively.

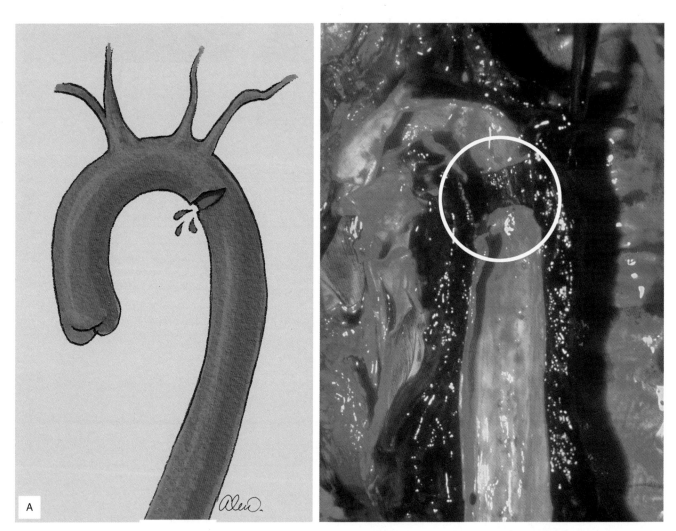

Figure 4.25 (A–D) Illustration and autopsy specimen of the typical site of blunt aortic rupture, distal to the left subclavian artery (A). Intraoperative photograph of a transected thoracic aorta found at emergency room thoracotomy (B). Intraoperative appearance of thoracic aortic rupture (RLN = Recurrent Laryngeal Nerve) (C). Surgical specimen of a contained aortic rupture. The outside layer of the aorta is intact (D). (E) Blunt thoracic aortic injury. Chest x-ray shows a widened mediastinum and deviation of the trachea to the right (left). CT image confirms thoracic aortic injury (right). (F) CT angiography with 3-D reconstruction shows a contained aortic rupture (left). Endoluminal view of the aortic pseudoaneurysm (right). (G) CT images of a blunt thoracic aortic injury with leak. This patient needs an emergency operation because of the risk of imminent free rupture. (H) Aortogram of traumatic aortic pseudoaneurysm, (left) treated with stent-graft deployment (right). Note the occlusion of the left subclavian artery by the device. (I–K) CT scan showing a rupture of the thoracic aorta (I). CT scan appearance of the deployed stent graft with occlusion of the rupture site (J, K).

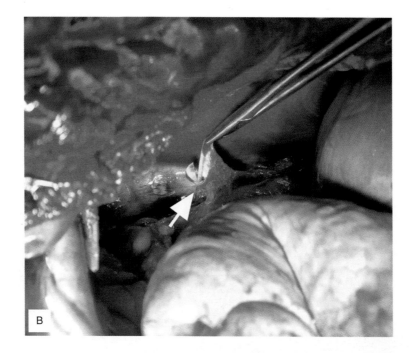

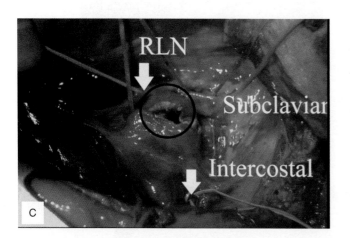

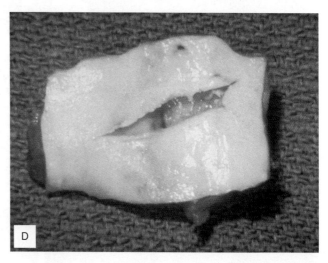

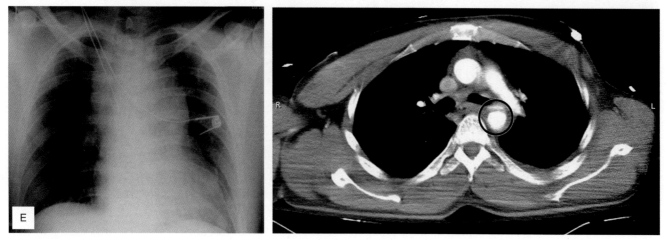

Figure 4.25 (cont.)

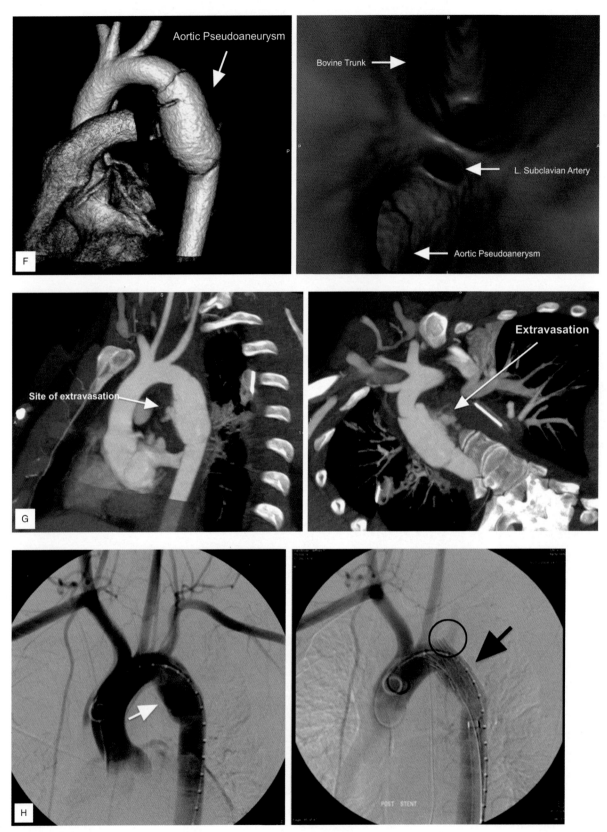

Figure 4.25 (*cont.*)

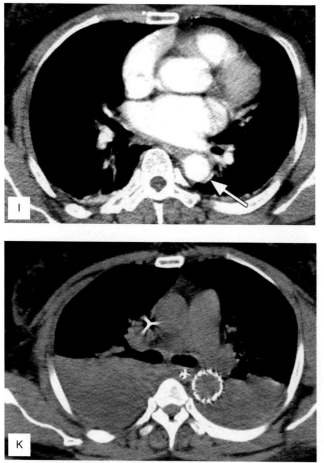

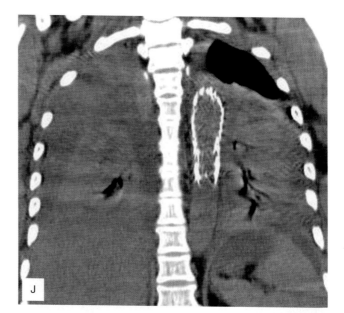

Figure 4.25 (*cont.*)

4.9 Penetrating Thoracic Outlet Injuries

The most important structures of the thoracic outlet are the aortic arch with its major branches (innominate artery, origin of left carotid artery, and left subclavian artery), the superior vena cava, the innominate vein, and the subclavian veins.

Hemodynamically stable patients with penetrating injuries in this anatomical area should be investigated for vascular injuries. CTA is an excellent investigation for suspected thoracic outlet vascular injuries. CFD is an alternative reliable investigation for suspected subclavian vascular injuries. Angiography should be reserved for cases with shotgun injuries or when the CFD evaluation is not definitive or endovascular stenting is a possibility. Injuries to the branches of the aortic arch require surgical repair, though angiographically placed endovascular stents can be used in selected cases with false aneurysms or arteriovenous fistulas.

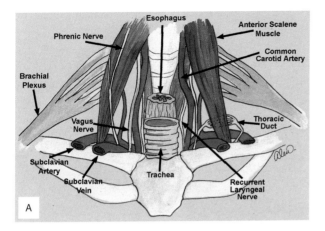

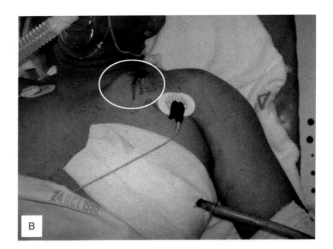

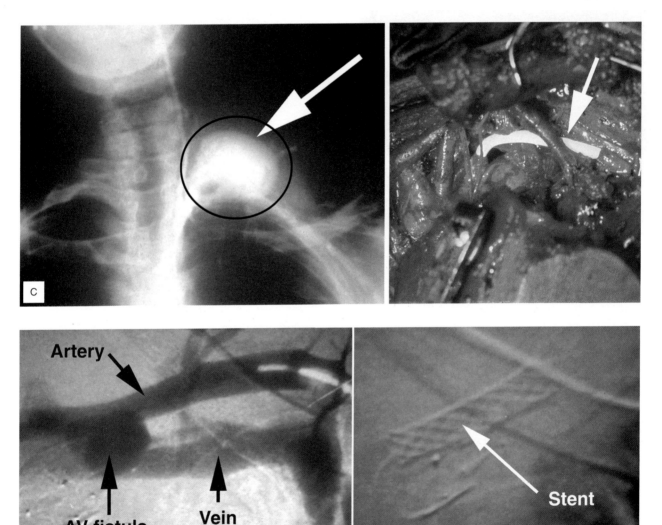

Figure 4.26 (A) Penetrating thoracic outlet injuries. Illustration of the anatomy of vital structures in the thoracic outlet. (B) Patient with a stab wound injury to the left supraclavicular area, presenting with a large pulsating hematoma. (C) Arteriography of the previous patient shows a false aneurysm of the left subclavian artery (left). Operative reconstruction of the left subclavian artery with prosthetic graft (right). (D) Patient with gunshot wound in the right clavicular region, presenting with a decreased peripheral pulse and a bruit below the clavicle. Arteriography shows an arteriovenous fistula between the subclavian artery and vein (left). The injury was successfully managed with angiographic stenting (right).

4.10 Transmediastinal Gunshot Wounds

Transmediastinal gunshot wounds are associated with a high incidence of major injuries to mediastinal structures. Hemodynamically unstable patients should have an emergency operation. About 70% of hemodynamically stable patients do not have significant injuries requiring surgical repair. These patients need evaluation of the mediastinal structures (heart, aorta, esophagus, tracheobronchial tree).

Besides the routine FAST and ECG for the evaluation of the heart, CTA and esophagography/esophagoscopy may be indicated. Chest CTA is very accurate in selecting patients who might benefit from aortography or esophageal or tracheobronchial studies. Patients with bullet tracks toward the aorta, the trachea, or the esophagus are candidates for further studies.

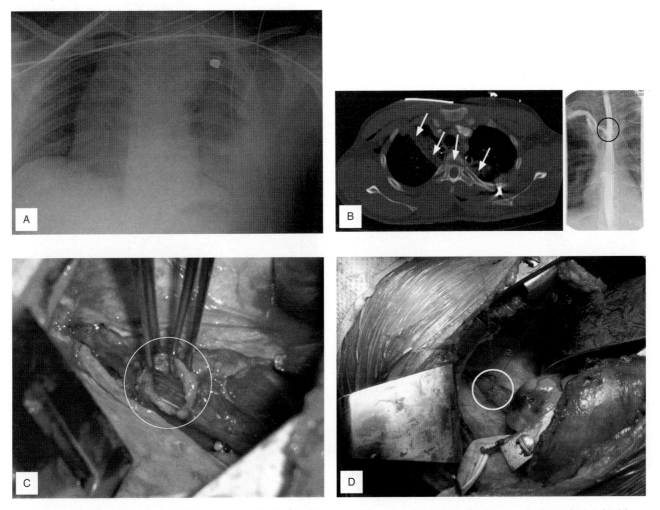

Figure 4.27 (A) Gunshot wound of the upper mediastinum. Chest x-ray shows a widened mediastinum, a finding which is highly suspicious for a vascular injury. This patient needs evaluation with CT angiography or conventional angiography. (B) CT scan of a victim with transmediastinal gunshot wound. The bullet tract is very close to the esophagus (arrows) (left). This is a strong indication for further esophageal evaluation. Esophagogram shows a leak from the upper thoracic esophagus (right). (C–D) Intraoperative photograph of the esophageal injury (C), which was repaired primarily (D).

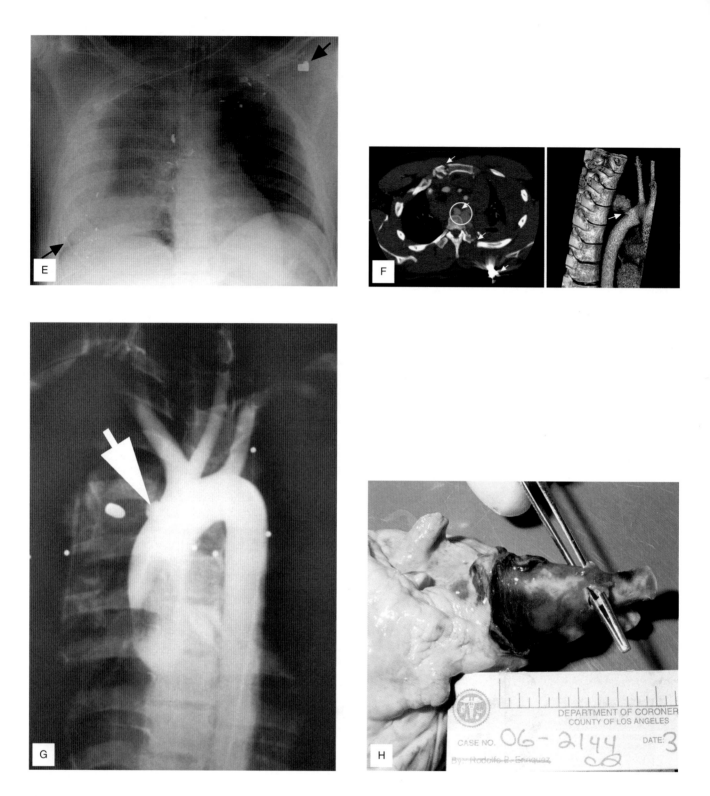

Figure 4.27 (*cont.*) (E–F) Chest x-ray of patient with a transmediastinal gunshot wound, with an entry at the right lower chest and fragments along the missile tract. The bullet is lodged in the left upper chest (E). CT scan with intravenous contrast shows an injury to the aorta (circle). Note the fracture of the sternum and the bullet in the subcutaneous tissues in the left upper back (F, left). CT image with 3-D reconstruction shows the aortic injury (F, right). (G) Low-velocity transmediastinal gunshot wound. Aortography shows a small aneurysm of the ascending aorta. (H) Autopsy specimen showing a through-and-through penetrating injury to the ascending thoracic aorta.

4.11 Diaphragmatic Injuries

Penetrating Diaphragmatic Injuries

About 60% of all gunshot wounds and 30% of all stab wounds to the left thoracoabdominal area (the area between the nipple and costal margin anteriorly and the tip of the scapula and lower ribs posteriorly) are associated with diaphragmatic injuries. About 10% of gunshot wounds and 30% of stab wounds to this area with no abdominal symptoms have diaphragmatic injuries. Unrecognized diaphragmatic injuries may result in diaphragmatic hernias, sometimes many months or years after the injury. To prevent this complication, early diagnosis and repair of all injuries to the left diaphragm is essential. Right diaphragmatic injuries, with the exception of anterior injuries, rarely result in hernias because of the protective presence of the liver.

The diagnosis of penetrating diaphragmatic injury should be suspected from the presence of a wound over the thoracoabdominal area. The chest x-ray is normal in the majority of patients with uncomplicated diaphragmatic perforations. An elevated hemidiaphragm is suspicious but not diagnostic of diaphragmatic injury. (Conditions that may be associated with an elevated diaphragm include atelectasis, hepatic or splenic hematoma, gastric dilatation, fractures of the lower ribs, and phrenic nerve injury.) CT scan and magnetic resonance imaging (MRI) are often not diagnostic in small,

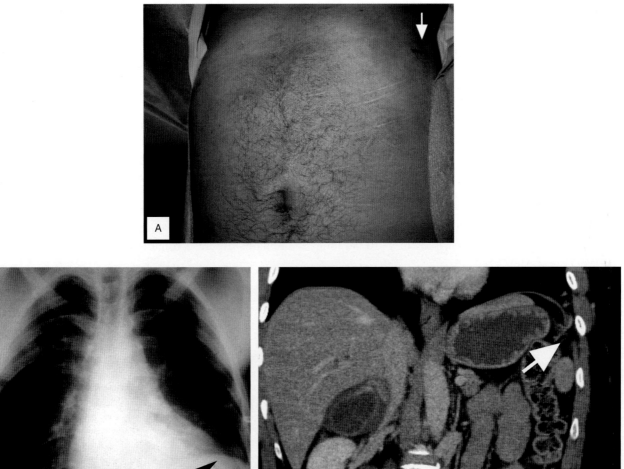

Figure 4.28 (A–B) Penetrating diaphragmatic injuries. (A) Photograph of stab wound to the left thoracoabdominal area (arrow). Penetrating trauma in this area is highly suspicious for diaphragmatic injury. (B) Chest x-ray shows an elevated left diaphragm, which is suspicious for diaphragmatic injury (left). CT scan shows a left diaphragm injury (right).

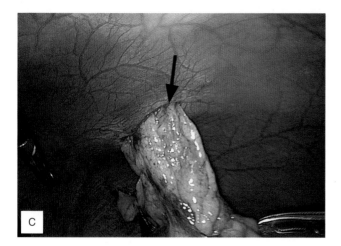

Figure 4.28 (*cont.*) (C) Laparoscopy shows a diaphragmatic perforation with omentum herniating into the left chest.

uncomplicated diaphragmatic injuries. The most reliable way to diagnose uncomplicated diaphragmatic injuries is routine laparoscopy for all asymptomatic patients with suspicious penetrating wounds in the left thoracoabdominal or anterior right thoracoabdominal regions. In the presence of a diaphragmatic hernia, the chest x-ray, CT scan, or MRI are almost always diagnostic.

Blunt Diaphragmatic Injuries

Rupture of the diaphragm is found in about 7% of all laparotomies for blunt trauma. The left diaphragm is involved in about 70% of the cases and the right diaphragm in about 30%. In 3% of cases, both diaphragms are ruptured. The tear is about 7–10 cm long as compared with 2–3 cm in penetrating trauma. Blunt abdominal trauma with a sudden increase of the intra-abdominal pressure (usually in belted car occupants) is the most common mechanism of diaphragmatic rupture, though fractured ribs may also cause tears. Deceleration injuries may cause detachment of the diaphragm from the ribs.

The chest x-ray, CT scan, or MRI are usually more diagnostic than in penetrating trauma because of the large size of the diaphragmatic tear in blunt trauma. In most patients there are major associated intra-abdominal injuries, and the diagnosis of diaphragmatic injuries is made intraoperatively. However, in some cases there is no associated abdominal trauma, and in the absence of herniation the diagnosis of diaphragmatic tear may be missed. Laparoscopy in suspected cases remains the most reliable investigation.

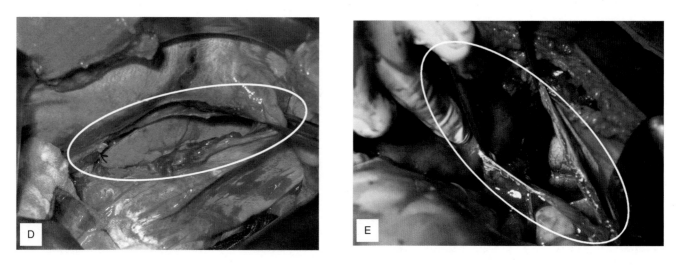

Figure 4.28 (*cont.*) (D) Blunt diaphragmatic rupture: high-speed motor vehicle crash with left diaphragmatic rupture. Note the lung through the tear (left). Post-repair of the injury (right). (E–F) Blunt versus penetrating diaphragmatic injuries. (E) Appearance of blunt diaphragmatic injuries through a thoracotomy (left) and through a laparotomy (right). Note the large size of the injuries.

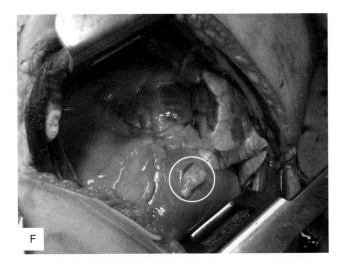

Figure 4.28 (*cont.*) (F) Appearance of penetrating a diaphragmatic injury through a thoracotomy. The injury is usually small (2–3 cm). Note the omentum herniating through the diaphragmatic defect.

Traumatic Diaphragmatic Hernias

Traumatic diaphragmatic hernias may appear within minutes, hours, days, weeks, or many years after injury to the diaphragm. In the vast majority of cases, the hernia is found in the left diaphragm, although right diaphragmatic hernias may occur as well. The most commonly herniating viscera are the omentum, stomach, and colon, followed by spleen, small bowel, liver, and tail of pancreas.

Many hernias remain asymptomatic and are discovered during routine chest x-rays. Other patients present with signs of gastrointestinal obstruction, respiratory distress, and sepsis due to a gangrenous viscus. The diagnosis is suspected from the chest x-ray and history of previous trauma and confirmed by CT scan, MRI, or contrast studies. A nasogastric tube may be seen curling into the left chest on x-ray and is pathognomonic of gastric herniation. The radiological appearance of a diaphragmatic hernia may be confused with many other pathologies such as lung laceration, bronchopneumonia, residual hemothorax, phrenic nerve injury, intrapulmonary abscess, and diaphragmatic eventration. The history of trauma and high index of suspicion remains the cornerstone of early diagnosis. Delayed diagnosis of a complicated diaphragmatic hernia (obstruction, ischemia or necrosis, or cardiorespiratory complication due to compression) is associated with high mortality. All diaphragmatic hernias require surgical repair through a laparotomy or laparoscopically.

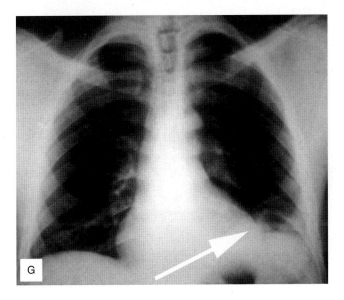

Figure 4.28 (*cont.*) (G–I) Radiological appearance of traumatic diaphragmatic hernias. (G) Chest x-ray with a suspicious shadow at the base of the left hemithorax following a stab wound many months earlier. Further investigations showed gastric herniation into the chest. (H) Chest x-ray shows the nasogastric tube curling into the left chest (arrow), pathognomic of gastric herniation. Chest x-ray shows significantly elevated right diaphragm following a motor vehicle crash two weeks earlier. (I) The entire liver (arrow) and hepatic flexure of the colon were found at laparotomy to be herniated into the right chest. (J) Chest x-ray and CT scan of patient, many months after a stab wound to the left thoracoabdominal area, shows a tension diaphragmatic hernia with significant deviation of the heart to the right chest (left). CT scan showing the stomach herniating into the chest (right). (K) Chest x-ray shows a tension diaphragmatic hernia a few weeks after a stab wound to the left lower chest (left). CT findings confirm the stomach, spleen, and colon herniating into the chest (right).

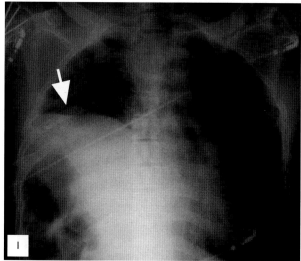

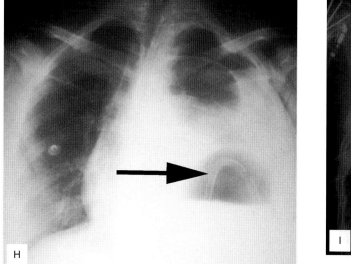

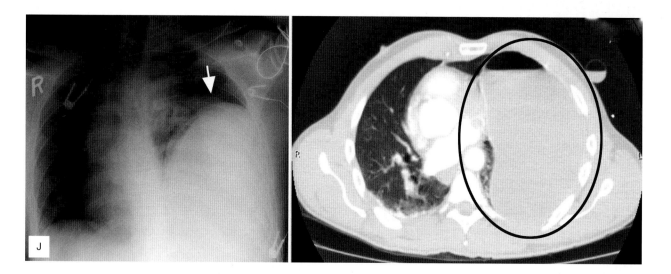

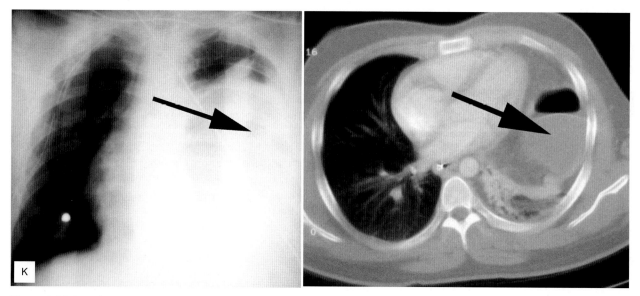

Figure 4.28 (*cont.*)

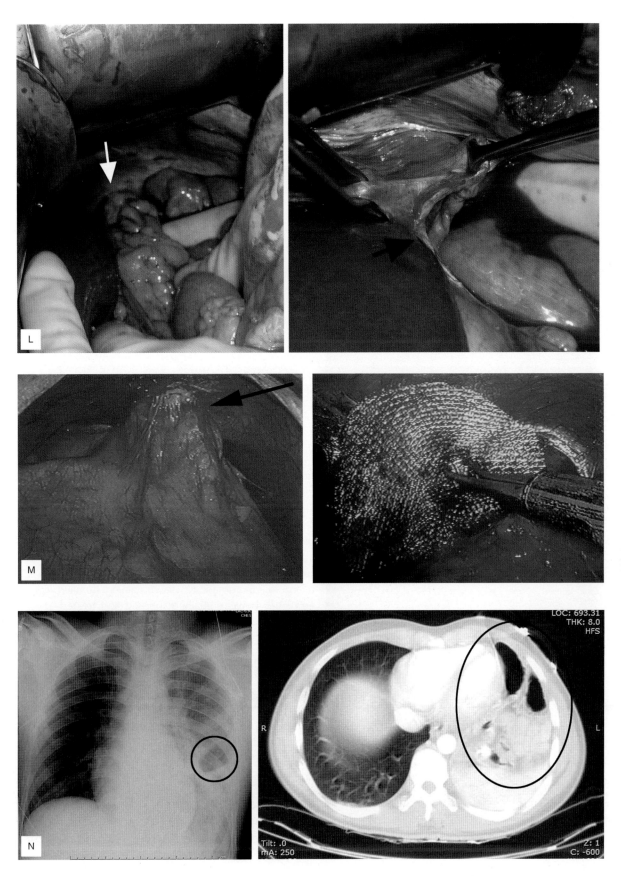

Figure 4.28 (*cont.*) (L) Operative appearance of left diaphragmatic hernia containing colon and omentum (left). Photograph of the diaphragmatic defect after reduction of the hernia contents (right). (M) Laparoscopic appearance of the stomach and omentum herniating into the chest (left) and successful repair with the mesh (right). (N) High-speed motor vehicle crash. The chest x-ray is highly suspicious for left traumatic diaphragmatic hernia (left). The CT scan shows herniation of the stomach, spleen, and bowel into the left chest (right).

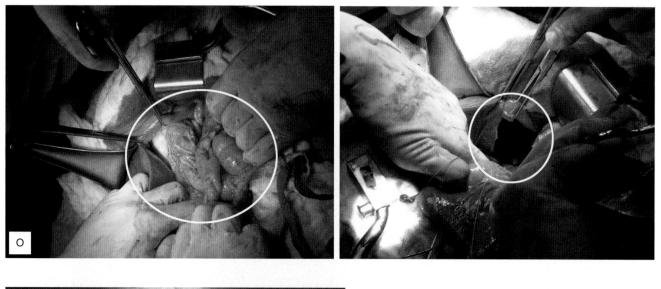

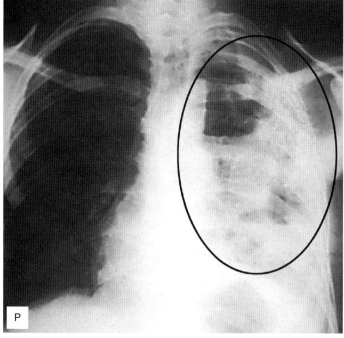

Figure 4.28 (*cont.*) (O) Intraoperative photograph showing a large diaphragmatic hernia with herniation of multiple abdominal contents (left). The photograph in the right shows the diaphragm defect after the reduction of the herniating viscera. (P) Chest x-ray of a large diaphragmatic hernia containing stomach, colon, and small bowel, initially diagnosed and treated as bronchopneumonia. The delay in diagnosis resulted in ischemic necrosis of the colon.

4.12 Esophageal Injuries

Esophageal injuries should be suspected in all penetrating proximity injuries, especially if the x-ray or CT scan shows mediastinal or subcutaneous emphysema in the neck. In suspected cases, esophagography and/or esophagoscopy should be performed. The combination of both investigations is highly sensitive in the identification of esophageal injuries. Early diagnosis and surgical repair are critical for good outcome. Delayed diagnosis is associated with a high incidence of sepsis and mortality.

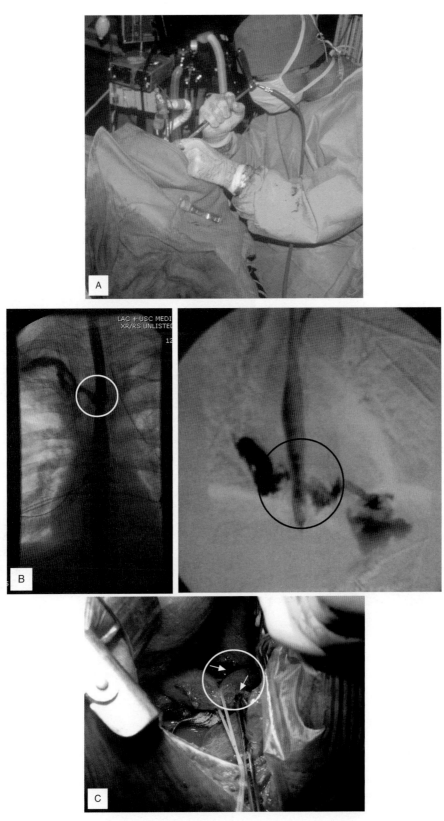

Figure 4.29 (A) Intraoperative rigid esophagoscopy for suspected esophageal injury. (B) Gastric swallow studies showing injuries to the upper thoracic (left) and lower thoracic esophagus (right), following gunshot injuries. (C) Intraoperative photograph showing through-and-through esophageal wound with suction tip passing through the esophageal perforations.

4.13 Thoracic Duct Injury

Rupture of the thoracic duct is usually due to penetrating trauma in the left supraclavicular region or the mediastinum and rarely due to blunt deceleration trauma. The diagnosis should be suspected in the presence of milky fluid in the pleural cavitity. Sometimes in patients who have not received any oral feeding for a few days, the fluid may be clear or blood-stained. The diagnosis is confirmed by the presence of many lymphocytes and the high concentration of lipids in the fluid.

Most thoracic duct leaks heal nonoperatively with a low-fat oral diet or total parenteral nutrition. In patients with high output (more than 500 ml per day) persisting for more than 2–3 weeks without any sign of improvement, a thoracotomy or thoracoscopy with thoracic duct ligation may be necessary.

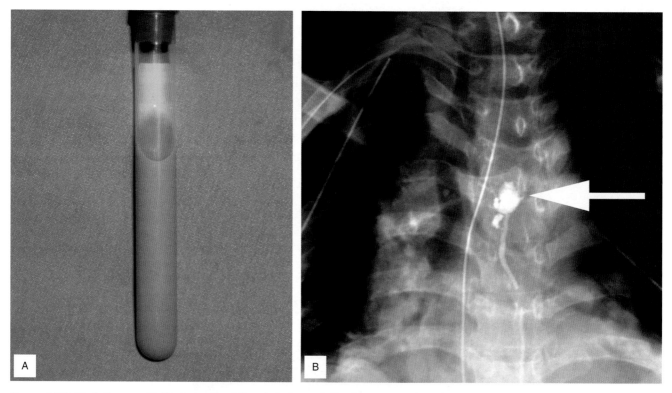

Figure 4.30 Chylothorax. (A) Photograph of the chylothorax following penetrating chest trauma. Note the milky appearance of the thoracic collection. (B) Lymphangiogram shows a significant leak from the thoracic duct.

4.14 Traumatic Asphyxia

Traumatic asphyxia is the result of severe crush injury to the chest. Because of the sudden increase of pressure in the venous and capillary systems, the victim develops extensive petechiae in the skin and conjunctivae. Similar microhemorrhages may develop in the brain and lungs, and the patient may present with central nervous or respiratory problems. The treatment is symptomatic.

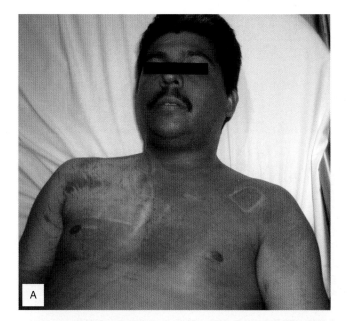

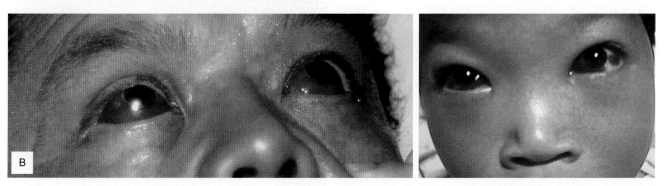

Figure 4.31 Traumatic asphyxia. (A) Photograph of a patient with crush trauma to the chest and traumatic asphyxia. Note the extensive petechiae on the face and chest. (B) Photographs of extensive petechiae on the face and conjuctival hemorrhages in an adult and a child with traumatic asphyxia.

4.15 Impaled Thoracic Foreign Bodies

Impaled thoracic foreign bodies should not be removed on the scene of injury. Impaled foreign bodies should be taped to the torso during the transportation and removed in the operating room if the foreign body appears to be in proximity of intrathoracic vessels, pulmonary hilum, or mediastinal structures. Removal of the foreign body in an uncontrolled environment may result in uncontrolled hemorrhage and death. The FAST to rule out pericardial tamponade in addition to the plain chest radiograph provides helpful imaging prior to removal of the foreign body.

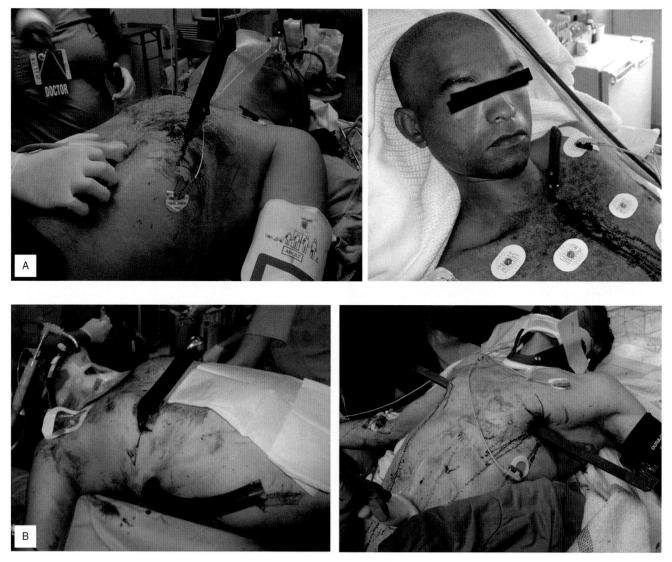

Figure 4.32 Retained thoracic foreign bodies. (A) Stab wounds to the chest with embedded knifes. (B) Photographs of patients sustaining penetrating injuries and impaled large rods. The impaled objects should be removed under the direct control of the surgeon, usually in the operating room.

5 Abdominal Injury

Demetrios Demetriades and Kenji Inaba

Blunt Abdominal Trauma

Introduction

Traffic accidents, followed by falls, are by far the most common cause of severe blunt abdominal trauma. Solid organs, usually the spleen and liver, are the most commonly injured organs. Hollow viscus perforations are fairly uncommon, and they are usually associated with seatbelts or high-speed deceleration.

There are five main mechanisms of injury with blunt trauma:

1. Direct crushing of organs between the anterior and posterior abdominal walls.
2. Avulsion injuries from deceleration forces, as in high-speed accidents or falls from heights.
3. Transient formation of a closed bowel loop with high intraluminal pressure and rupture of the hollow viscus.
4. Lacerations by bony fragments (e.g., pelvis, lower ribs).
5. Sudden and massive elevation of the intra-abdominal pressure (usually seatbelted individuals involved in high-speed accidents) may cause diaphragmatic or even cardiac rupture.

Clinical Examination

The clinical evaluation of blunt abdominal trauma is often complicated by associated soft tissue contusion, fractures of the lower ribs or pelvis, head injuries with depressed level of consciousness, and spinal injuries. These conditions make clinical examination difficult and unreliable, and significant hollow viscus injuries may be missed with potentially lethal consequences.

Most preventable deaths due to trauma are the result of delayed diagnosis of intra-abdominal injuries. Despite these limitations, physical examination remains the cornerstone of abdominal evaluation. Of particular importance is the "seatbelt sign" on the abdominal wall. Its presence is associated with a high incidence (about 20%) of significant intra-abdominal injuries.

Investigations

1. Chest x-rays should be obtained in all major trauma cases. Pelvic x-rays should be obtained selectively. Thoracic trauma is a commonly associated problem. Fractures of the lower ribs, an elevated diaphragm, and free intraperitoneal air are important radiological signs suggestive of intra-abdominal trauma.
2. Trauma ultrasound: Portable ultrasound or bedside ultrasound has become one of the most valuable emergency department investigations in the evaluation of abdominal trauma or the multitrauma patient. The ultrasound should be performed by emergency physicians or trauma surgeons. The study determines the presence or absence of free intraperitoneal fluid, mainly in the hepatorenal, splenorenal, and suprapubic spaces. It is quick, noninvasive, safe, portable, and fairly accurate. Its most important weaknesses are the inability to identify the source of free intraperitoneal fluid or to detect injuries to the bowel, retroperitoneum, and diaphragm and its accuracy is operator-dependent. The presence of free fluid on ultrasound in a hemodynamically unstable patient is an indication for urgent laparotomy. However, in

hemodynamically stable patients, an abdominal CT scan is the most appropriate next step.

3. Diagnostic peritoneal lavage (DPL): DPL has largely been replaced by the trauma ultrasound. However, diagnostic peritoneal aspirate (DPA) has an important role in the evaluation of the abdomen in a hemodynamically unstable patient, if the ultrasound is not definitive or not available. The procedure can be performed with the open or percutaneous closed technique; the closed one uses a guidewire technique, as in central venous line insertion, and is faster and less invasive. The aspiration of gross blood during a DPA has major significance and is a strong indication for laparotomy in the hemodynamically unstable multitrauma patient. The role of intraperitoneal fluid infusion and lavage is rarely necessary or useful.

4. CT scan: Contrast CT scan has become the most important and useful investigation in the evaluation of suspected blunt abdominal trauma. It is very sensitive in diagnosing solid organ injuries. In addition to the site and size of solid organ injury, it may give valuable information about the presence of active bleeding or false aneurysms, provided intravenous contrast has been administered. The role of CT scan in the diagnosis of hollow viscus perforation is rather limited, and up to 30–40% of injuries may be missed. CT scan findings suggesting bowel injury include pneumoperitoneum, thickened bowel wall, extravasation of oral contrast, fat stranding and free intraperitoneal fluid in the absence of solid organ injury.

5. Intravenous pyelogram (IVP): One-shot IVP in the emergency department has little or no role in the evaluation of abdominal trauma. Formal IVP has largely been replaced by contrast CT scan, though it may still have a role in suspected ureteric injuries.

6. Angiography: This is an important diagnostic and therapeutic tool in selected cases of abdominal trauma, such as in suspected bleeding from pelvic fractures or complex liver injuries.

7. Magnetic resonance cholangiopancreatography (MRCP): This is a good test for evaluation of the integrity of the pancreatic duct in suspected pancreatic trauma.

8. Urinalysis: All patients should be evaluated for hematuria. Gross or symptomatic microscopic hematuria should be evaluated by means of contrast CT scan and cystogram. Asymptomatic microscopic hematuria does not need further evaluation.

9. Serum amylase and lipase: They may be useful laboratory tests for suspected pancreaticoduodenal trauma, although the sensitivity and specificity are fairly low. Normal levels do not reliably exclude pancreatic trauma, and they are elevated in only about 70% of cases with proven pancreatic trauma. Serial measurements are more useful than the initial values.

General Management

The initial evaluation and management should follow standard advanced trauma life support (ATLS) guidelines. Trauma ultrasound studies should be part of the standard evaluation of all suspected abdominal blunt trauma. Hemodynamically unstable patients or those with signs of peritonitis should be taken to the operating room with no delay. Time-consuming investigations should be reserved only for the patient who is hemodynamically stable and whose diagnosis is uncertain.

In the multitrauma patient, there is often combined abdominal and head trauma. The timing of evaluation and management of the injuries of these anatomical areas is important and can have a major effect on outcome. In the presence of hemodynamic instability, the abdomen should be evaluated by trauma ultrasound or DPA. If there is evidence of free intraperitoneal fluid, the patient should have a laparotomy first and a head CT scan postoperatively. If there are localizing neurological signs, burr holes should be considered during laparotomy before CT evaluation. In the hemodynamically stable patient with peritonitis and GCS ≤12 or localizing signs, a CT scan of the head should precede laparotomy, under close monitoring. It is rare that both a laparotomy and a craniotomy are required simultaneously.

Many carefully selected patients with solid organ injury (liver, spleen, kidney) can safely be managed nonoperatively, provided that they are hemodynamically stable and have no signs of peritonitis. Overall, about 70% of blunt liver injuries, about 80% of splenic injuries, and about 90% of renal injuries can be managed nonoperatively.

Common Mistakes and Pitfalls

1. Delayed diagnosis of hollow viscus perforation in a clinically unevaluable patient (e.g., associated head injury, spinal cord injury, or intoxication) is a common problem. The presence of a seatbelt sign should raise the index of suspicion. Look for subtle

CT scan findings, such as bowel edema, intraperitoneal gas, and free intraperitoneal fluid in the absence of a solid organ injury. They are highly suspicious findings, and exploratory laparotomy should be considered. Repeat abdominal CT scan should be considered in suspicious cases.

2. Missed pancreaticoduodenal injuries are notorious for their fairly silent clinical presentation. The initial CT scan may miss the injury, and the serum amylase or lipase may be normal. In suspicious cases, repeat the CT scan 6–10 hours later and perform serial enzyme determinations.

Penetrating Abdominal Trauma

Introduction

The initial evaluation of penetrating abdominal trauma is usually very different from evaluation of blunt trauma. Penetrating trauma, especially gunshot wounds, is much more likely to be associated with life-threatening major vascular injuries than blunt trauma.

Knife injuries to the anterior abdomen are associated with significant intra-abdominal injuries in about 50% of patients. In gunshot wounds, about 80% of cases have major injuries requiring surgical repair.

Clinical Examination

Physical examination is usually reliable in identifying patients with significant intra-abdominal injuries. The physician must remember that patients with a short prehospital time may seem hemodynamically stable despite severe active intra-abdominal bleeding, and thus serial examinations are critical in the initially asymptomatic patient. Tachycardia and elevated diastolic pressure (narrow pulse pressure) are suspicious markers of bleeding, and these patients should be re-evaluated every few minutes during admission.

Investigations

Very few investigations are needed in the evaluation of penetrating abdominal trauma. Radiological studies should be reserved for stable patients.

1. Chest x-ray should be obtained in selected patients with stab wounds or gunshot wounds with suspected thoracic involvement. The x-ray may show hemopneumothoraces, an elevated diaphragm, free air under the diaphragm, and foreign bodies.
2. Abdominal x-rays have no role in stab wounds to the abdomen, and they should not be obtained.

However, if time permits, they should be obtained for all torso gunshot wounds with no exit and in patients with suspected spinal or pelvic fractures.
3. CT scan with intravenous contrast studies may be useful in evaluating patients with gunshot wounds who are hemodynamically stable and have a soft abdomen. The CT scan may show a bullet tract away from any major structures and avoid an unnecessary operation. Some trauma centers practice nonoperative management of gunshot wounds to the liver, kidney, or spleen in carefully selected patients who are hemodynamically stable and have a soft abdomen. CT scanning of these patients can demonstrate the extent of the solid organ injury and may identify false aneurysms or active bleeding.
4. Bedside trauma ultrasound (FAST) can identify patients with hemoperitoneum. However this is not a contraindication for nonoperative management. In addition, the pericardium should be examined in all patients with proximity wounds.
5. Angiography may play an important diagnostic and therapeutic role in patients with liver, kidney, or spleen injuries when the CT scan is suspicious for false aneurysms, arteriovenous fistula, or active bleeding. Similarly, in patients who have undergone damage control operations for severe liver injuries, angiographic embolization of any remaining bleeding vessels may be life-saving.
6. Diagnostic laparoscopy has a definitive role in the evaluation of suspected diaphragmatic injuries (see Chapter 4).

General Management

One of the most important goals in managing penetrating abdominal injuries is to avoid nontherapeutic laparotomies and yet not miss any significant injuries. Patients presenting with hemodynamic instability or signs of peritonitis require an emergency operation without any delay. Patients with minimal or equivocal abdominal signs should be monitored with serial clinical examinations and continuous hemodynamic recordings. Further investigations, such as CT scanning, serial white blood cell count, or diagnostic laparoscopy, should be performed in appropriate cases. If the patient develops hemodynamic instability or signs of peritonitis, an exploratory laparotomy should be performed. Patients who remain asymptomatic are discharged after 48–72 hours of observation. The selective nonoperative management policy can be applied in both stab wounds and gunshot wounds, provided the patient is clinically evaluable.

Common Mistakes and Pitfalls

1. Patients with short prehospital times may seem hemodynamically stable on admission, despite significant active intra-abdominal bleeding. Once a decision for laparotomy has been made, no time should be wasted for further investigations.
2. Penetrating injuries to the diaphragm are usually clinically and radiologically silent. All patients with left or anterior right thoracoabdominal injuries who are asymptomatic should be evaluated by diagnostic laparoscopy.
3. Patients with associated severe head or spinal cord injuries and those undergoing general anesthesia for an extra-abdominal operation cannot be evaluated clinically. In these groups of patients, the presence of a deep penetrating abdominal wound should be an indication for laparotomy, irrespective of signs or symptoms.
4. Patients selected for observation and nonoperative management should not receive analgesics or prophylactic antibiotics because of the risk of masking important signs and symptoms.

Blunt Abdominal Trauma

5.1 Mechanism of Injury

Intra-abdominal injuries may occur by three mechanisms:

1. Crushing of an organ against the spine, pelvis, or ribs and the abdominal wall.
2. Deceleration, such as high-speed accidents or falls from heights.
3. Sudden increase of the intraluminal pressure and bursting of a hollow viscus, commonly seen with seatbelt injuries.

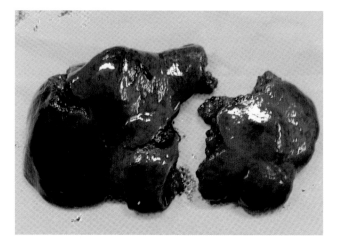

Figure 5.1 Direct crushing injury to spleen.

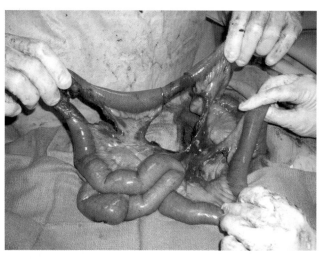

Figure 5.2 Mesenteric "bucket handle" avulsion injury to small bowel from deceleration injury following a high-speed car accident.

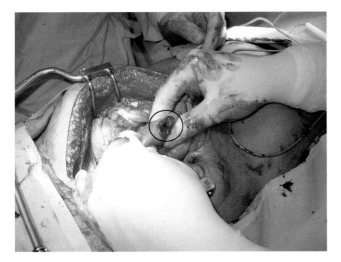

Figure 5.3 Small bowel rupture due to closed loop and increased intraluminal pressure.

Seatbelts have significantly decreased deaths in motor vehicle accidents. Although the incidence of intra-abdominal injuries has not changed with the use of seatbelts, the nature of the injuries has changed: seatbelt wearers are more likely to suffer hollow viscus perforation.

The presence of seatbelt marks on the abdominal wall is an important physical finding because of the high incidence of associated intra-abdominal injuries (22% with seatbelt marks versus 3% in patients wearing seatbelts but without a seatbelt mark).

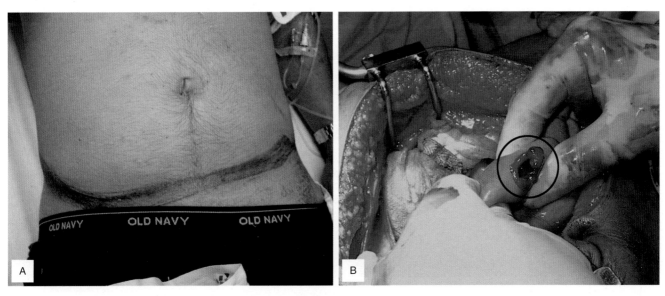

Figure 5.4 Seatbelt mark in a car accident patient. (A) The presence of this sign is a marker of significant intraabdominal injury. (B) Intraoperative photograph of the same patient showing perforation of the small bowel.

5.2 Diagnosis of Hemoperitoneum

Hemoperitoneum by itself often does not give peritoneal signs. Thus, the clinical diagnosis, especially in the presence of multitrauma, can be difficult. Trauma ultrasound (FAST), performed in the emergency department by emergency physicians or surgeons, is a fast, usually reliable, and noninvasive method of detecting intraperitoneal bleeding. The hepatorenal, splenorenal, and suprapubic spaces are examined for free fluid during the trauma ultrasound exam. However, ultrasound does not identify the source of the bleeding and cannot evaluate the retroperitoneum, hollow viscera, or the diaphragm.

DPL has largely been replaced by ultrasound. However, DPA has a definitive role in the evaluation of an unstable patient when the ultrasound is not diagnostic or not available. It can be performed with the open technique or the closed guidewire technique.

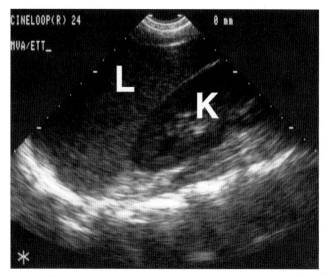

Figure 5.5 Normal FAST: right upper quadrant window depicts liver and right kidney with no free fluid. (K, kidney; L, liver.)

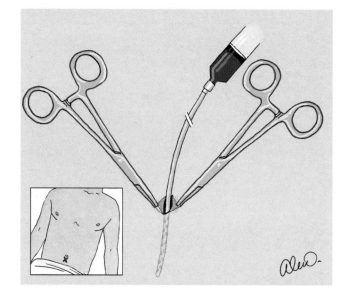

Figure 5.7 Open diagnostic peritoneal lavage/aspiration technique. This technique is rarely used.

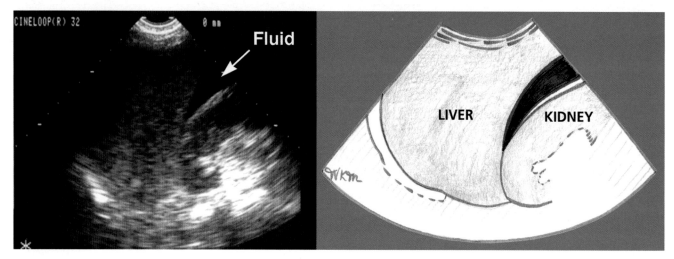

Figure 5.6 FAST exam with free fluid between liver and kidney (arrow).

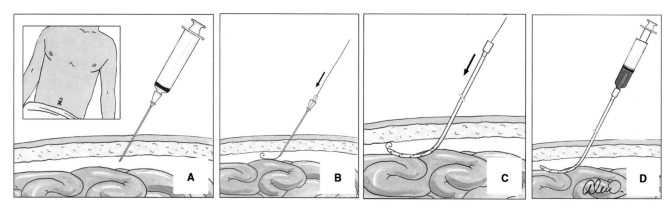

Figure 5.8 Closed diagnostic peritoneal lavage/aspiration technique. (A) A small (3–4 mm) skin incision is made about 1 cm below the umbilicus. A needle, attached to a syringe, is introduced intraperitoneally. (B) A guidewire is introduced through the needle and the needle is removed. (C) The catheter is introduced over the wire, aiming towards the pelvis. (D) The guidewire is removed and aspiration for blood is performed.

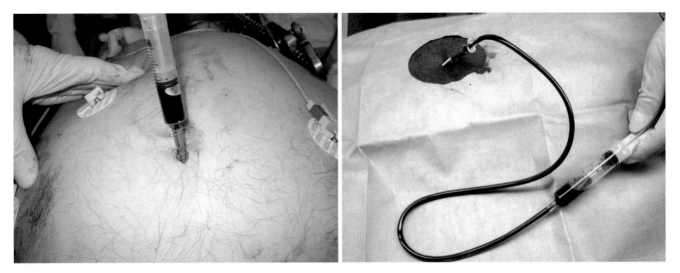

Figure 5.9 Aspiration of gross blood from catheter during DPA.

CT scan should be considered in hemodynamically stable patients. Under these circumstances, it is the most valuable investigation. It can also identify the source of the bleeding and visualize the retroperitoneum.

5.3 Splenic Injuries

The clinical presentation of a splenic rupture may vary from mild left hypochondrial pain to severe hypovolemic shock. The diagnosis is suspected from the clinical examination (pain in left upper abdomen often radiating to the left shoulder, signs of hypovolemia) or trauma ultrasound showing free intraperitoneal fluid and confirmed by CT scan or laparotomy.

Most isolated minor or moderate severity (grades I–III) splenic injuries can safely be managed nonoperatively (about 90% in children, 70% in adults). The criteria for nonoperative management are

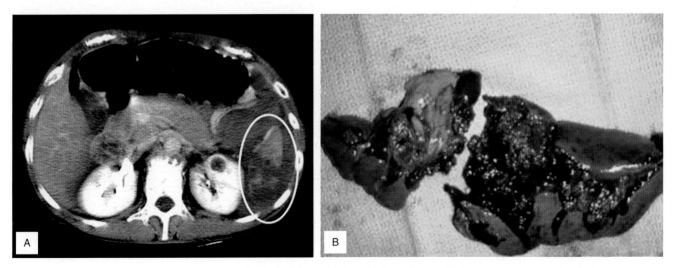

Figure 5.10 (A) Abdominal CT with a grade IV spleen injury. (B) Surgical specimen of the removed ruptured spleen.

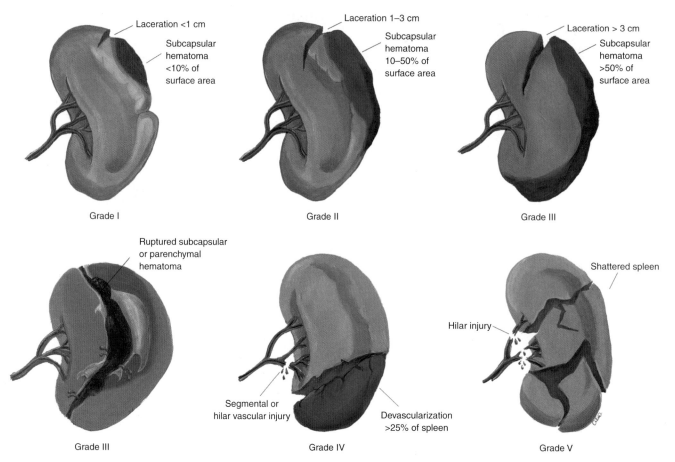

Figure 5.11 Grades of splenic injuries, according to the American Association for the Surgery of Trauma classification. Most grade I–III injuries can safely be managed nonoperatively. The majority of grade IV or V injuries require operative management.

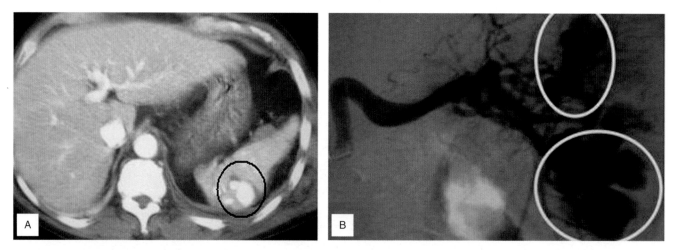

Figure 5.12 (A) CT scan showing a large intrasplenic aneurysm. (B) Angiography showing multiple intrasplenic pseudoaneurysms. These injuries can be managed with angioembolization.

hemodynamic stability, a soft abdomen, and no other indications for laparotomy. The abdominal CT scan may be very helpful in determining the need for surgical intervention: severe injuries (grades IV or V) often fail nonoperative management. The presence of blushing (extravasation of contrast) on CT scan is suggestive of active bleeding or a false aneurysm. In these cases, depending on the clinical

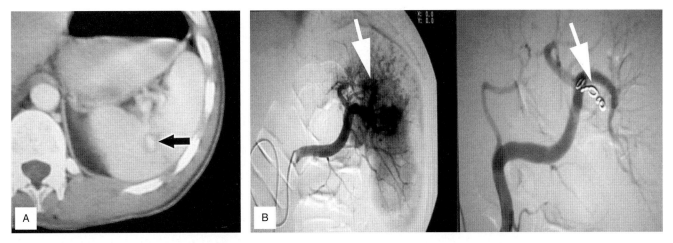

Figure 5.13 (A) CT demonstrating splenic injury with pseudoaneurysm (arrow). (B) Angiogram before (left) and after successful embolization of the pseudoaneurysm (right).

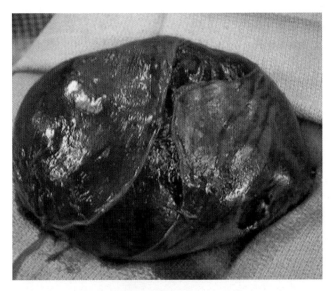

Figure 5.14 Operative specimen of a subcapsular splenic hematoma which ruptured many weeks after the injury.

condition of the patient, operative intervention or angiographic embolization should be considered. Caution should be exercised in the selection of patients for nonoperative management in the presence of multiple associated severe injuries. Severe splenic injuries treated nonoperatively should be followed up by serial CT scans until there is satisfactory healing or absorption of any large hematomas. Subcapsular hematomas may rupture and bleed dangerously many days or weeks after injury.

Postsplenectomy complications may be systemic (postsplenectomy sepsis or thrombocytosis) or local (subdiaphragmatic abscess, pancreatic pseudocyst or fistula, gastric dilatation, necrosis of the fundus of the stomach, thrombosis of the splenic vein, left pleural effusion, and atelectasis). To avoid postsplenectomy sepsis, vaccines targeting *Neisseria meningitidis*, *Haemophilus influenzae*, and *Streptococcus pneumoniae* should be administered to all patients. The vaccines are most effective if given a few days before splenectomy. It is advisable that patients with high-grade injuries selected for nonoperative management receive the vaccine, in case the management fails and a splenectomy is needed, although this policy not widely practiced. The splenectomized patient should be advised that medical care should be sought with the first signs or suspicion of any infections.

5.4 Liver Injuries

The clinical presentation of a liver injury may vary from minor pain in the right upper abdomen to peritonitis or hypovolemic shock. The diagnosis is suspected from the physical examination and

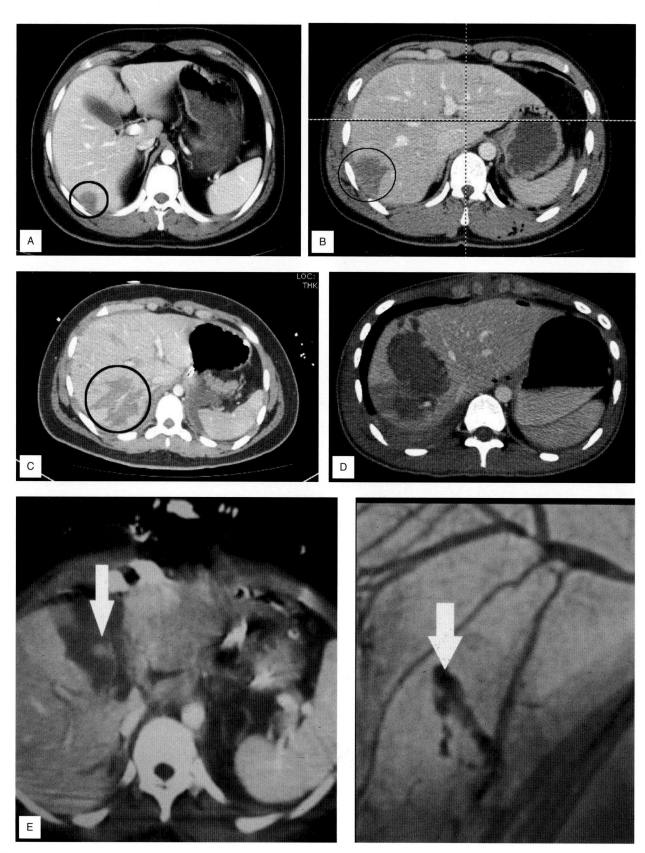

Figure 5.15 CT scans of various grades of blunt liver trauma: (A) grade I, (B) grade II, (C) grade III, (D) grade IV. (E) CT scan shows liver pseudoaneurysm confirmed by angiography (left). The patient was successfully embolized (right).

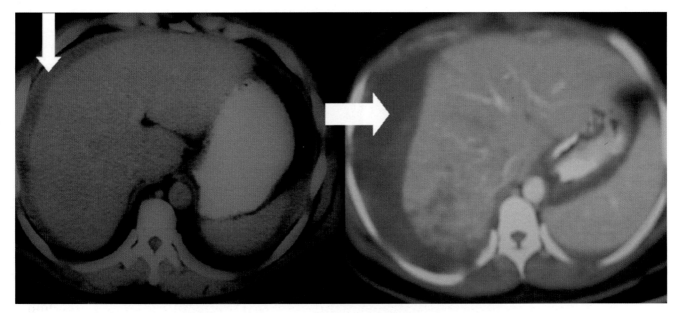

Figure 5.16 CT scans of a small (left) and a large (right) subcapsular liver hematomas following blunt trauma.

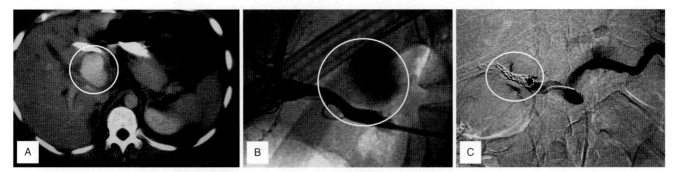

Figure 5.17 (A) CT scan shows a large pseudoaneurysm of the hepatic artery. (B) The finding is confirmed by angiography and (C) the lesion is successfully managed with angioembolization.

Figure 5.18 CT scan shows a grade IV liver injury (circle) with a "blush" suggestive of active bleeding or pseudoaneurysm. The patient was successfully managed with embolization.

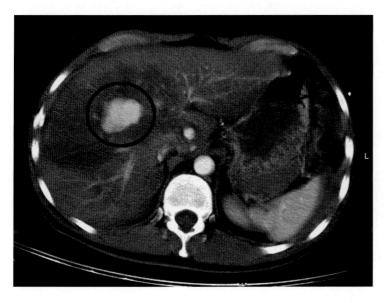

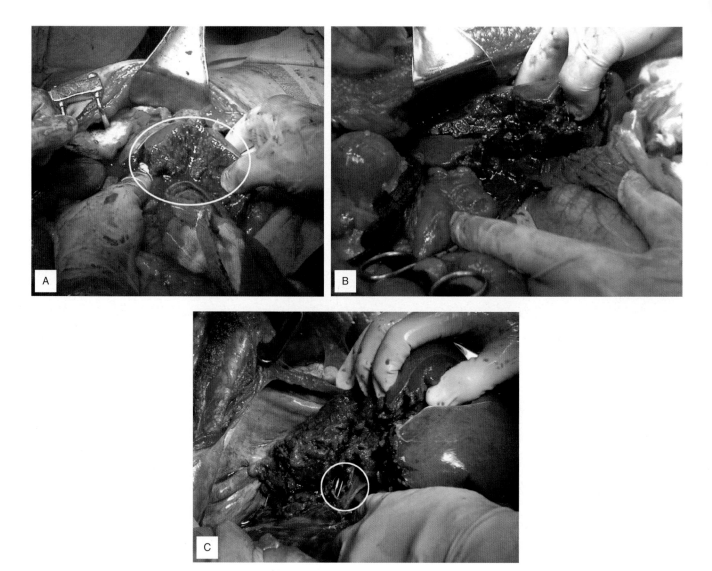

Figure 5.19 Intraoperative appearance of severe liver injuries. (A) grade III, (B) grade IV, (C) grade V. In the grade V injury there is avulsion of the hepatic veins and tear of the inferior vena cava (circle).

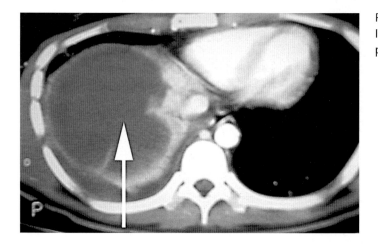

Figure 5.20 Large biloma many weeks after a grade IV liver injury. The patient was successfully managed with percutaneous drainage.

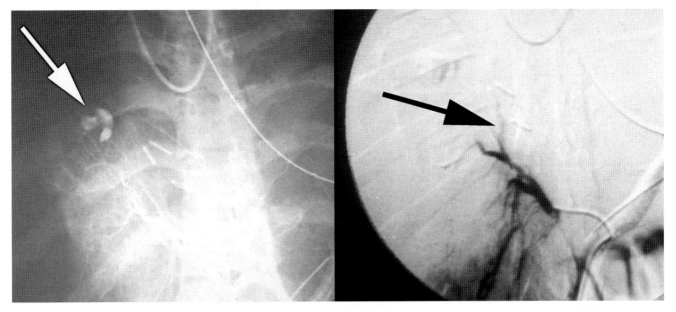

Figure 5.21 This patient presented with a copious amount of blood in the nasogastric tube soon after a grade IV liver injury. This finding is highly suspicious of hemobilia. Angiogram confirming pseudoaneurysm and hemobilia (left) which was successfully embolized (right).

trauma ultrasound and confirmed by CT scan or laparotomy. Most minor and moderate liver injuries (grades I–III) and even some severe injuries (grades IV and V) may be successfully managed nonoperatively, provided the patient is hemodynamically stable and the abdomen is soft. Hemodynamically stable patients with extravasation of contrast on CT scan (blush), indicating bleeding or false aneurysm, are excellent candidates for angioembolization. The operative management may vary from simple suturing and draining to liver packing or nonanatomical lobectomy. In addition, postoperative angiographic embolization is a very effective adjuvant modality in complex cases.

Post-traumatic liver complications include liver abscess, biloma, false aneurysms, and hemobilia (bleeding into the biliary tree). Most of these complications can be managed with percutaneous drainage or angiographic embolization.

5.5 Pancreatic Injuries

Most pancreatic injuries due to blunt trauma occur at the neck of the pancreas, caused by crushing of the organ against the spine. The clinical presentation may vary from mild epigastric pain to obvious peritonitis. The diagnosis is suspected from the history of abdominal trauma and confirmed by specific investigations or at operation. The initial serum amylase or lipase may be elevated in about 70% of patients, and serial measurements should be performed in suspected cases. The CT scan is usually diagnostic, although the early CT scan may not show the injury. It is essential that in suspected cases a repeat CT scan be performed 6–8 hours after the initial investigation. Endoscopic retrograde cholangiopancreatography (ERCP) or MRCP may be useful in determining any damage to the duct. The MRCP does not require endoscopy and is well tolerated by patients.

Many superficial pancreatic injuries not involving the duct may be managed successfully without

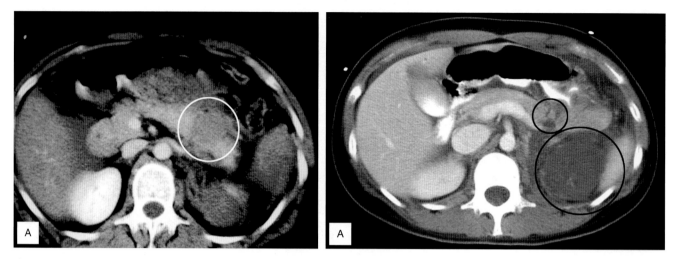

Figure 5.22 (A) CT demonstrating distal pancreatic transection (circle). (B) CT scan shows distal pancreatic injury (small circle) and no contrast uptake by the left kidney, due to thrombosis of the left renal artery (large circle).

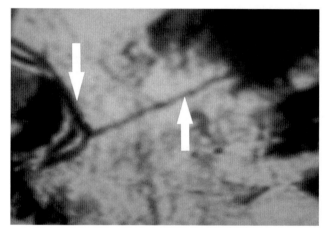

Figure 5.23 Normal magnetic resonance cholangio pancreatography (MRCP) demonstrating the common bile duct (left arrow) and the pancreatic duct (right arrow).

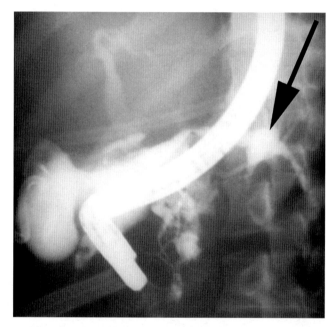

Figure 5.24 Endoscopic retrograde cholangio pancreatography (ERCP) demonstrates distal pancreatic injury with partial transection and extravasation (arrow).

operation. However, in cases with proven ductal injury or clinical signs of peritonitis, an operation should be performed. In the presence of distal ductal injury (to the left of the superior mesenteric vessels), a distal pancreatectomy is the procedure of choice. In severe injuries to the head of the pancreas or severe combined pancreatoduodenal injuries, a Whipple's pancreatoduodenectomy may be necessary. In injuries to the head of the pancreas when the integrity of the duct cannot be determined by inspection or intraoperative pancreatography, simple drainage of the area is safer than major resections.

Local complications directly related to the injury include pancreatic pseudocyst, pancreatitis, abscess, and fistula. Many of these complications can be managed nonoperatively or by percutaneous drainage.

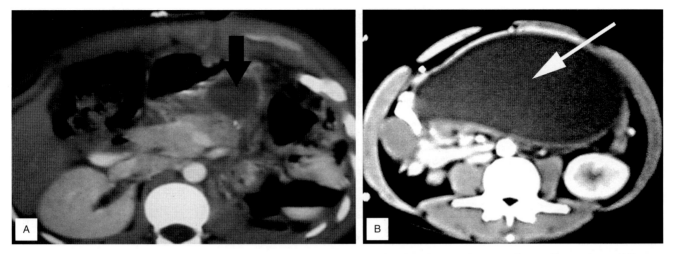

Figure 5.25 Post-traumatic pancreatic pseudocysts presenting many weeks after the initial injury. The small pseudocyst (A) was successfully observed, while the large one (B) needed percutaneous drainage.

5.6 Renal Injuries

A kidney injury may manifest clinically with pain in the flank and gross hematuria. Ancillary investigations should be reserved for only hemodynamically stable patients with a soft abdomen. An abdominal CT scan with intravenous contrast is the most useful investigation and has largely replaced the intravenous pyelography (IVP). The CT scan provides information about the site and size of parenchymal injuries, and shows vascular thrombosis or evidence of active bleeding or false aneurysm. The IVP is rarely used and is reserved for evaluation of the ureters when the CT is equivocal. Angiographic evaluation is useful in cases with suspected false aneurysms or arteriovenous fistula on CT scan or in patients with persistent gross hematuria or post-traumatic hypertension.

The vast majority of blunt renal injuries can be safely managed nonoperatively. Any attempt to

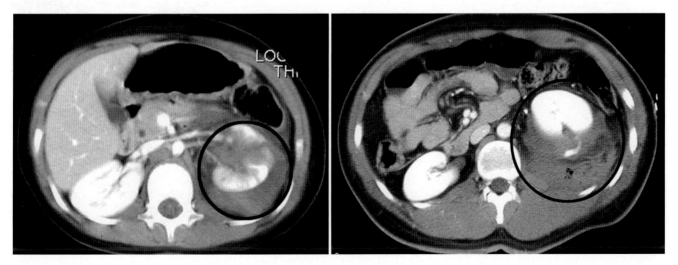

Figure 5.26 CT scans demonstrating high-grade kidney injuries following blunt trauma. Note the extensive hematomas around the kidney.

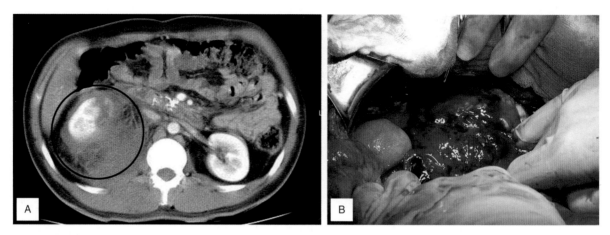

Figure 5.27 (A) CT scan shows a severe right kidney injury with a large surrounding hematoma. (B) Intraoperative appearance of the renal hematoma.

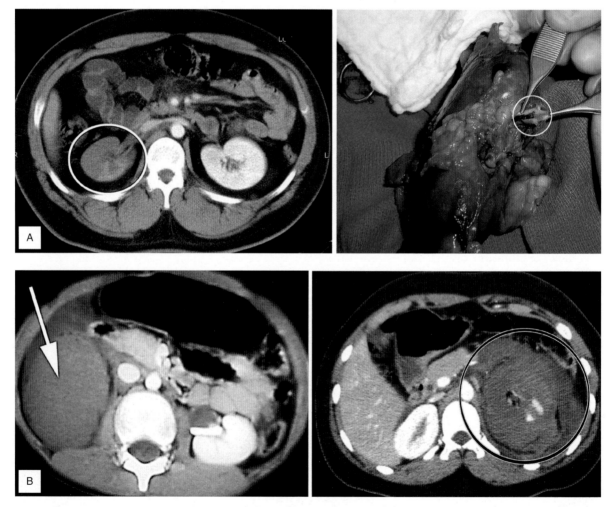

Figure 5.28 (A) CT scan of patient with blunt renal artery injury (no contrast uptake). There is isolated renal artery thrombosis without any parenchymal injury (left). The operative specimen (right) shows a clot in the renal artery. (B) Patients with renal artery thrombosis, associated parenchymal injuries (left), and extensive perirenal hematomas (right). These cases are less likely to be managed successfully with endovascular stenting.

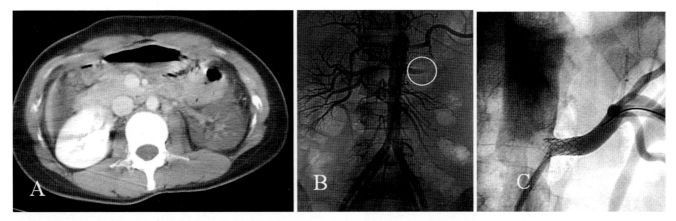

Figure 5.29 (A) Blunt trauma with left renal artery thrombosis. (B) Angiography confirms the injury. (C) The artery was successfully restored with an angiographically placed stent.

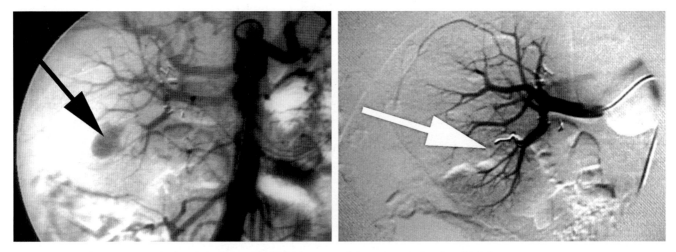

Figure 5.30 False aneurysm in the right kidney (left) with successful angioembolization (right).

explore and repair all renal injuries may result in loss of the kidney. Exploration of the kidney should be reserved for patients with intraoperative expansion of the perirenal hematoma or hemodynamic instability.

Renal artery thrombosis is almost always diagnosed on CT scan and shows as lack of contrast uptake by the kidney. If the diagnosis is made within a few hours of the injury, the injured artery can successfully be managed with an angiographically placed stent. However, prolonged ischemia causes permanent damage to the kidney and precludes revascularization.

Complications related to renal injury include false aneurysm, arteriovenous fistula, urinoma, late hematuria, and late hypertension.

5.7 Bladder Injuries

Bladder injuries are usually due to pelvic fractures or blunt abdominal trauma with a full bladder. The rupture may occur intraperitoneally or extraperitoneally. The patient may present with hematuria or inability to pass urine, and the diagnosis is confirmed by plain or CT cystogram.

All intraperitoneal ruptures need operation and repair. Most extraperitoneal ruptures can be managed nonoperatively with transurethral catheter drainage for about 10 days.

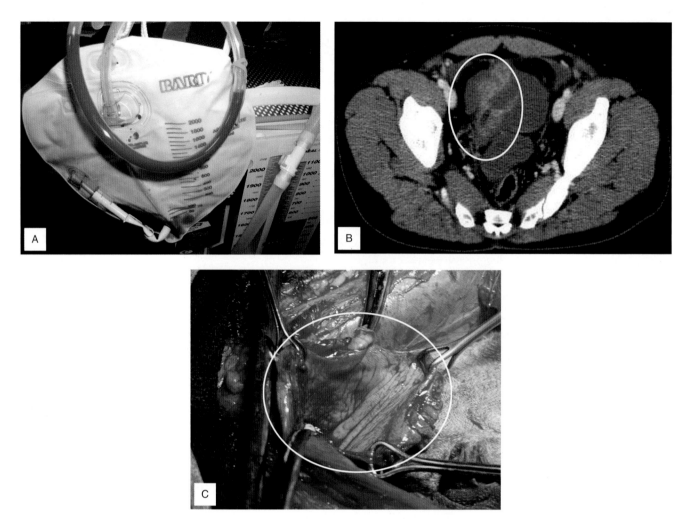

Figure 5.31 Intraperitoneal rupture of the bladder. (A) The patient presented with lower abdominal pain and gross hematuria following blunt trauma. (B) CT cystogram showing intraperitoneal bladder rupture. (C) Intraoperative appearance of the bladder rupture.

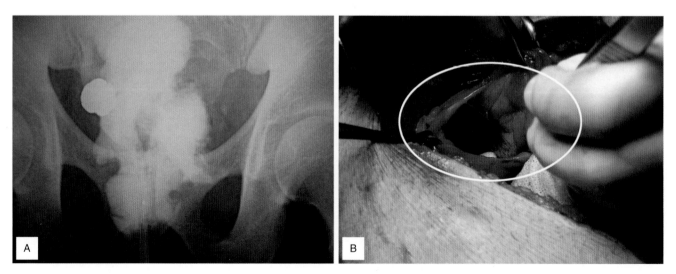

Figure 5.32 Intraperitoneal rupture of the bladder. (A) Voiding cysto-urethrogram shows significant intraperitoneal rupture of the bladder. (B) Intraoperative appearance of the bladder rupture.

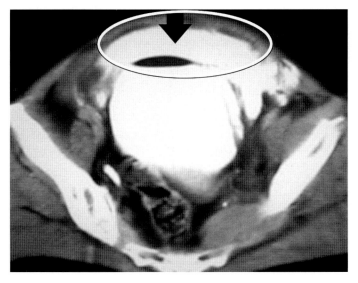

Figure 5.33 CT cystogram showing extraperitoneal rupture. This type of injury can safely be managed with Foley's catheter drainage of the bladder for 10–14 days.

5.8 Urethral Injuries

Urethral injuries occur almost exclusively in males, and they are usually associated with anterior pelvic fractures or falls resulting in straddle injuries. The clinical presentation may include blood at the urethral meatus, a scrotal or perineal hematoma, inability to pass urine, floating prostate on rectal examination, and urine extravasation in the scrotum. The diagnosis is confirmed by urethrogram.

In suspected urethral injuries, avoid transurethral catheterization until a retrograde urethrogram shows integrity of the urethra. Experienced physicians may attempt careful insertion of the urethral catheter without using any force. In the majority of cases, drainage of the bladder with a transurethral or suprapubic catheter provides the definitive management. An alternative is immediate endoscopic realignment, with a Foley catheter placement by a urologist. Emergency operative repair of the urethra is not advocated because of the inferior results.

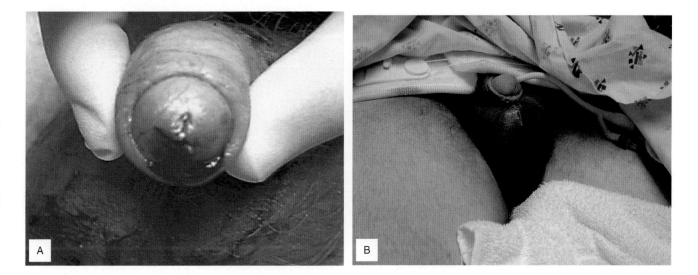

Figure 5.34 (A–C) Clinical signs of rupture of the urethra: blood at the meatus (A) or scrotal hematoma (B,C) in patients with pelvic fractures or after straddle injury are highly suspicious of urethral rupture. These patients should be evaluated by urethrogram.

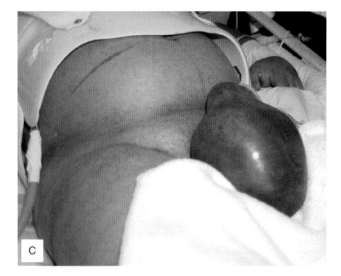

Figure 5.34 (*cont.*)

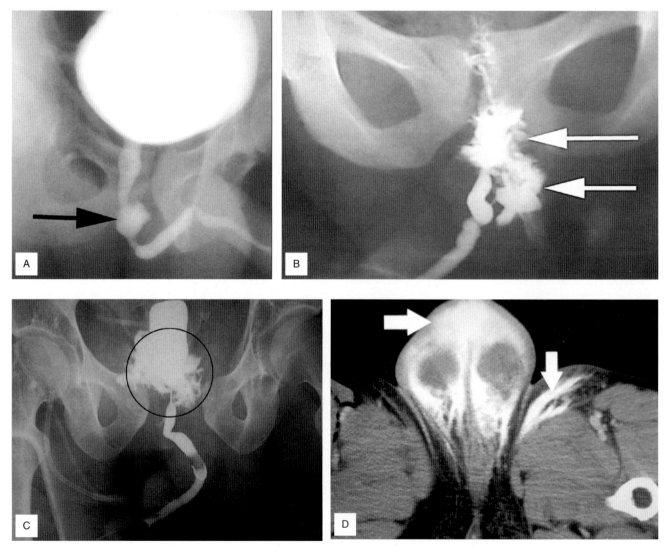

Figure 5.35 (A–C) Voiding cysto-urethrograms showing rupture of the urethra. (D) CT cystogram showing massive extravasation of contrast in the scrotum and extraperitoneal tissues secondary to posterior urethral disruption.

5.9 Duodenal Injuries

Blunt duodenal trauma may occur as a result of direct trauma to the abdomen that compresses the duodenum against the vertebral column or following deceleration injuries. The injury usually involves the retroperitoneal part of the duodenum. The clinical examination may be difficult due to subtle signs and symptoms because of the retroperitoneal location of the rupture. The initial presentation may include minor epigastric tenderness and tachycardia, and signs of peritonitis may appear a few hours later.

Laboratory tests are of little help in the early diagnosis of duodenal rupture. The serum amylase may be elevated and should be monitored at 4–6-hour intervals. Plain films may show retroperitoneal air, especially around the upper pole of the right kidney. CT scan with oral contrast is the imaging modality of choice.

Early diagnosis and surgical repair remain the cornerstones for a good outcome. Common postoperative complications include local infection and fistula formation.

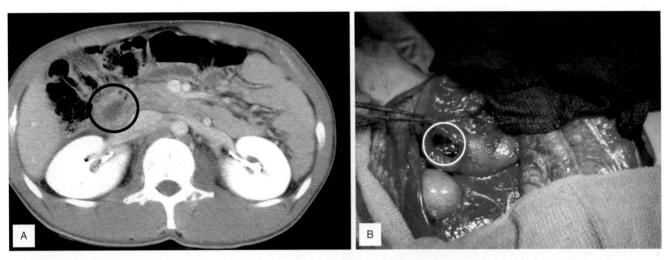

Figure 5.36 Blunt trauma to duodenum. (A) CT demonstrates duodenal wall thickening with intramural air. (B) Intraoperative appearance of duodenal perforation.

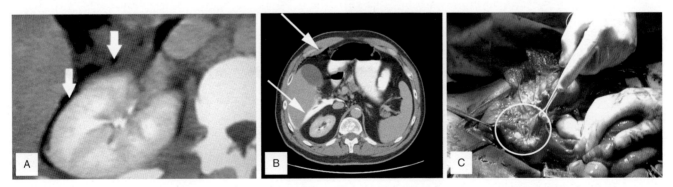

Figure 5.37 (A) CT scan shows free air around the right kidney, due to retroperitoneal rupture of the duodenum. (B) CT scan with oral contrast shows contrast extravasation between the kidney and the liver (lower arrow). Note the tiny bubble of free gas under the anterior abdominal wall (upper arrow). (C) Operative appearance of a near complete transection of the duodenum.

5.10 Small-Bowel Injuries

Small-bowel perforation occurs in about 3% of blunt abdominal trauma patients. The diagnosis can be difficult, especially in unevaluable multitrauma patients, and is one of the most commonly missed injuries. A seatbelt sign is a highly suspicious finding that should alert the physician to the possibility of bowel injury.

The plain abdominal x-ray is usually of little help because in most cases it is nondiagnostic and fails to show any free intraperitoneal air. The abdominal CT scan may be diagnostic in about 70% of cases, as it may show small amounts of free air or thickening of the bowel wall or mesentery. The presence of free fluid without evidence of solid organ injury is a highly suspicious finding, and requires careful close monitoring and a low threshold for exploration. In suspicious cases, serial clinical examinations, white blood cell monitoring, and a follow-up CT scan should be carried out. DPL at the early stages is nonspecific and of very little value, though delayed DPL may show an elevated white blood cell count in the fluid.

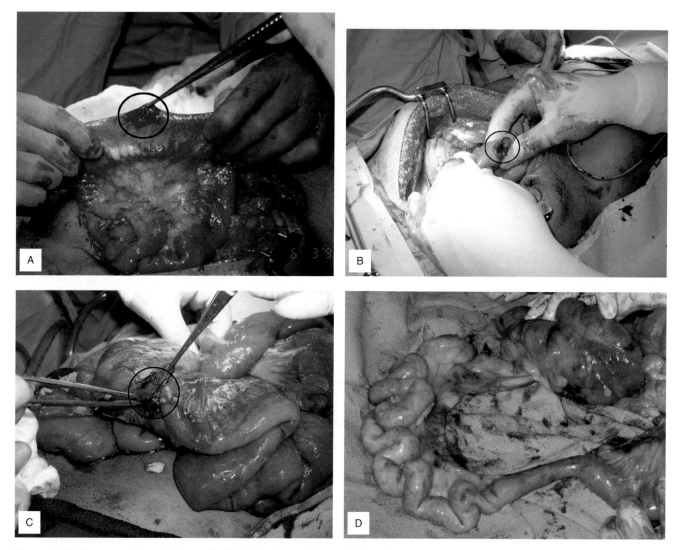

Figure 5.38 Blunt small bowel injury. (A–C) Perforation of the small bowel, usually at the antimesenteric border, is the result of transient closed loop formation and high intraluminal pressure. Note the inflammation and pseudomembranes (arrows) in delayed diagnosis (C). (D) Small bowel mesenteric tear, "bucket handle" type injury, is the result of rapid deceleration forces.

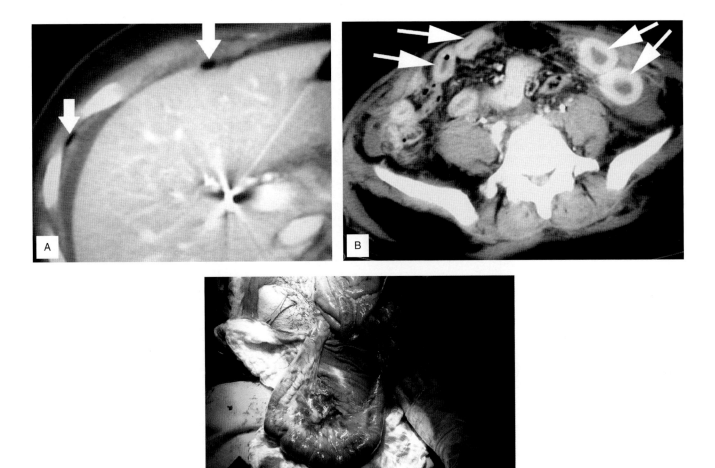

Figure 5.39 CT scan findings in small bowel injury. (A) Small amounts of free intraperitoneal gas (arrows) may be found in many cases. (B) Thickening of the small bowel wall (arrows) may be found, especially if the CT scan is taken a few hours after the injury. (C) Intraoperative photograph of small bowel "bucket handle" avulsion injury with ischemia, following high-speed motor vehicle collision.

5.11 Colorectal Injuries

Blunt colorectal trauma may occur in high-speed deceleration accidents or in association with pelvic fractures. Deceleration injuries usually cause avulsion of the mesocolon and ischemia of the colon, while in pelvic fractures there is often free perforation of the rectosigmoid. The diagnosis is usually easy in intraperitoneal injuries because of the presence of peritonitis. However, in extraperitoneal rectal injuries, the physical findings may be unremarkable, and the diagnosis may be delayed. The diagnosis of rectal injury should be suspected in severe pelvic fractures, especially in the presence of blood on rectal examination. A Gastrografin enema and a careful sigmoidoscopy without excessive insufflation can confirm the injury. Abdominal CT scan usually shows large amounts of free intra-abdominal gas. Early operation is essential to reduce the possibility of sepsis.

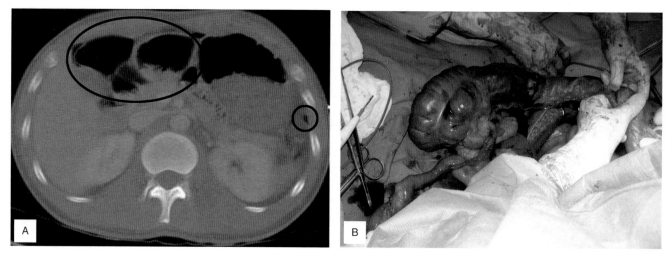

Figure 5.40 (A) Abdominal CT shows a large amount of free intraperitoneal gas following a car accident. (B) Intraoperative appearance of colonic "bucket handle" avulsion injury with ischemia and perforation.

Penetrating Abdominal Trauma

5.12 Mechanism of Injury

A distinction should be made between low-velocity and high-velocity penetrating abdominal injuries because the severity of the injury, the treatment, and the prognosis are different. High-velocity injuries

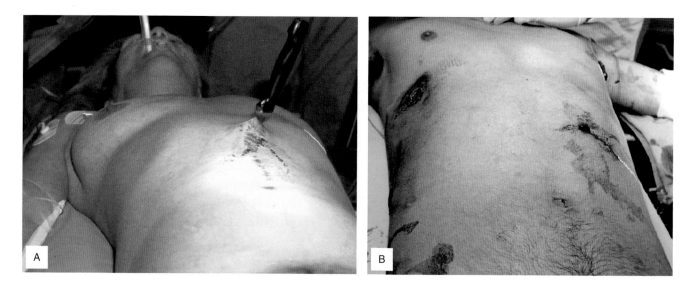

Figure 5.41 (A) Stab wound to the abdomen with impaled knife. These objects should only be removed in the operating room. Only about 50% of anterior abdominal stab wounds have significant injuries requiring surgical repair. (B) Low-velocity gunshot wound. About 75% of these wounds have significant injuries requiring surgical repair. (C) Shotgun wound to the abdomen. At close range, these are highly destructive with extensive tissue loss.

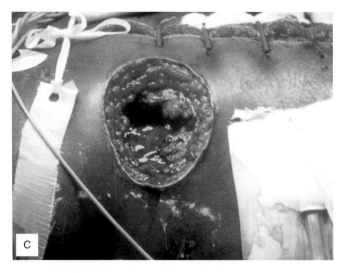

Figure 5.41 (*cont.*)

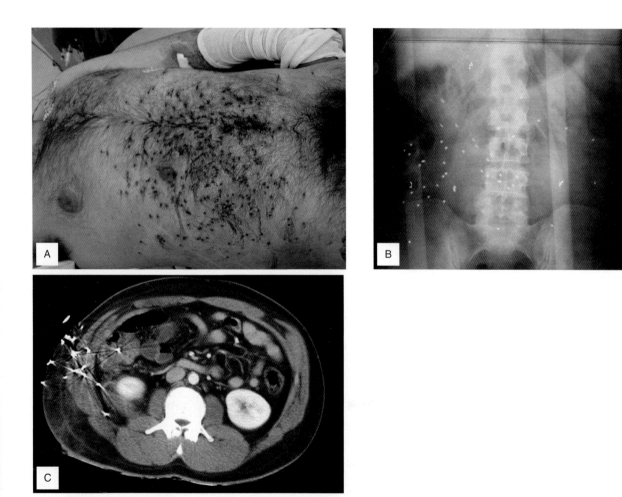

Figure 5.42 Shotgun wound to the abdomen, from about 6 meters distance. From this distance the ability of the projectiles to penetrate the soft tissues is limited. (A) Note the minor soft tissue damage. (B) The plain x-ray shows significant scatter of the pellets. (C) The CT scan shows that most of the pellets remained in the soft tissues, outside the peritoneal cavity.

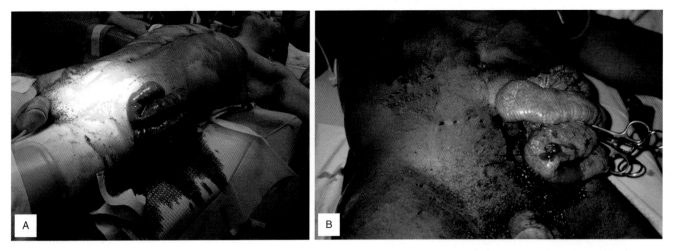

Figure 5.43 (A–B) Evisceration of bowel following stab wounds to the abdomen. If the operating room is not immediately available an attempt should be made to return the bowel into the peritoneal cavity preoperatively. Patient coughing and straining may aggravate the evisceration.

cause extensive damage by direct laceration, production of a shock wave, and transient cavitation (see Chapter 10, Ballistics). Although rare in the civilian sector, almost all cases require a laparotomy. Low-velocity injuries (knives, most civilian handguns) cause damage only by direct laceration, and often there is no significant intra-abdominal injury requiring surgical repair. Although many centers recommend routine laparotomy, many others practice selective nonoperative management for select low-velocity injuries. Criteria for nonoperative management are hemodynamic stability and an examinable patient without evidence of peritonitis. These patients are closely monitored with frequent hemodynamic and abdominal examinations and serial white blood cell counts for 24–48 hours.

Omental or bowel evisceration is associated with significant intra-abdominal injuries requiring surgical repair in about 75% of cases.

5.13 Investigations in Penetrating Abdominal Injury

Investigations should be reserved for only fairly stable patients. Chest and abdominal films are important in gunshot wounds for localization of any missiles or fragments. Also, they may identify any fractures, especially of the spine. Abdominal x-rays are of no value in knife injuries and should not be performed. In hemodynamically stable patients with minimal or no abdominal signs, abdominal CT scan may be helpful in identifying the bullet tract or any solid organ injuries. If the bullet tract is extraperitoneal, the patient may avoid an unnecessary operation. For solid organ injuries, the CT scan provides information about the injury grade and the presence of active bleeding or false aneurysm, and it is helpful in planning the optimal treatment.

Laparoscopy is useful in the evaluation of penetrating injuries of the left thoracoabdominal and anterior right thoracoabdominal regions to exclude diaphragmatic injuries. This procedure is discussed extensively in Chapter 4, Thoracic Injury.

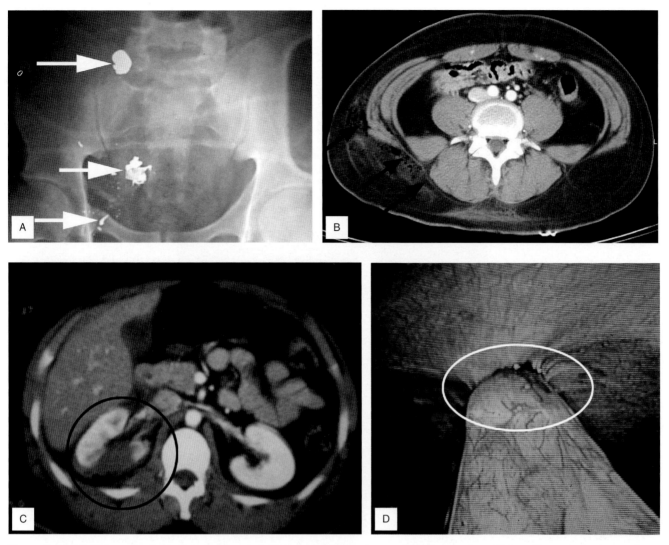

Figure 5.44 (A) Plain radiograph showing two missiles and small fragments. (B) CT scan of a patient with a gunshot wound to the abdomen. The missile tract is extraperitoneal (arrows). This patient can be safely managed nonoperatively. (C) CT scan is useful in identifying the extent of solid organ injuries. In this case it shows a right kidney injury but no other significant injuries. This patient may be managed nonoperatively. (D) Laparoscopy is a valuable diagnostic tool in the evaluation of the diaphragm in patients with left thoracoabdominal injuries. In this case, it shows a diaphragm injury with omental herniation.

5.14 Transpelvic Gunshot Injuries

About half of all transpelvic gunshot injuries are associated with significant injuries requiring surgical repair. The selection of patients for operation or observation should be based on clinical examination and appropriate diagnostic tests. The presence of an acute abdomen, hemodynamic instability, rectal bleeding, or gross hematuria is an absolute indication for an operation. Injuries to extraperitoneal organs (rectum, urethra) may not give peritoneal signs. Asymptomatic patients should be evaluated by rigid endoscopy and Gastrografin enema. A CT scan with thin cuts may be useful in delineating the bullet track and identifying patients who may benefit from further investigations.

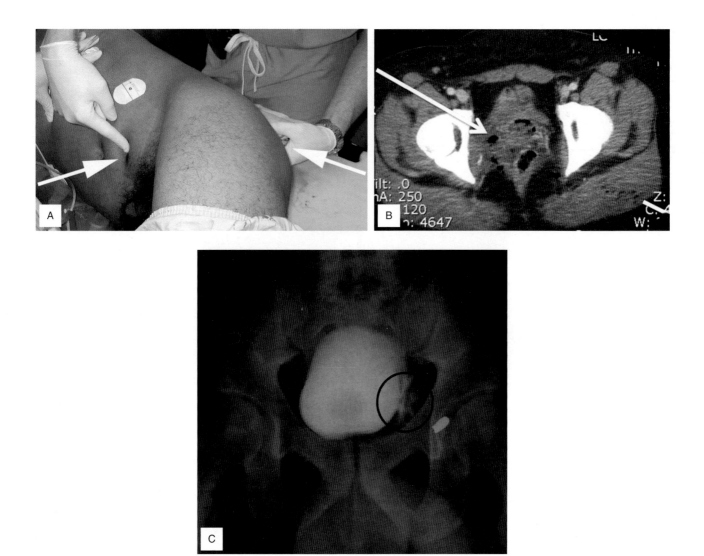

Figure 5.45 Transpelvic gunshot wound. (A) Significant injuries are found in about 50% of the cases. (B) CT demonstrating transpelvic trajectory through rectum and extraluminal gas. (C) Transpelvic gunshot wound with gross hematuria: cystogram showing bladder injury with contrast extravasation.

5.15 Penetrating Injuries to the Liver

About 30% of all knife wounds to the liver may be managed nonoperatively. Although most trauma centers practice routine laparotomy for all gunshot wounds to the liver, recent studies have suggested that carefully selected cases (about 10% of all cases or 20% of isolated gunshot wounds to the liver) can be safely managed nonoperatively. The criteria for nonoperative management are hemodynamic stability and a soft abdomen. A CT scan with intravenous contrast should be performed to assess the extent of the injury and identify any evidence of

active bleeding or false aneurysms, which may benefit from angiographic embolization. Hemodynamic instability, the presence of peritonitis, and the need for multiple blood transfusions are indications for laparotomy.

Complications of penetrating liver injuries include bleeding, false aneurysm, arteriovenous fistula, hemobilia, biloma, and liver abscess. Most of these complications can be managed successfully with interventional radiology (angiographic embolization or percutaneous drainage).

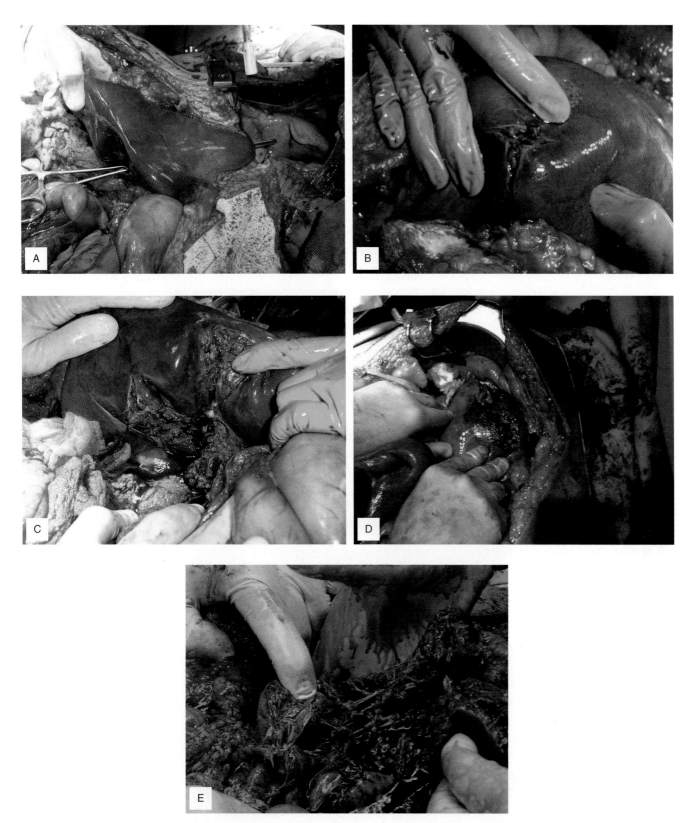

Figure 5.46 (A–D) Low-velocity gunshot wounds to the liver. (E) High-velocity gunshot wound to the liver.

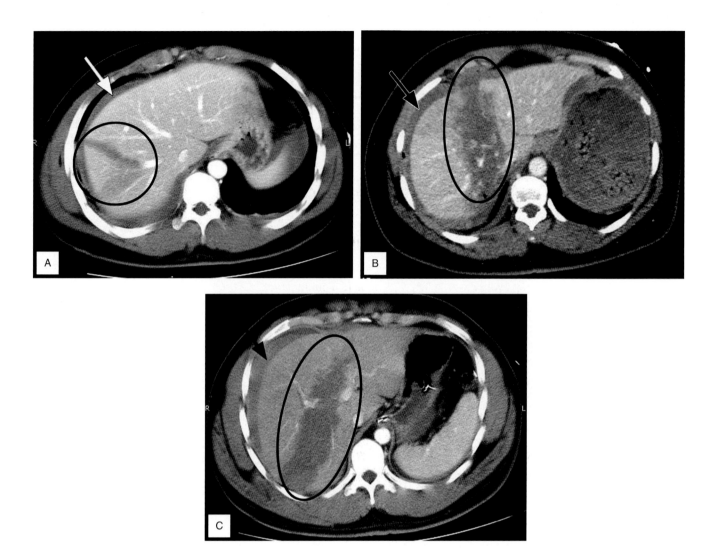

Figure 5.47 Many penetrating liver injuries can safely be managed nonoperatively, provided the patient is hemodynamically stable and has no peritonitis. A CT scan should always be performed: (A) CT scan of stab wound (B, C) and gunshot wounds to the liver successfully managed nonoperatively.

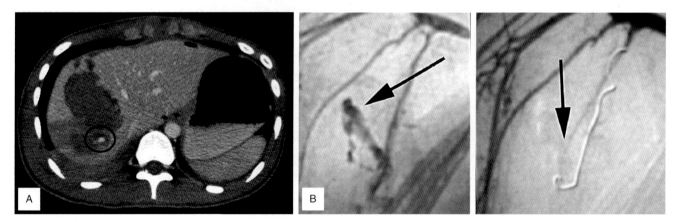

Figure 5.48 (A) CT scan of a patient with a gunshot wound shows a significant liver injury with a pseudoaneurysm (circle). (B) Angiography confirms the aneurysm and successful embolization was performed. The patient was managed nonoperatively.

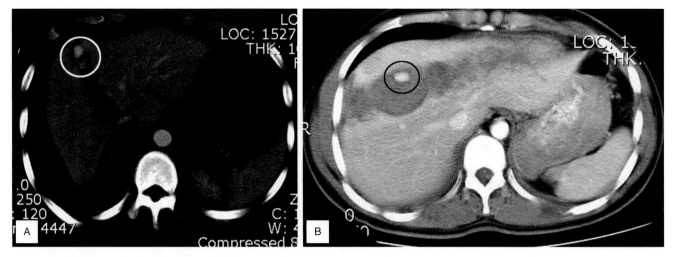

Figure 5.49 (A) CT scan of patient with grade III liver injury due to a gunshot wound shows an arteriovenous fistula. (B) Patient with grade IV gunshot to the liver shows a pseudoaneurysm. Both patients were successfully managed nonoperatively with angioembolization.

5.16 Penetrating Splenic Injuries

Some penetrating injuries to the spleen can be safely managed nonoperatively, provided the patient is hemodynamically stable, is evaluable and does not have peritonitis. However, in the majority of cases there are associated intra-abdominal injuries or significant bleeding, and the patient needs an emergency laparotomy. Investigations should be reserved for stable patients and should include abdominal CT scanning with intravenous contrast. Laparoscopy should be considered in appropriate cases to exclude diaphragmatic injury.

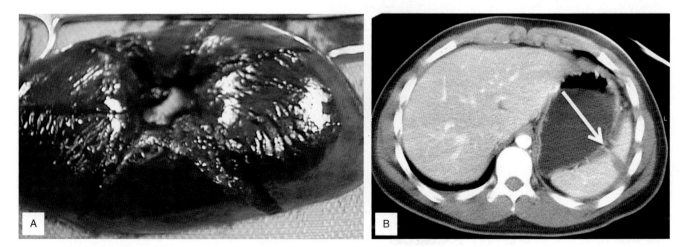

Figure 5.50 (A) Gunshot wound to spleen with extensive damage requiring emergency splenectomy. (B–C) Low-grade splenic injuries due to (B) a stab wound and (C) a gunshot wound, successfully managed nonoperatively.

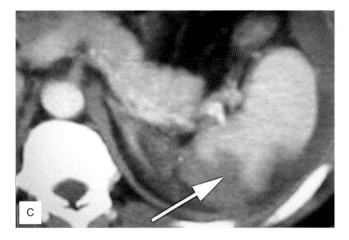

Figure 5.50 (*cont.*)

5.17 Penetrating Pancreatic Injuries

Almost all penetrating pancreatic injuries require operation because of the severity of the injury and the presence of other associated injuries. The man-agement of the pancreatic injury may vary from simple drainage to distal pancreatectomy or pancreatoduodenectomy.

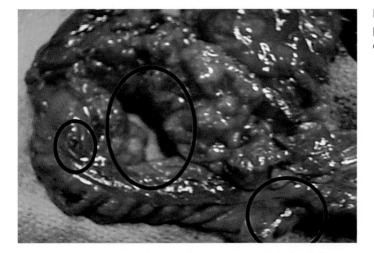

Figure 5.51 Operative specimen following pancreatoduodenectomy for extensive injury to the head of the pancreas and duodenum from a gunshot wound.

5.18 Penetrating Renal Injuries

Many isolated penetrating kidney injuries can be managed nonoperatively, provided the patient is hemodynamically stable and has a soft abdomen. A CT scan with intravenous contrast is to assess the

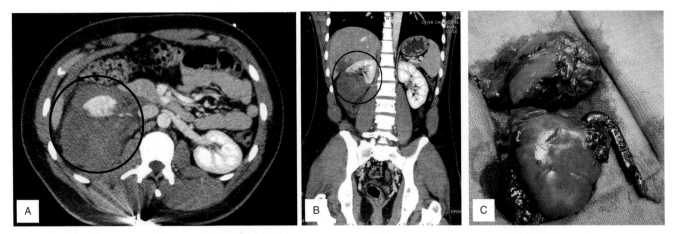

Figure 5.52 Gunshot injury to kidney. (A–B) CT scan shows severe injury and a large perinephric hematoma. A nephrectomy was performed. (C) Note the complete transection of the kidney.

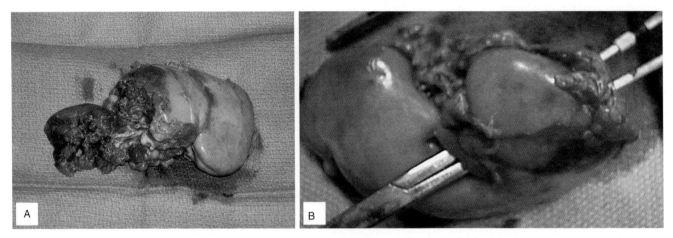

Figure 5.53 (A–B) Nepherectomies for severe penetrating renal trauma.

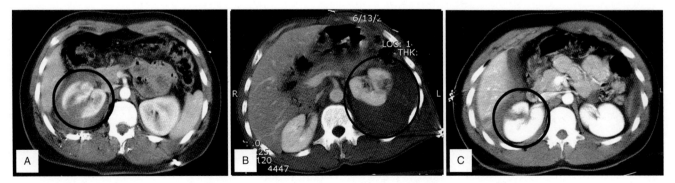

Figure 5.54 (A–C) CT scans demonstrating penetrating injuries to the kidney managed nonoperatively.

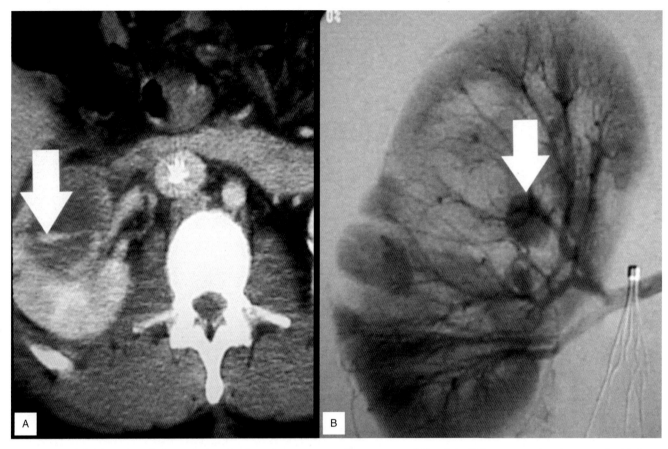

Figure 5.55 (A) CT scan and (B) angiography demonstrate a pseudoaneurysm of the right kidney secondary to a gunshot injury.

extent of parenchymal injury and the presence of pelvicaliceal system leak or vascular lesions such as false aneurysm or arteriovenous fistula. Angiography is recommended in cases with persistent gross hematuria or suspected aneurysm or arteriovenous fistula in which CT findings are not diagnostic.

Post-traumatic complications include urinoma, false aneurysm, arteriovenous fistula, abscess, and hypertension. Most of these complications can be managed with interventional radiology.

5.19 Penetrating Colorectal Injuries

Almost all intraperitoneal colorectal injuries give early signs of peritonitis, and they are easy to diagnose. However, small retroperitoneal colonic or extraperitoneal rectal injuries may not give any early clinical signs. Rectal examination may show blood in the stool. Abdominal CT scan with intravenous and rectal contrast may be helpful in diagnosing the

injuries. A carefully performed sigmoidoscopy may show blood in the rectum or even the actual perforation.

Early surgical intervention is important to reduce the risk of septic complications. Most colon injuries can be managed safely with primary repair or resection and primary anastomosis. Colostomy is reserved for

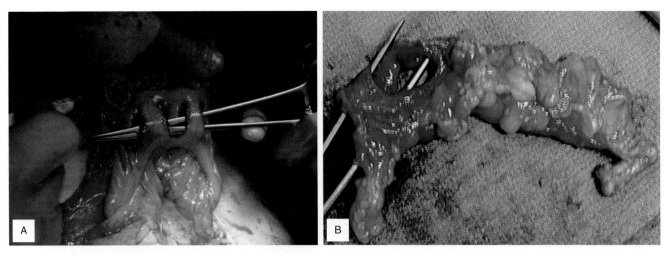

Figure 5.56 (A–B) Gunshot injuries with destructive trauma to the colon requiring resection. These injuries are associated with a very high incidence of septic complications.

cases with edematous bowel or in the damage control setting. Small rectal injuries may be managed by primary repair, and large injuries require a proximal colostomy.

The most common complications are abdominal sepsis (intra-abdominal abscess, wound sepsis) and colonic fistula. More than 20% of patients with colonic resection develop severe abdominal septic complications.

5.20 Abdominal Vascular Injuries

Most patients with penetrating abdominal vascular injuries present in shock, although in some cases retroperitoneal containment may prevent rapid exsanguination and early shock. Peritonitis due to associated hollow viscus perforations is a common finding. The diagnosis of vascular injury should be suspected in the presence of severe hemodynamic instability or a rapidly distending abdomen. A trauma ultrasound is often very helpful, although it cannot detect retroperitoneal bleeding.

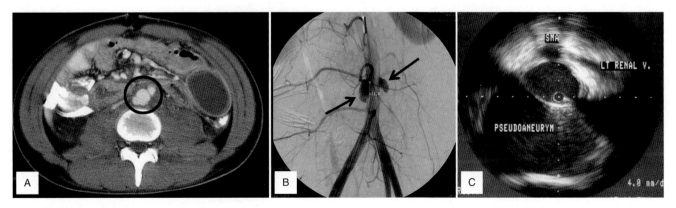

Figure 5.57 Gunshot wound to the abdominal aorta with leak and pseudoaneurysm below the renal arteries. (A) CT scan, (B) angiography, and (C) endovascular ultrasound.

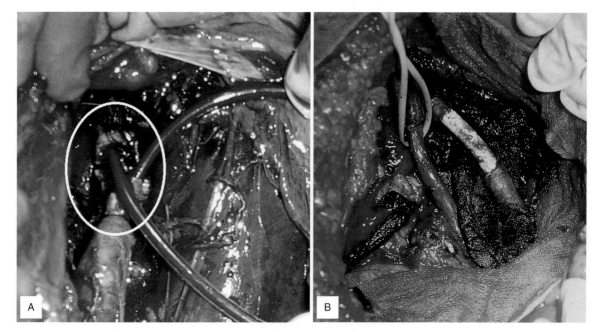

Figure 5.58 Gunshot wound to the common iliac artery: (A) with temporary shunting and (B) after definitive repair with a prosthetic graft.

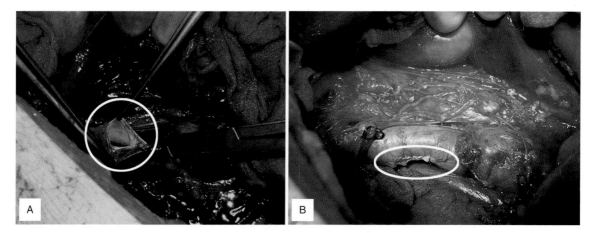

Figure 5.59 Stab wound to the infrarenal inferior vena cava: (A) before and (B) after primary repair.

5.21 Abdominal Trauma in Pregnancy

Anatomical and Physiological Changes in Pregnancy

About 7% of all pregnant women suffer traumatic injuries during pregnancy and trauma is the leading cause of death in this population. Many anatomical and physiological changes occur during late pregnancy:

(a) The blood volume increases by about 50% during the last trimester, and the trauma victim may lose

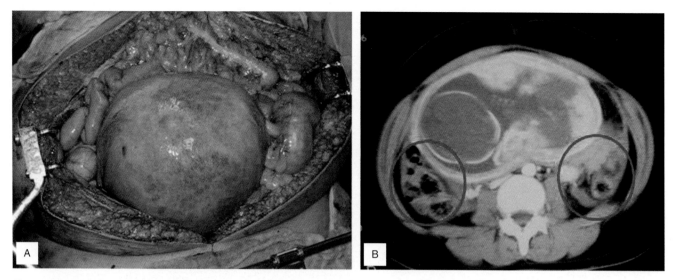

Figure 5.60 In advanced pregnancy the enlarged uterus displaces the intra-abdominal organs and may alter the injury patterns and the clinical presentation. Note the displaced intestine, (A) intraoperatively and (B) on CT scan.

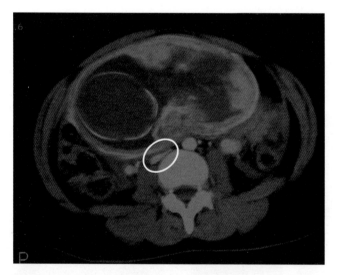

Figure 5.61 CT scan showing compression of the inferior vena cava by the enlarged uterus (circle). To prevent this problem, the patient or the spinal board should be tilted to the left by about 20 degrees.

up to one-third of blood volume without any significant hemodynamic changes.

(b) The enlarged uterus during the last trimester compresses the inferior vena cava and impairs venous return. In addition it displaces the intra-abdominal organs, resulting in changes of the injury patterns and clinical signs.

(c) The elevated diaphragm increases the respiratory rate and reduces the functional residual capacity, resulting in reduced respiratory reserves.

(d) Hematological changes occur during the second and third trimester of pregnancy. They include "anemia of pregnancy," mild leucocytosis, and hypercoagulability.

Clinical Examination and Investigations

In addition to the routine clinical examination and tests according to ATLS principles, all pregnant patients should undergo vaginal examination with sterile gloves in order to evaluate the cervix and vagina and look for amnionic fluid, or bleeding. FAST exam and fetal ultrasound should be performed in all patients. The gestation age is assessed from the history, clinical examination, and ultrasound. A fetal ultrasound performed by an obstetrician can assess the gestation age, the fetal heart rate (fetal heart rate can be detected by 7–8 weeks) and evaluate for possible placenta abruption.

Abdominal CT scan should be performed only if it is absolutely necessary, having in mind the potential risks of the irradiation to the fetus, especially during the first trimester. Magnetic resonance imaging (MRI) studies may replace CT scanning in selected stable patients. There is no evidence that MRI has any adverse effects on the fetus. Cardiotocography (monitoring of the fetal heart rate and uterine contractions) should be initiated as soon as possible in cases with viable fetus.

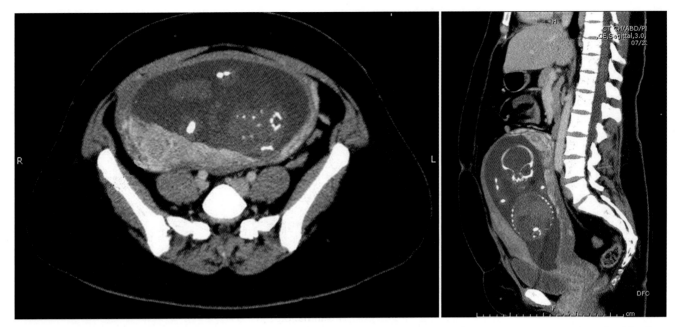

Figure 5.62 CT scan evaluation in pregnancy should be performed only in carefully selected cases because of the risk of fetal irradiation, especially in early pregnancy.

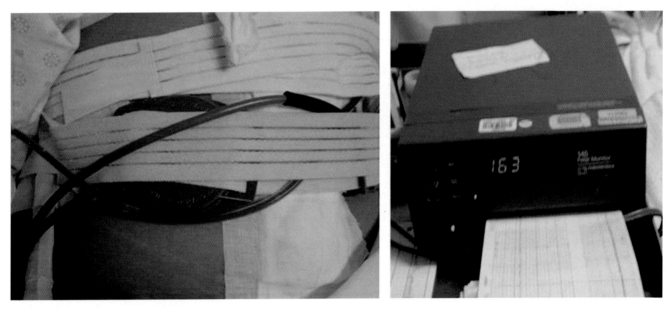

Figure 5.63 Monitoring of the fetal heart rate and uterine contractions with cardiotocography should be performed in all pregnancies with viable fetus (>24 weeks).

Pregnancy-Related Complications

(a) Placenta abruption is the most common complication and has been reported in up to 5% of minor trauma and up to 65% in major. Most cases present within the first 6 hours of injury. The usual clinical presentation includes vaginal bleeding, pain, and fetal distress. The fetal mortality in the presence of placenta abruption is as high as 70%.

(b) Fetomaternal bleeding in Rhesus-negative mothers may cause erythroblastosis fetalis in subsequent pregnancies. Immunoglobulin (Rho-Gam) should be administered routinely to all Rhesus-negative injured pregnant patients. A mini dose (50 mcg) should be given in early pregnancy and a standard dose (300 mcg) after the first trimester.

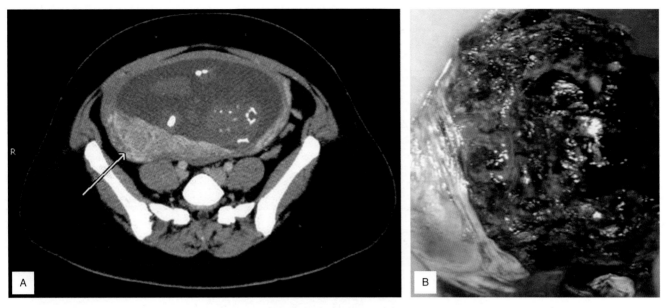

Figure 5.64 Placenta abruption is a common complication after trauma. Ultrasound is not very sensitive in the diagnosis. (A) CT scan is more reliable but it has the disadvantage of fetal irradiation. (B) Placenta abruption after a cesarian section.

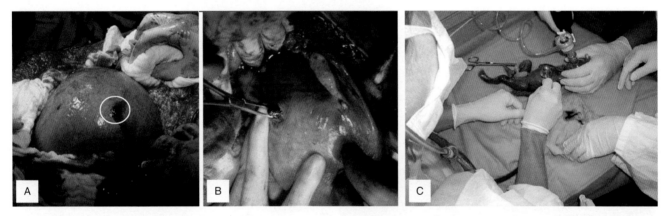

Figure 5.65 (A–B) Gunshot wound to the pregnant uterus. (C) A cesarian section was performed but the fetus did not survive.

(c) Amniotic fluid embolization is a fairly rare but highly lethal complication with a maternal mortality of up to 80%. It is usually complicated by acute respiratory distress syndrome and disseminated intravascular coagulopathy.

(d) Premature rupture of membranes.

(e) Fetal loss: Fetal mortality is high, even in fairly moderate maternal injuries. Even in seemingly stable patients it is possible that there is fetal hypoperfusion and increased risk of fetal death. The mother may be compensating at the expense of the fetus with uterine vasoconstriction. Pelvic fractures in pregnancy pose special problems and the overall fetal mortality is about 35%.

(f) Uterine rupture occurs in about 1% of pregnant women involved in motor vehicle injuries. It is a life-threatening condition because of excessive bleeding and immediate laparotomy is indicated.

Management

The trauma team should include the obstetrician and a neonatologist teams.

All pregnant patients should receive supplemental oxygen, irrespective of SaO_2, because the fetal hemoglobin oxygen dissociation curve is to the left of the

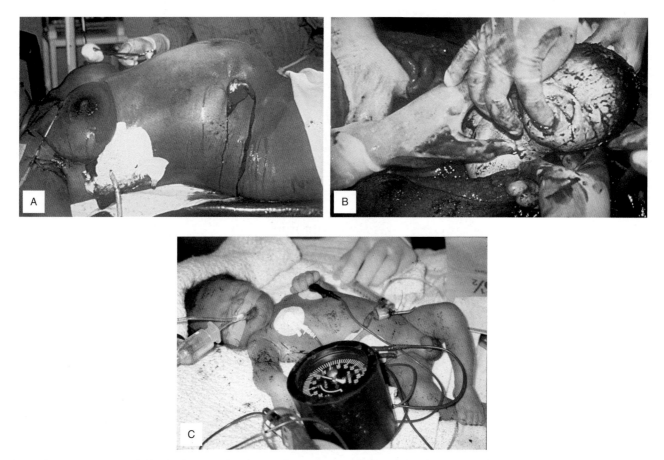

Figure 5.66 Penetrating abdominal trauma in advanced pregnancy. (A) The patient had signs of peritonitis. (B) A cesarean section was performed during the exploratory laparotomy. (C) The baby survived after many weeks in neonatal ICU.

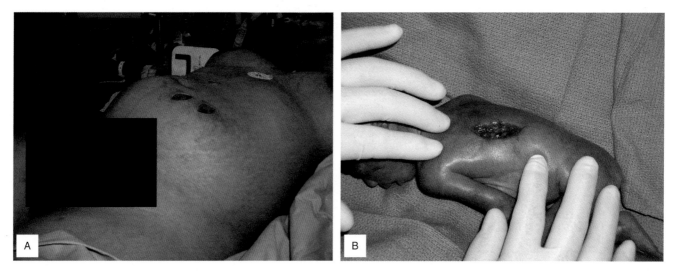

Figure 5.67 (A) Stab wounds to the anterior abdominal wall of a pregnant patient. An emergency laparotomy and cesarean section were performed. (B) The fetus also sustained a stab wound to the back and did not survive.

adult, resulting in fetal hypoxia despite normal maternal oxygenation.

In advanced pregnancy the patient or the spinal board should be tilted about 20 degrees to the left in order to reduce the compression of the inferior vena cava by the uterus and improve venous return.

All Rhesus-negative patients should receive R(D) Immunoglobulin, in order to prevent isoimmunization and erythroblastosis fetalis in future pregnancies.

In severe trauma, with nonviable fetus (<24 weeks) no efforts should be made to stop contractions or deliver the fetus by cesarean section. If the mother needs surgery, it should not be delayed because of the pregnancy.

Indications for Cesarean Section

Cesarean section should be performed in the presence of fetal distress if the fetus is viable (>24 weeks), if maternal death occurs and the fetus is viable, in the presence of major maternal complications (eclampsia, DIC, amniotic fluid embolization), or during laparotomy if the exploration and management of maternal injuries is difficult due to the presence of the enlarged uterus.

Perimortem Cesarean Section

This desperate procedure should be performed in cases of maternal death or imminent death if the fetus is potentially viable (>24 weeks). The best results are achieved if the fetus is delivered within 5 minutes of maternal death. Fetal survival with cesarean sections 15–20 minutes after maternal death has been reported, although the incidence of hypoxic brain damage is high.

Musculoskeletal Injury

Edward J. Newton

Introduction

Orthopedic injuries are found in approximately 85% of blunt trauma victims, and thus good knowledge in their emergency care is important. Many injuries are also acutely life-threatening or limb-threatening and need to be evaluated in an expedited fashion. Despite the importance of early treatment, the standard primary survey evaluation with the advanced trauma life support (ATLS) approach is necessary to detect other injuries that have a higher priority. During the primary survey, the only attention to musculoskeletal injury is acute hemorrhage control with direct pressure.

Clinical Examination

The physical exam is an integral component of detecting acute orthopedic injuries. The overlying skin should be examined for contusions and lacerations. Lacerations need a more detailed evaluation for neurovascular injury, tendon injury, foreign bodies, and proximity to fracture sites. Cool, pale skin may indicate acute vascular insufficiency. Capillary refill and peripheral pulses are checked and compared with the unaffected limb. In some cases Doppler ultrasound may be required to detect poor pulses. The muscle compartments are palpated for firmness that may indicate an acute compartment syndrome. General range of motion and areas of tenderness help guide necessary radiographs. Careful peripheral nerve exam is also important, as nerve injury may be part of the injury complex.

Investigations

1. Plain radiographs are necessary for most orthopedic injuries. Fractures are usually evident on plain radiographs, but occasionally the fracture is occult, requiring further imaging guided by the clinical exam. X-rays should view the affected bone in at least two perpendicular planes and provide a full view of the involved bone, including the joints above and below. Depending on the spectrum of injuries, full radiographic imaging may need to be delayed to stabilize the patient from life-threatening injuries.

2. Computed tomography (CT) scanning is useful in evaluating patients with continued pain and with normal plain radiographs, such as in acute hip injuries. CT scan provides much more detail of an identified injury and allows 3-D reconstruction.

3. Magnetic resonance imaging (MRI) is rarely needed to acutely evaluate musculoskeletal injury. It is useful in detecting occult fractures, as in hip injuries, and is also useful in delineating ligamentous and cartilaginous injury, such as may be seen with acute knee trauma. It has a prominent role in spinal injuries.

4. Bone scanning at 72 hours is occasionally used to follow up patients who may have occult fractures of the scaphoid.

5. Doppler ultrasound, CT angiography or conventional arteriography, in conjunction with the ankle–brachial index (ABI), are used to evaluate patients with possible vascular injury.

6. Intracompartment pressure can easily be measured with portable equipment and can help guide the management of patients with possible compartment syndrome.

General Management

Life-threatening injuries receive priority, and thus many orthopedic emergencies may receive more extensive evaluation and treatment in the postoperative phase. Some orthopedic injuries require special mention as they are life-threatening and need similar prioritization. Major pelvic fractures are associated with significant retroperitoneal hemorrhage which is difficult to control. Liberal blood transfusions, expedited stabilization of the fracture, and emergency angiography with embolization may be necessary to hemodynamically stabilize the patient. Major arterial injury with exsanguination may occur with penetrating injury or by blunt force with fracture or dislocation-induced vessel laceration. Depending on the involved vessel and the clinical status of the patient, emergency operative therapy may be necessary to control bleeding. Acute crush syndrome causes traumatic rhabdomyolysis that will lead to acute renal failure if not promptly managed with vigorous intravenous hydration, diuretics, and alkalinization.

Open fractures and open joints are limb-threatening and need irrigation, tetanus immunization, and parenteral antibiotics. Formal operative debridement is done on an emergent basis. Traumatic amputations will need to be considered for emergency reimplantation, and the amputated part appropriately cooled and carefully cared for. Compartment syndrome may develop over hours, and thus high-risk injuries need serial physical examinations and compartment pressures evaluated. Dislocations need prompt reduction with deep sedation and neurovascular status checked before and after the reduction. Closed fractures need at least gross alignment with splinting in the emergency department to decrease bleeding and pain and prevent further displacement and injury of the adjacent neurovascular structures. Definitive closed or open reduction can be completed once the patient has been stabilized from other injuries.

Common Mistakes and Pitfalls

1. Significant occult blood loss can occur with fractures of large bones such as the femur and pelvis and can often account for acute hemorrhagic shock. Anticipate large blood loss with these injuries while excluding other causes of hemorrhage,
2. Compartment syndrome may insidiously develop in the multitrauma patient, and thus repeat clinical examination is paramount for early diagnosis of this condition. Pain out of proportion to the apparent injury is an early symptom and will need to be evaluated by assessing compartment pressures. Segmental fractures in long bones such as the tibia are especially susceptible to compartment syndrome.
3. Neurovascular injury complicates many fractures and needs to be carefully sought. ABI, Doppler ultrasound, or CT arteriography may be needed to delineate acute vascular injury.
4. Occult fractures should be suspected in patients with significant pain but with normal radiographs. Further radiographs, CT scanning, MRI, or bone scan may be necessary for fracture identification.
5. Pediatric radiographs are inherently more difficult to interpret because of osseous growth plates and incomplete ossification. At times, comparison views of the other extremity will be necessary, and occult fractures should be suspected in children with tenderness over the physis.
6. Long bone fractures should be splinted before transferring the patient to the radiology suite. Immobilization of the fracture reduces pain and bleeding and prevents further damage to the neurovascular structures.

6.1 Classification of Fractures

Correct terminology is necessary and allows clear communication when describing orthopedic injuries. Fractures are first described by anatomic location, and long bones are usually divided in thirds describing the location of the injury. Open or compound fractures refer to fractures with a break in the overlying skin, in contrast to closed fractures which have normal skin integrity.

The fracture line or pattern is then described and follows the following common convention:

1. Transverse: fracture line perpendicular to the long axis of the bone.
2. Oblique: fracture line oblique to the long axis of the bone.
3. Spiral: fracture line curved in a spiral fashion.
4. Comminuted: fracture with two or more pieces.

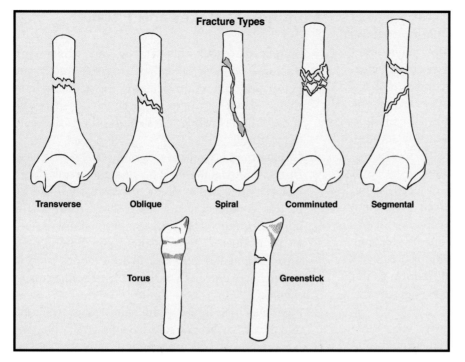

Fracture Types

Transverse   Oblique   Spiral   Comminuted   Segmental

Torus   Greenstick

Figure 6.1 Illustration of fracture pattern types.

5. Segmental: fracture at two distinct levels.
6. Torus: wrinkling or buckling of bone cortex seen in pediatrics.
7. Greenstick: incomplete fracture, seen in pediatrics.

Displacement refers to the degree of offset of the bone ends relative to one another, and completely displaced fractures tend to be more unstable injuries. Displacement is described by outlining the position of the distal bone relative to the proximal end. A bayonet deformity refers to injuries with 100% displacement and overriding of the bone ends with shortening of the affected extremity.

Angulation refers to the angle between the longitudinal axes of the main fracture segments. Fractures with significant angulation generally require reduction to maintain good function.

6.2 Open Fractures

Open or compound fractures are true orthopedic emergencies. They are defined as fractures in contact with the outside environment and thus require a break in the skin covering the fracture site. The skin break may be large and obvious or a small puncture wound injury, and thus determination if a fracture is open can sometimes be difficult.

The Gustilo classification is often used when describing open fractures:

Type I: Puncture wound <1 cm and relatively clean.
Type II: Laceration longer than 1 cm but without extensive soft tissue damage, flaps, or avulsion and with a minimal to moderate crushing component.

Type IIIA: Adequate soft tissue coverage of the fracture despite extensive soft tissue laceration or flaps, or high-energy trauma irrespective of the size of the wound.
Type IIIB: Extensive soft tissue loss with periosteal stripping and bone exposure.
Type IIIC: Open fracture associated with arterial injury requiring repair.

Staphylococcus aureus, often resistant to methicillin (MRSA), commonly causes osteomyelitis and thus antibiotic therapy is guided against this organism. Emergency therapy includes covering the wound with sterile saline dressings, along with the appropriate tetanus immunization and pain management. All

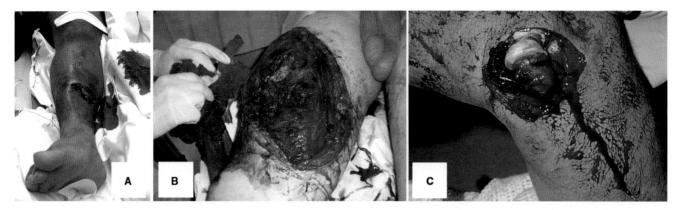

Figure 6.2 Open fracture of (A) mid-tibia, (B) elbow, and (C) knee.

open fractures of large bones require early operative irrigation and debridement. Patients needing emergent operation for severe associated injuries can have external fixation performed whereas stable patients are eligible for internal fixation. Mangled extremities may require amputation.

6.3 Mangled Extremity

This condition is the result of severe crush trauma, high-velocity missiles, or shotgun injuries. There is a combination of orthopedic trauma, extensive soft tissue damage, and injury to the neurovascular structures. The most immediate priority is to control bleeding, often by the use of tourniquets in the appropriate cases. The initial clinical evaluation should include assessment of the extent of skeletal and soft tissue injury, the presence of peripheral pulse and skin perfusion, and motor–sensory function. Patients with obvious nonsalvageable limbs should be transferred to the operating room for bleeding control and amputation. Investigations should be reserved only for cases with possibly salvageable limbs. In these cases, plain

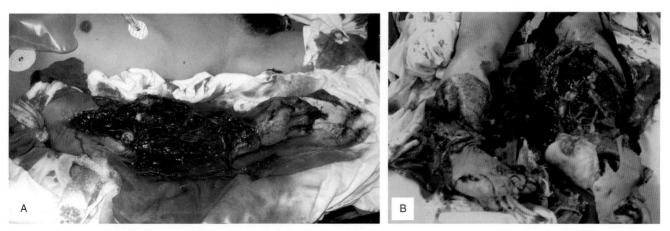

Figure 6.3 (A) Mangled right arm with severe crush injury. This patient accidentally placed his arm into an industrial mixer. Amputation was required. (B) Mangled lower legs bilaterally, following a train accident. The patient required bilateral amputations.

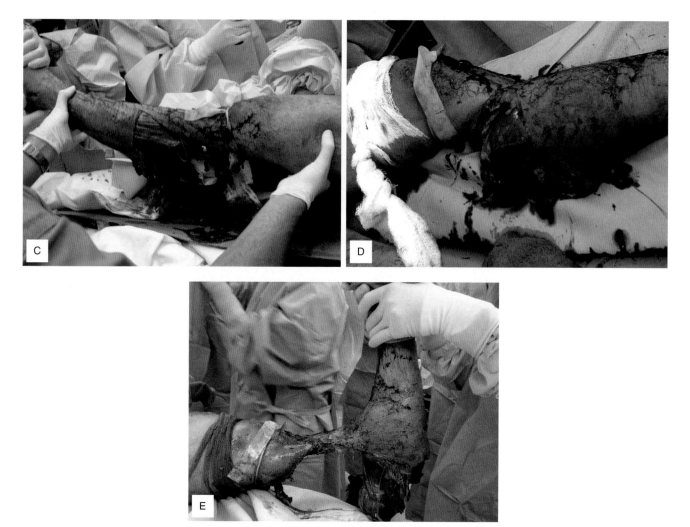

Figure 6.3 (*cont.*) (C) Mangled leg following a motorcycle accident. There is extensive soft tissue loss with neurovascular injury. The patient required amputation. (D) Mangled lower leg with fairly limited crushing and loss of skin and muscle. The popliteal vessels were transected. Note the tourniquet above the knee which was placed to control severe bleeding. The patient underwent successful reconstruction. (E) Near complete amputation of the leg following a motorcycle accident. There is only a bridge of skin holding the leg in one piece.

films should be obtained to determine the extent of the fractures. Color flow Doppler (CFD) studies, CT angiography, or conventional angiography may be necessary to assess the vascular structures and plan any vascular reconstruction.

The severity of the mangled extremity and the prediction of the need for amputation are commonly assessed with the Mangled Extremity Severity Score (MESS), which takes into account the extent of the skeletal/soft tissue injury, the presence and duration of limb ischemia, the presence of shock on admission and the age of the patient. High scores are predictive of the need for amputation. Although this scoring system is a useful tool, it has significant limitations and should not be the sole criterion in determining the need for amputation or salvage operations.

6.4 Open Joint Injury

Open joint injuries are serious orthopedic emergencies with septic arthritis and osteomyelitis being common complications. Detection may be straightforward on physical exam or may be subtle, requiring adjunctive testing. Any deep wound in proximity to a joint should be considered as entering the joint.

Plain x-rays can show an associated fracture, air, or a foreign body within the joint but may be normal. Careful exploration under sterile conditions may reveal a wound track directly penetrating the joint capsule. In questionable cases, a saline or methylene blue arthrogram may provide the answer by revealing dye leakage through the wound site. Emergency therapy includes parenteral antibiotic coverage and tetanus immunization. All major open joints require formal exploration and irrigation.

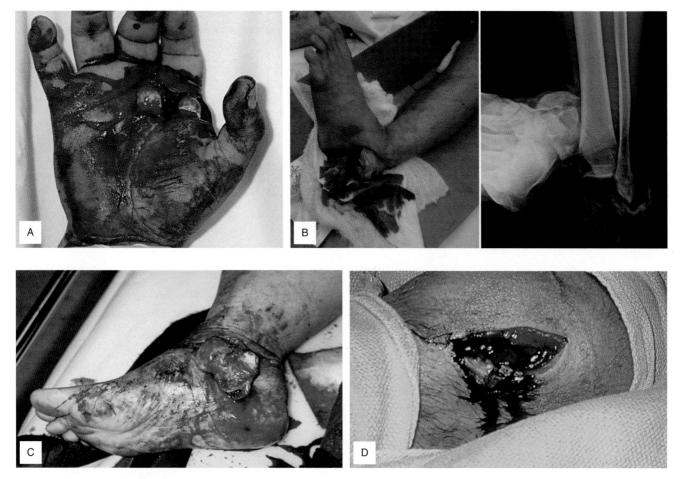

Figure 6.4 (A) Open volar dislocation of the metacarpal joint. (B) Photograph (left) and radiograph (right) of an open joint and fracture of the ankle. (C) Open joint and fracture of the ankle following a motorcycle accident. (D) Photograph of a methylene blue arthrogram of the knee with leakage through the proximal wound signifying an open joint.

6.5 Epiphyseal Injuries

In a growing child, the epiphyseal plate is a weak cartilaginous structure and is predisposed to injury. Injuries most often occur in the zone of hypertrophic cartilage cells, and the germinal cells are usually undamaged; thus, fortunately growth is often not affected.

The most commonly used classification of epiphyseal injuries is the Salter–Harris classification. In this

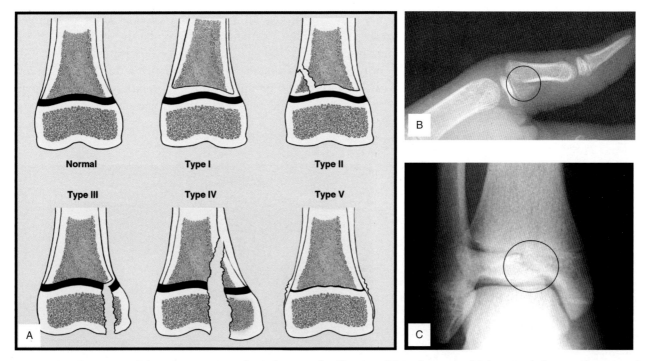

Figure 6.5 (A) Illustration of the Salter–Harris pediatric fracture classification. (B) Radiograph of Salter–Harris fracture involving the proximal phalanx of the thumb. (C) Radiograph of a juvenile Tillaux fracture. This is a Salter–Harris III fracture of the ankle.

classification, prognosis becomes progressively worse with higher numerical order.

Type I: A very common slip through the zone of provisional calcification without fracture. No germinal layer is involved, and the fracture usually heals without consequence. Comparison radiographs are often necessary for diagnosis.

Type II: An epiphyseal plate slip with an associated fracture through the metaphysis, forming a triangular fragment. This is a very common type and forms three-quarters of all epiphyseal injuries. Prognosis is good.

Type III: An epiphyseal plate slip with a fracture through the epiphysis involving the articular surface. This fracture involves the germinal

layer, and thus accurate reduction is necessary but does not guarantee avoidance of growth complications.

Type IV: Epiphyseal fracture involving both the plate and metaphysis. These fractures are complicated, and significant growth disturbance can occur unless good anatomic reduction is achieved. Operative intervention is often needed in this type of fracture.

Type V: Impaction injury in which the epiphyseal plate is destroyed. They are rare and difficult to diagnose. Unfortunately, growth arrest is the rule in this injury.

As with any pediatric injury consideration should be given to the possibility of nonaccidental trauma.

6.6 Torus and Greenstick Fractures

Pediatric bones are much less brittle than adult bones and thus are less likely to have complete fractures through the bone. A torus fracture is an incomplete fracture with a small fold in the cortex. It is often seen at the end of long bones. A greenstick fracture is an incomplete angulated fracture of a long bone recognized by a bowing appearance. These pediatric variants are common and can be easily missed.

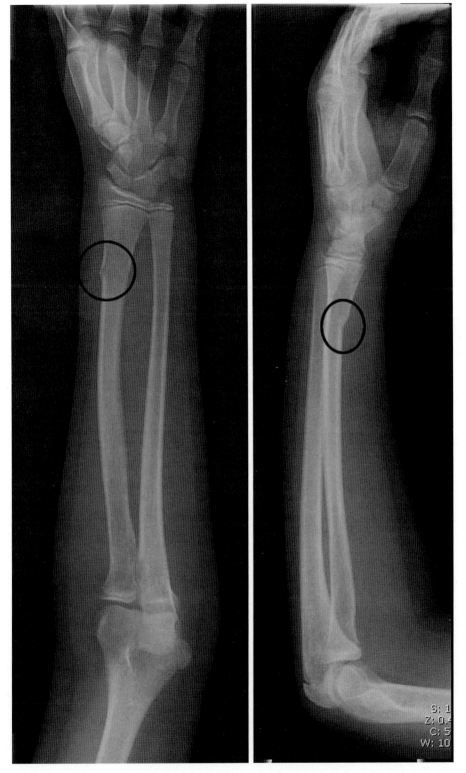

Figure 6.6 Anteroposterior and lateral radiograph of a distal radius torus fracture.

6.7 Supracondylar Fracture

Distal humerus fractures that are proximal to the epicondyles are termed supracondylar fractures, and most of these fractures occur in children aged 5–10 years. In children, the ligaments and joint capsule are

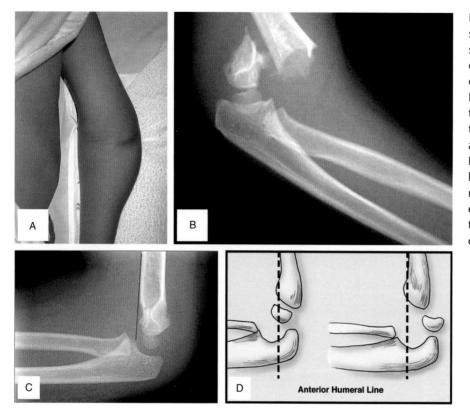

Figure 6.7 (A) Photograph of a swollen elbow of a child suffering a supracondylar fracture. (B) radiograph of the elbow shows displaced extension supracondylar fracture. (C) Radiograph of a minimally displaced transverse supracondylar fracture with the anterior humeral line passing anterior to the capitellum. (D) Illustration of the anterior humeral line. Normally this line intersects the middle of the capitellum. With an extension fracture, this line intersects the anterior one-third of the capitellum or passes entirely anteriorly.

Anterior Humeral Line

stronger than the bone, and thus hyperextension injury often causes bone fracture while adults often suffer a posterior dislocation of the elbow with a similar mechanism.

Supracondylar fractures are of two common types: flexion and extension, with extension fractures the overwhelming majority. These extension injuries are often the result of a fall on an arm with the elbow fully extended. On exam, the elbow will be swollen, often with a joint effusion and with significant pain and tenderness. In addition, the olecranon will be more prominent as it is attached to the posteriorly displaced distal fragment. Careful neurovascular examination of the arm is necessary as many of these fractures are complicated by brachial artery and median, radial, or ulnar nerve injury. In addition, compartment syndrome can be seen with displaced fractures and needs

to be considered. If compartment syndrome continues unchecked, ischemic necrosis of muscle and nerves can result in Volkman's contracture which causes permanent dysfunction of the arm and hand.

Radiographically, these fractures are often detected on the lateral view of the elbow. Because many of these fractures are transverse they may not be readily visible on the anteroposterior view. In addition, up to 25% of these are fractures of the greenstick variety with the posterior cortex remaining intact. The only abnormality seen may be a posterior fat pad sign or an abnormal anterior humeral line. Supracondylar fracture must be suspected in any child with acute elbow trauma, swelling, and pain, in spite of normal radiography. Most undisplaced fractures are treated nonoperatively with casting, and most displaced fractures undergo percutaneous pinning.

6.8 Amputations

Amputations are devastating injuries and require expert knowledge in the care of the patient and the

amputated part. The area affected is important in the decision to consider reimplantation. Lower extremity

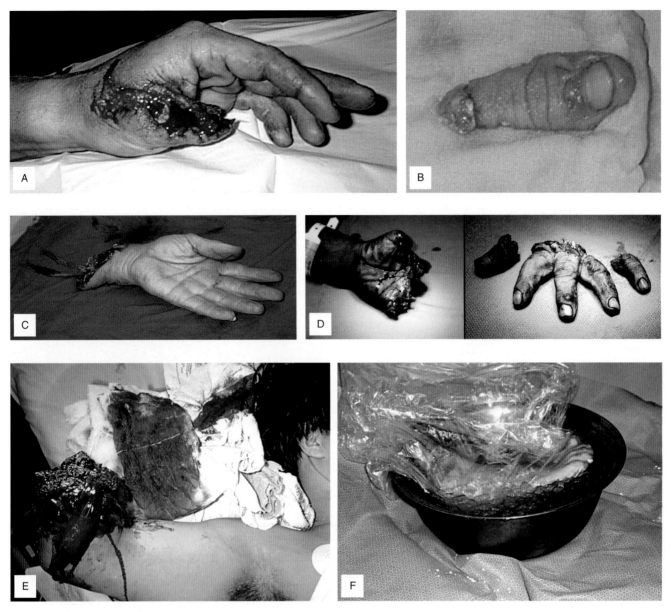

Figure 6.8 (A–B) Extremity amputations. (A) Photograph of a hand with thumb amputated secondary to a power saw injury; (B) the amputated part in saline-soaked gauze. Reimplantation was performed. (C–D) Amputated hand and multiple fingers (secondary to the hand being caught in a gear mechanism). Reimplantation was performed. (E) Proximal tor. Reimplantation was performed. (F) Amputated foot being cooled in ice water slurry.

reimplantation is rarely indicated, given the frequency of associated crush injury and the efficacy of current prostheses. In contrast, upper extremity amputations, especially involving the thumb, are often reimplanted, given the severe disability that occurs with the loss of that single digit. Time elapsed since the injury is also an important consideration. Reimplantation is less likely to be successful if the warm ischemia (room temperature) time has been more than 6–8 hours. If the part has been properly cooled and cared for, then this window of time may be

successfully extended to 12–24 hours. In addition, clean, sharp amputations are more likely to be successful than crush injuries. In general, amputated parts should be considered as candidates for reimplantation, and even severely crushed parts can be used for skin coverage.

The amputated part must be cared for properly to maximize the chance of successful reimplantation. The part should be handled minimally with no antiseptics. In addition, no debridement should occur. The part should be irrigated with normal saline and then wrapped loosely in sterile soaked gauze. It should then be placed in a watertight plastic bag and the bag placed in an ice water mixture.

The patient's stump should also be irrigated with normal saline and direct pressure used to control any bleeding. No antiseptics are used, but prophylactic systemic antibiotics and tetanus immunization should be administered.

6.9 Tendon Injury

Tendon lacerations are important injuries to detect, and full examination of the hand will usually detect complete lacerations. Diagnosis of partial injuries is more difficult, as tendon function is usually still intact. A careful examination of the laceration through the full range of motion is necessary, as the injured area of tendon may retract out of the field of view.

Flexor tendon repair in the hand is difficult and fraught with complications. Flexor tendon repair should be performed by an experienced hand surgeon, often in an operating room setting, although extensor tendon injury over the hand and fingers can be repaired in the emergency department. Prophylactic antibiotic, tetanus immunization, and splinting are essential components of emergency management.

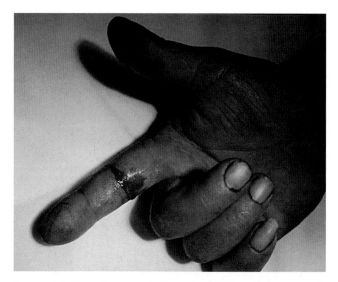

Figure 6.9 This photograph illustrates the classic position of extension in a patient with finger flexor injury.

6.10 Peripheral Vascular Injury

Most peripheral vascular injuries occur as a result of acute penetrating trauma, with gunshot wounds being more damaging than stab wounds. Fortunately, blunt trauma rarely causes vascular injury except with markedly displaced fractures and dislocations. Prompt identification and repair is important, given the relatively short "golden period" of about 6 hours, after which irreversible ischemic insult will occur.

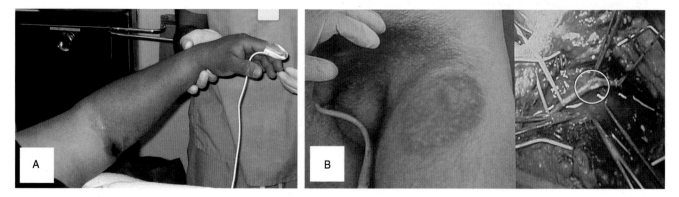

Figure 6.10 (A) Photograph of a patient with a gunshot wound of the elbow with obvious demarcation of cyanosis distally and absent distal pulses. Pulse oximetry is being used but is not sensitive for detecting vascular injury. (B) Gunshot

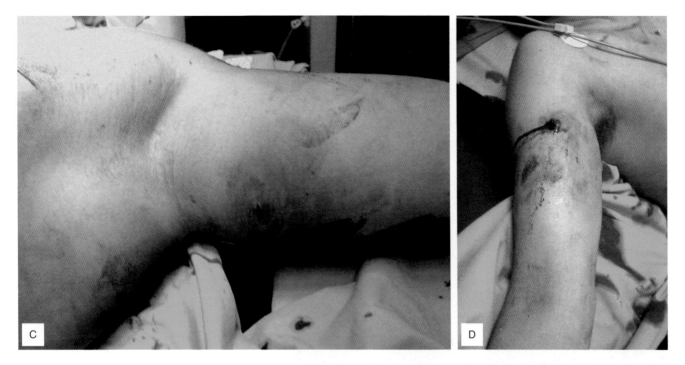

Figure 6.10 (*cont.*) wound with an entry in the posterior thigh and a large groin hematoma anteriorly. Left foot is cool and pale (left). Operative view revealing associated femoral artery injury (right). (C–D) Patients with gunshot wounds to the arm with large hematomas and diminished peripheral pulses. Both patients had injury to the brachial artery.

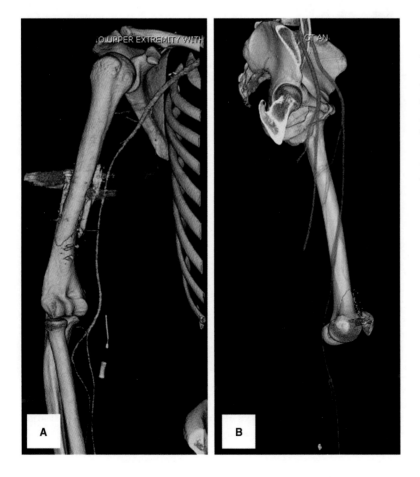

Figure 6.11 (A) Gunshot wound to the arm with a bullet tract near the brachial vessels. CT angiogram with 3-D reconstruction shows a normal brachial artery. (B) Gunshot wound to the thigh with a stable hematoma. CT angiogram with 3-D reconstruction shows a normal superficial artery. (C–D) Patients with gunshot wounds to the upper thigh. In both patients, CT angiography with 3-D reconstruction shows transection and thrombosis of the superficial femoral artery (arrow).

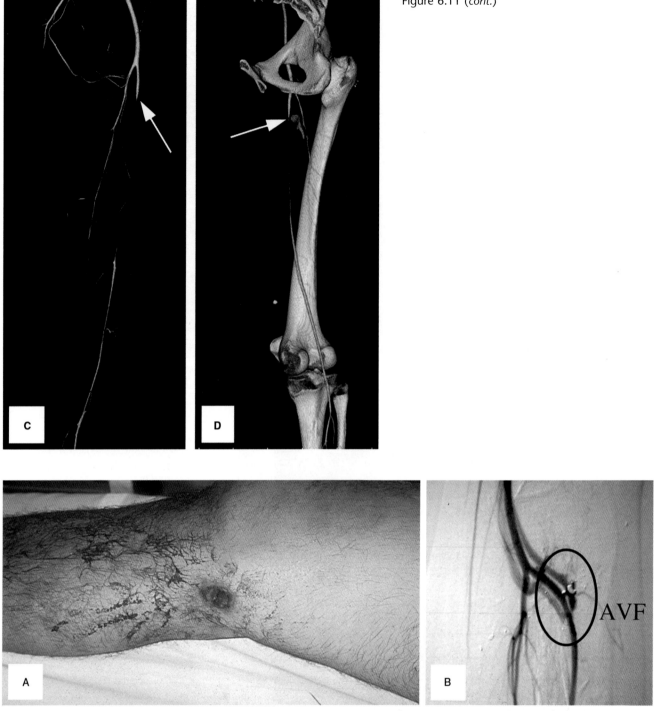

Figure 6.11 (*cont.*)

Figure 6.12 Gunshot wound to the knee. (A) The patient had diminished peripheral pulses and a bruit on auscultation. (B) Angiography shows an arteriovenous fistula.

Physical examination is important for early diagnosis, and most authors divide examination findings into "hard" and "soft" signs. Hard signs of vascular injury include the following: pulsatile bleeding, unexplained hypotension, absent peripheral pulse, expanding hematoma, palpable thrill, audible bruit, or evidence of regional ischemia such as a pale, cool extremity.

In the presence of any of these signs, operative exploration is usually recommended.

Soft signs include moderate hematoma formation, injury in proximity to major neurovascular tracts, peripheral nerve injury, and diminished but palpable pulses. To assist the evaluation of diminished pulses, the API (Doppler-determined arterial pressure in the

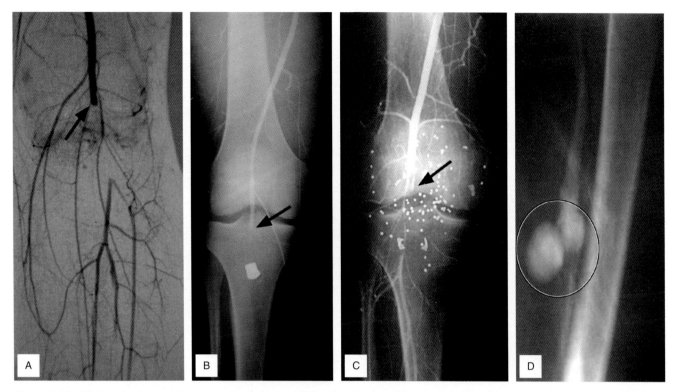

Figure 6.13 (A) Gunshot wound to the knee and no peripheral pulse on palpation. Angiography shows transection and thrombosis of the popliteal artery (arrow). Collateral vessels provide a satisfactory peripheral perfusion. (B) Gunshot wound to the popliteal fossa with no peripheral pulse. The leg was cold. Angiography shows transection and thrombosis of the popliteal artery (arrow). Note the absence of collateral circulation. (C) Shotgun injury to the knee with absent peripheral pulses. Angiography shows transection and thrombosis of the popliteal artery (arrow). (D) Gunshot wound to the mid-thigh. The patient had diminished peripheral pulses and a bruit on auscultation. Angiogram shows injury to the superficial femoral artery and a pseudoaneurysm (circle).

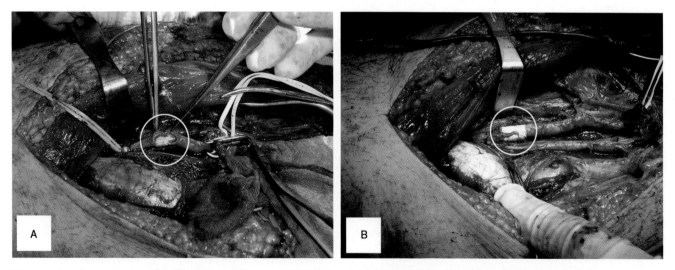

Figure 6.14 Gunshot wound to the thigh with severe active bleeding. (A) Intraoperative photograph shows an injury to the superficial femoral artery (circle). (B) The vessel was repaired with a synthetic graft.

affected limb divided by the pressure in the unaffected limb) is often used to screen for injury. An index of >0.9 generally excludes significant injury, and an index of <0.9 mandates further investigation. Though there are variations in the stepwise approach, all patients with soft signs should undergo further diagnostic testing such as CFD ultrasound or arteriography to exclude serious injuries requiring operative

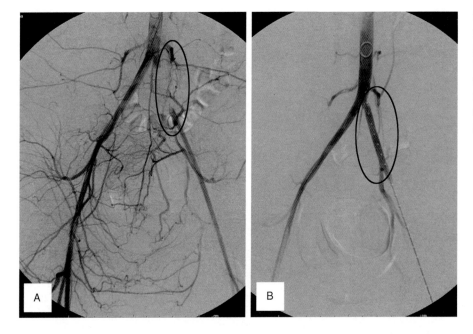

Figure 6.15 Patient with complex pelvic fractures and absent femoral pulse. (A) Angiography shows thrombosis of the left common iliac artery (circle). (B) The thrombosis was successfully managed with an angiographically placed stent-graft (circle).

attention. CT angiography has become the investigation of choice and has replaced conventional angiography in most cases. It is highly specific and sensitive, not invasive, and can be performed during routine CT scanning.

Besides acute limb loss, patients with these injuries are also at risk for acute compartment syndrome. Late complications of missed injuries include pseudoaneurysm formation, delayed thrombosis, arteriovenous fistula, and intermittent claudication.

6.11 Peripheral Nerve Injury

Peripheral nerve injuries, though not life-threatening, can cause significant long-term disability. Nerve injuries are generally classified in the following three groups:

1. Neuropraxia: Mild transient nerve dysfunction without gross anatomic disruption to the nerve, often secondary to contusion, local ischemia, or prolonged local pressure.
2. Axonotmesis: More extensive injury with interruption of axons but with preservation of the neural sheath. Complete loss of motor and sensory function is seen distal to the site of injury. Spontaneous recovery is possible and is dependent on the distance between the site of injury and the peripheral muscles to be reinnervated.
3. Neurotmesis: Complete severance of the nerve or damage to the point where spontaneous regeneration is impossible. This injury is often seen following direct lacerations, severe contusions, crushing or ischemic compressive injuries, electrical and thermal burns, and chemical injuries.

Physical examination can exclude peripheral nerve injury in a conscious, cooperative patient. Diagnosis of peripheral nerve injury in a comatose or intoxicated patient is extremely difficult and is often delayed. Penetrating injury proximal to a nerve will need careful examination and exploration. In addition, these injuries may have coexistent vascular or tendon injury to be excluded. Certain orthopedic injury complexes are more likely to harbor coexistent nerve injuries and the following tables outline common injury patterns.

Completely severed nerves will need microsurgical repair. In clean, sharp wounds, such as from a knife or glass, ideally this repair can be done early. If the injury is from a missile or crushing injury the paralysis is often due to neuropraxia and expectant management for 4–6 weeks is recommended before operative repair is attempted. If the wound is grossly contaminated, then nerve repair should be delayed.

Upper Extremity Patterns	
Nerve Injury	Upper Extremity Injury
Ulnar	Elbow injury
Distal median	Wrist dislocation
Median, anterior interosseous	Supracondylar fracture
Musculocutaneous	Anterior shoulder dislocation
Radial	Distal humeral shaft fracture, anterior dislocation of shoulder
Axillary	Anterior shoulder dislocation, proximal humeral fracture

Lower Extremity Patterns	
Nerve Injury	Lower Extremity Injury
Femoral	Pubic rami fracture
Obturator	Obturator ring fracture
Posterior tibial	Knee dislocation
Superficial peroneal	Fibular neck fracture, knee dislocation
Deep peroneal	Fibular neck fracture, compartment syndrome
Sciatic	Posterior hip dislocation
Superior and inferior gluteal	Acetabular fracture

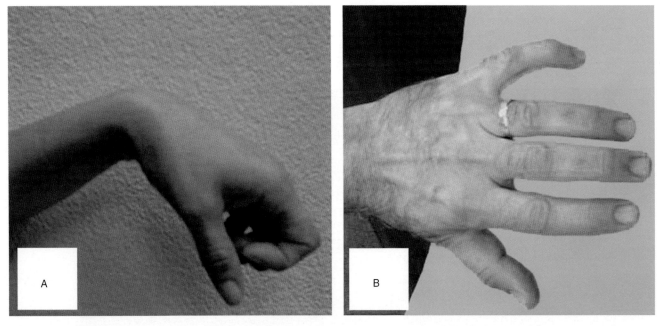

Figure 6.16 Peripheral nerve injuries in the upper extremity. (A) Proximal radial nerve injury with the characteristic wrist drop. (B) Ulnar nerve injury with the characteristic abduction and slight flexion of the small finger.

Common Peripheral Nerve Injuries

Radial Nerve
1. Proximal Injury:
   (a) Motor: Inability to extend the forearm, wrist, and fingers. Characteristic wrist drop.
   (b) Sensory: Anesthesia over the dorsum of the forearm and the back of the hand at the base of the thumb and first interosseous space.
2. Distal Injury: No motor problems. Area of anesthesia over the base of the thumb, dorsally.

Median Nerve
1. Proximal Injury:
   (a) Motor: The patient cannot make a fist. Inability to flex the index and middle fingers, while the ring and small fingers can be flexed (by the part of the flexor profundus digitorum which is innervated by the ulnar nerve). This is the "benediction" or "Pope's" hand. Loss of abduction, flexion, and a position of the thumb.
   (b) Sensory: Anesthesia over the radial 3½ fingers.

Ulnar Nerve
1. Proximal Injury:
   (a) Motor: Inability to abduct and adduct the fingers. If the patient tries to grip a card between the thumb and finger, this is only possible by flexing the terminal phalanx of the thumb (Froment's sign). The small finger is in abduction and slight flexion.
   (b) Sensory: Anesthesia over the ulnar 1½ fingers.

2. Distal Injury: Roughly the same problems as in proximal injuries, except that the flexor carpi ulnaris and part of the flexor profundus digitorum retain their innervation.

Circumflex or Axillary Nerve
Paralysis of the deltoid muscle results in inability to abduct the arm.

Musculocutaneous Nerve
Inability to flex the forearm.

Sciatic Nerve
1. Motor: Foot drop, weakness of the knee flexion.
2. Sensory: Complete sensory loss below the knee, except a narrow strip along the inner surface of the leg and foot, which gets innervation from the long saphenous nerve.

Lateral Popliteal Nerve
1. Motor: Paralysis of the extensor and peroneal groups of muscles, resulting in foot drop.
2. Sensory: Anesthesia of the lateral leg, lower two-thirds.

Medial Popliteal Nerve
1. Motor: Paralysis of the calf muscles.
2. Sensory: Anesthesia of the sole.

Femoral Nerve
1. Motor: Paralysis of the quadriceps and inability to extend the knee.
2. Sensory: Anesthesia over a strip along the inner surface of the leg and foot.

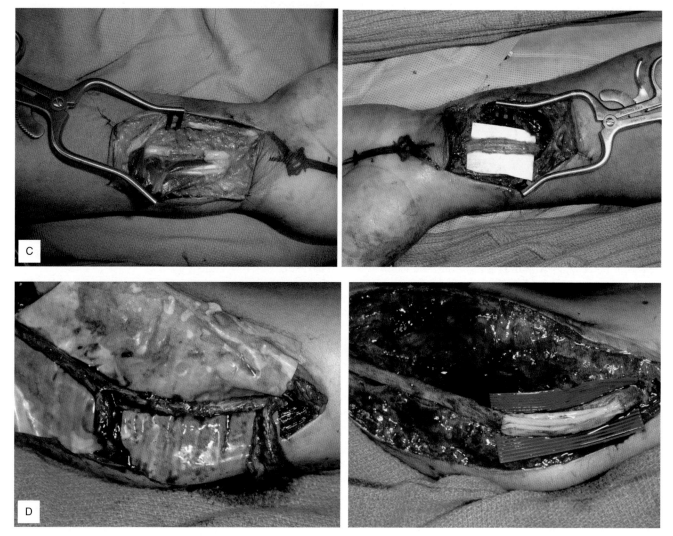

Figure 6.16 (*cont.*) (C) Operative view of a transected median nerve before (left) and after repair (right) (photograph courtesy of Dr. Milan Stevanovic). (D) Operative view of a partially transected ulnar nerve before (left) and after repair (right) (photograph courtesy of Dr. Milan Stevanovic).

6.12 Metacarpal Fractures

Metacarpal fractures are commonly seen in the emergency department and are often secondary to direct force, such as a clenched fist injury. Fourth and fifth metacarpal neck fractures of this nature are often referred to as "boxer's fractures." Metacarpal fractures can be classified in four types:

1. Head fracture: Rare injury.
2. Neck fractures: Very common fracture with the apex of the fracture being dorsal. Second and third metacarpal fractures require accurate reduction for good hand function, while the fourth and fifth fractures can heal with angulation up to 35 and 45 degrees respectively.

3. Shaft fractures: Can be transverse, oblique, spiral, or comminuted. Rotational deformities can occur especially with oblique and spiral fractures, and will need identification and correction. This is best evaluated clinically by having the patient flex the fingers into a fist. Rotational deformities will be recognized by an abnormal lie of the affected digit. Normally the fingers of the flexed hand all point toward the scaphoid bone at the wrist.
4. Base fractures: Uncommon fractures that are usually stable.

Most metacarpal fractures will have closed reduction, although comminuted, spiral, and oblique fractures may need operative fixation.

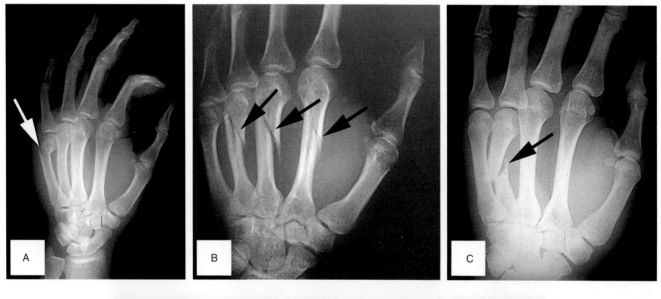

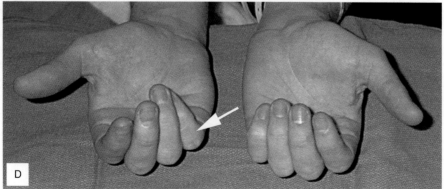

Figure 6.17 Metacarpal fractures. (A) Radiograph of a boxer's fracture of the fifth metacarpal bone. (B) Radiograph of oblique fractures of the metacarpal bones. (C) Radiograph of a displaced oblique fracture of the fourth metacarpal. (D) Photograph of a rotational fracture of the right fifth metacarpal. All fingertips should normally point toward the scaphoid.

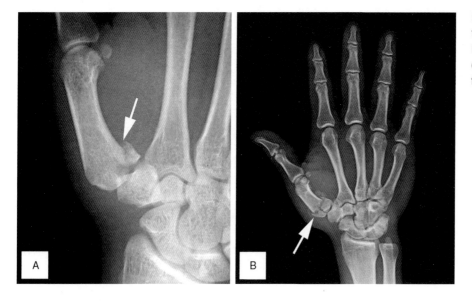

Figure 6.18 First metacarpal fractures. (A) Radiograph of a Bennett's fracture (arrow). (B) Radiograph of a Rolando's fracture (arrow).

First Metacarpal Fractures (Bennett's and Rolando's Fractures)

First metacarpal fractures are classified as articular or, less commonly, nonarticular, with the latter being either transverse or oblique. Articular fractures are further described in two common patterns.

Bennett's fracture is an oblique fracture which involves the carpometacarpal joint. It is usually due to direct axial force on a partially flexed thumb, such as in a fist-fight. The characteristic finding is a small triangular proximal fragment that remains anatomically correct while the shaft is displaced in a dorsal–radial fashion by the pull of the abductor pollicis longus and the abductor pollicis. Anatomic reduction is important, and these fractures are usually treated with percutaneous pinning or even open reduction.

Rolando's fracture is a comminuted fracture at the base of the first metacarpal. It is a relatively rare fracture often caused by a similar mechanism to a Bennett's fracture. The treatment is controversial and may vary from closed to open reduction, depending on the degree of comminution and displacement.

6.13 Scaphoid Fractures

Fractures of the scaphoid bone are common and usually occur from a fall on an outstretched hand. Pain as well as tenderness is usually demonstrated in the anatomic snuffbox. Pain with axial force along the first metacarpal will also help identify scaphoid injury.

Scaphoid fractures are classified as proximal one-third, middle third, and distal third fractures. The proximal third does not have its own blood supply, and thus these fractures are particularly at high risk for avascular necrosis if treatment is delayed or improper. Plain radiographs are often diagnostic, but up to 20% may present with normal radiographs initially. Patients with scaphoid tenderness and normal radiographs are placed in a thumb spica cast and will need a follow-up exam. A bone CT scan may be done in 3 days, or the patient may have repeat radiographs in 10 days to detect occult fractures. Nondisplaced scaphoid fractures are treated with thumb spica immobilization, and displaced or unstable fractures often need open reduction.

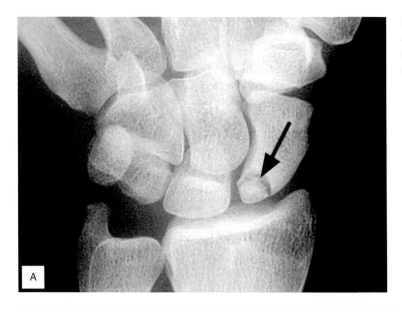

A

Figure 6.19 (A) Radiograph of a proximal one-third scaphoid fracture (arrow). This fracture is particularly at high risk for avascular necrosis if treatment is delayed.

6.14 Scapholunate Dislocation

Scapholunate ligamentous injury is often secondary to forced dorsiflexion of the wrist, as occurs in a fall on an outstretched hand. There is pain and tenderness on the radial aspect of the wrist, just distal to Lister's tubercle.

This injury is commonly missed, and radiographs should be carefully examined for an abnormal gap between the scaphoid and lunate on the posteroanterior view. This joint space is normally less than 3 mm, and any widening of this space is representative of a scapholunate ligamentous injury. This injury may be treated with closed reduction and percutaneous pinning or may require open reduction. Missed scapholunate injuries often cause chronic arthritis and pain or may cause ischemic necrosis of the lunate (Keinbock's disease).

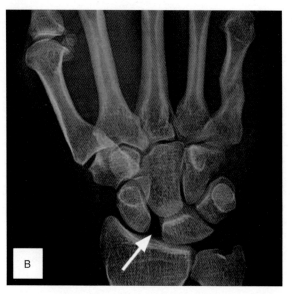

B

Figure 6.19 (cont.) (B) Scapholunate dislocation (arrow). Note the widening of the joint space between the scaphoid and the lunate.

6.15 Lunate and Perilunate Dislocation

Lunate and perilunate dislocation are relatively uncommon injuries that can easily be missed if the treating physician is not familiar with normal carpal relationships. The injury often involves high energy, such as a fall or a motor vehicle crash, which causes extreme hyperextension, ulnar deviation, and midcarpal dorsiflexion.

In the normal wrist, the lateral view reveals that the distal radius, lunate, and capitate align themselves forming three Cs atop each other. This relationship is significantly altered with a lunate or perilunate dislocation, and thus a lateral radiograph usually reveals the injury pattern.

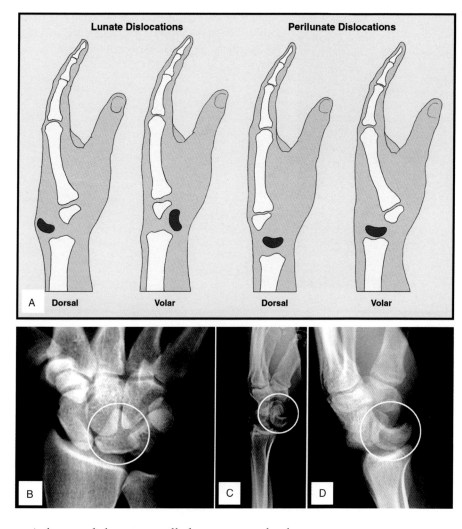

Figure 6.20 (A) Illustration of types of lunate and perilunate dislocations. (B) Anteroposterior x-ray of the wrist showing a lunate dislocation with a "piece of pie" lunate bone. (C) Lateral radiograph view of the wrist with a volar lunate dislocation. (D) Lateral radiograph view of the wrist with a dorsal perilunate dislocation.

A lunate dislocation will demonstrate the lunate pushed off the distal radius in a "spilled teacup" sign on the lateral view. On the anteroposterior view, the lunate will appear as a "piece of pie" sign. A perilunate dislocation demonstrates a capitate that is posterior or anterior to the lunate, while the lunate maintains contact with the distal radius. The anteroposterior view is less specific and shows an obliterated joint space between the lunate and the capitate. Treatment involves anatomical alignment with closed reduction, though open reduction may be necessary.

6.16 Wrist Fractures

1. Colles' Fracture

A Colles' fracture is the most common fracture of the wrist. It is a transverse fracture of the distal radius metaphysis, which is dorsally displaced and angulated. The fracture may also be intra-articular and can involve the ulnar styloid.

The usual mechanism is a fall on an outstretched hand, and the wrist may demonstrate the classic "dinner fork" deformity on exam. The treatment is usually closed reduction, though more comminuted and displaced fractures will need open reduction and fixation.

2. Smith Fracture

A Smith fracture is often referred to as a "reverse Colles'" fracture in which there is volar displacement of the distal fracture fragment. It results from a fall on a flexed wrist or a direct blow to the dorsum of the wrist. Closed reduction will usually yield acceptable

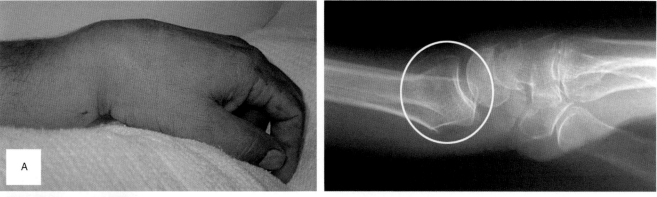

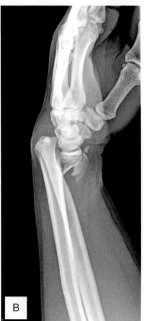

Figure 6.21 (A) Colles' fracture. Photograph of the classic "dinner fork" deformity seen with dorsal radius fractures (left). Lateral wrist radiograph of a Colles' fracture (right). (B) Radiograph of a volar Barton fracture. The carpus displaces anteriorly with the distal radius fragment.

results although intra-articular Smith fractures often undergo open reduction.

3. Barton Fracture

Barton fracture is a distal radius fracture in which the carpus displaces volarly with the radial fragment.

A reverse Barton fracture is actually more common in which the carpus displaces dorsally with a fragment of the distal radius. Open reduction internal fixation (ORIF) is usually performed for both these fractures because both involve intra-articular fractures.

6.17 Forearm Fractures

When evaluating forearm fractures, it is important to remember that isolated fractures in this area are rare. Injuries may encompass two fractures at similar or separate sites or may involve a single fracture with ligamentous injury, with or without dislocation. Careful examination of the wrist and elbow joints is imperative, as these are commonly involved sites. Some common patterns are seen in forearm fractures and thus knowledge of these injury patterns is important.

Both bones fractures (involving both the radius and ulnar shafts) are often seen in children secondary to falls on an outstretched hand. They are only rarely seen in adults and are then from high-energy mechanisms or severe direct impact. In a child, radiographs can reveal buckle or torus fractures, incomplete fractures, complete fractures, or a combination. Closed reduction is often successful in children because small amounts of residual angulation will resolve with bone remodeling. Complete fractures are more common in adults, and open reduction is often required.

The Monteggia fracture complex, first described in 1814, is a proximal ulnar fracture with an associated radial head dislocation. It is uncommon, representing about 7% of all forearm fractures. The injury is caused by forced pronation of the forearm during a fall on an outstretched hand. The radial nerve should be examined as it is commonly injured. Radiographs easily reveal the proximal ulnar fracture, and in these cases the radial head should be carefully evaluated. In the normal position, the radial head should align with the capitellum when a line is drawn through the radial shaft. Monteggia fractures are treated with open reduction.

The Galeazzi fracture complex is a distal fracture of the radius with an associated dislocation or subluxation of the distal radial–ulnar joint. The injury occurs with a fall on an outstretched hand with wrist in extension and the forearm forcibly pronated, or with a direct blow to the dorsoradial aspect of the wrist. This injury is relatively rare and accounts for only 7% of all forearm fractures. The anteroposterior radiograph reveals a fracture of the radius at the junction of the middle and distal thirds, and an increase in the joint space between the distal radius and ulna may be seen. The lateral view will demonstrate dorsal

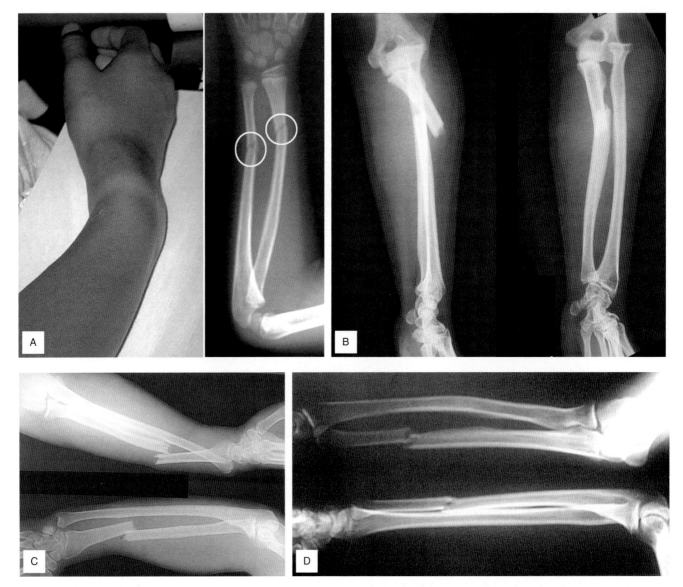

Figure 6.22 (A) Photograph and radiograph of a child with a "both bones" fracture. (B) Anteroposterior and lateral radiographs of a Monteggia fracture. (C) Anteroposterior and lateral radiographs of a Galeazzi fracture. (D) Anteroposterior and lateral radiographs of a nightstick fracture.

angulation of the radial fracture, and the head of the ulna will be displaced dorsally. Galeazzi fractures are unstable and require operative fixation.

Isolated ulnar shaft fractures or nightstick fractures are relatively common. They occur as a result of direct force to the ulna, often happening when raising one's arm in natural defense to a blow from an object such as a stick. In proximal ulnar fractures, the radial head should be carefully examined to exclude the presence of a Monteggia fracture. Associated injuries are rare but include compartment syndrome and vascular injury. Most undisplaced fractures are treated with plaster immobilization, while displaced fractures (>50% of width of ulna) may need open reduction.

6.18 Elbow Dislocation

Elbow dislocations account for about 20% of all dislocations and are the next most common dislocation after the shoulder and fingers. They are usually the result of a fall on an outstretched hand with arm extended and abducted. Most elbow dislocations (>90%) are posterior, and the patient will present with the elbow in 45 degrees of flexion, with a prominence of the olecranon process posteriorly. The collateral ligaments are torn, and careful neurovascular assessment is important as brachial artery and median nerve injuries can complicate this injury.

Radiographs will reveal a dislocation. Most often the coronoid process will slip posteriorly, but occasionally a fracture of the process will be noted. Reduction is performed under conscious sedation by countertraction with flexion of the elbow.

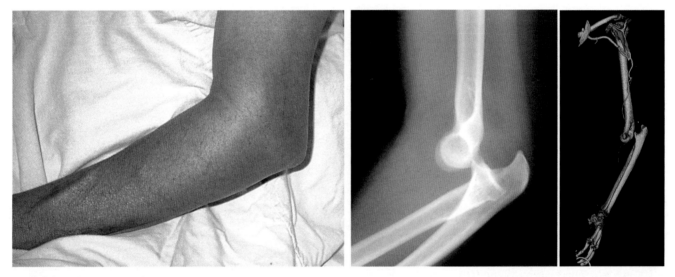

Figure 6.23 Posterior elbow dislocation: patient, plain film, and 3-D reconstruction of patient with posterior elbow dislocation.

6.19 Radial Head Fracture

Radial head fractures are common injuries of the elbow that usually occur with a fall on an outstretched hand or by direct trauma. The injury can result in damage to the articular surface, depression of the radial head, or an angulated fracture of the radial head and neck. Often a fracture is seen on radiographs, but they may reveal only a fat pad sign indicative of an effusion and an occult fracture. Nondisplaced or minimally displaced fractures are treated with a sling or posterior splint. Fractures that are displaced more than 3 mm or involve more than one-third of the joint surface are usually treated operatively with the insertion of small screws. Comminuted fractures are treated conservatively, though the treatment of severely comminuted and displaced fractures is controversial and includes excision of fragments and / or the radial head with or without the insertion of Silastic implants. Early mobilization of the elbow is important to reduce residual stiffness.

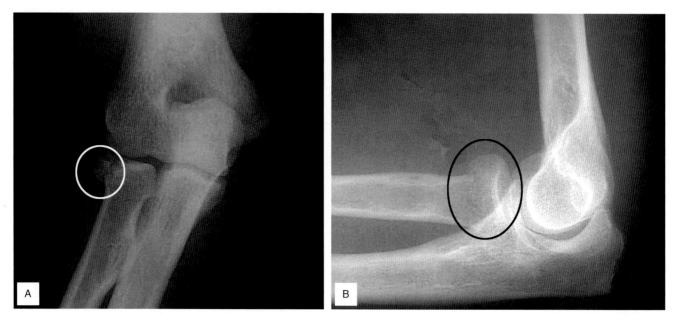

Figure 6.24 Radial head fractures. (A) Radiograph of a radial head fracture involving the articular surface. (B) Radiograph of an impacted radial head fracture.

6.20 Humeral Fracture

Humeral shaft fractures are often the result of direct blows to the arm, motor vehicle crashes, or minor falls in the elderly. Physical exam reveals severe tenderness localized to the fracture area. Radial nerve injuries complicate up to 20% of humerus fractures, though median and ulnar nerves are rarely injured.

Plain radiographs are most often diagnostic, and conservative treatment is used for the majority of closed injuries. The sugar-tong splint and hanging cast are good techniques for immobilization. Open fractures, severely comminuted fractures, and fractures that are not adequately aligned by closed reduction are treated with open reduction.

Fractures of the humeral head most often occur in older patients after minor falls. Associated rotator cuff tears and fracture–dislocation of the humeral head are common complications. Initial management is with a sling and swathe and the ultimate decision regarding open or closed treatment is based on the patient's age, the number and displacement of fracture fragments, the quality of bone, and the presence of associated injuries.

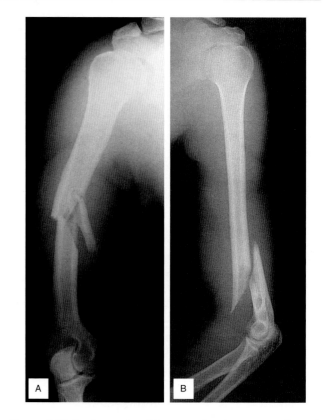

Figure 6.25 Radiographs of humerus fractures: comminuted mid-shaft humerus fracture. (A) This fracture is at high risk for radial nerve injury. (B) This injury is often associated with brachial artery injury.

6.21 Shoulder Dislocation

The shoulder is the most commonly dislocated joint. Shoulder dislocations can be classified as anterior, posterior, or inferior (luxatio erecta).

Anterior dislocations constitute >90% of all shoulder dislocations. They are usually the result of a fall on an outstretched hand with the arm abducted, extended, and externally rotated. On examination, the arm is held in slight abduction and external rotation. The humeral head is palpable anteriorly, and a slight hollow is noticed in the shoulder laterally. Axillary nerve injury complicates shoulder dislocation in up to 10% of cases.

Standard radiography includes anteroposterior and lateral views and either a transscapular Y view or an axillary view. Radiographs may reveal a compression fracture in the humeral head termed a Hill–Sachs deformity. In addition, a small anteroinferior glenoid rim fracture called a Bankart lesion may be seen. Recurrent dislocation is common especially with concomitant rotator cuff tears.

Multiple techniques that use traction, leverage, or a combination can be used to reduce this injury, including traction–countertraction, external rotation, Stimson technique, scapular rotation, and the Hippocratic technique. Closed reduction is successful in the majority of cases, though operative repair is used in irreducible cases, unstable joints, large glenoid rim fractures, >5–10 mm of displacement of avulsed greater or lesser tuberosity fractures, intrathoracic dislocations, and many posterior dislocations.

Posterior dislocations are rare injuries, about 5% of all dislocations. They can be difficult to diagnose, and up to 50% are thought to be initially misdiagnosed. The injury occurs with an axial load on an adducted internally rotated and forward flexed arm, direct blow to the shoulder, or severe muscular contractions as from a seizure or electrical injury. The arm is usually internally rotated on exam, and the patient is unable to elevate the arm above 90 degrees. The anteroposterior radiograph may look nearly normal, and thus the transscapular Y view or the axillary view is necessary to exclude the diagnosis. There are four important radiographic findings associated with posterior shoulder dislocation: the "light bulb" sign (rotation of the trochanters into an anteroposterior plane leaving the humeral head with the appearance of a light bulb), the deep sulcus sign (>6 mm distance between the humeral head and the glenoid rim), the "trough" sign (compression fracture of the humeral head resulting in two vertical parallel lines), and the rim or ellipse sign (loss of the usual elliptical overlap of the humeral head and the glenoid rim). Not all signs are present in a single patient but the presence of any of these signs suggests a posterior dislocation. Reduction is accomplished by slow in-line traction, usually with general anesthesia.

Inferior dislocation, also known as luxatio erecta, is a very rare dislocation forming <1% of all shoulder dislocations. The injury occurs with forced abduction of the arm, and the patient presents with a fully abducted arm and the elbow flexed with the forearm on or behind the head. Neurovascular compromise is common because these structures are inferior to the joint. Plain radiographs easily demonstrate the dislocation, and closed reduction is usually successful with a two-stage procedure. First the dislocation is rotated downward with in-line traction and converted into a simple anterior dislocation. Then reduction proceeds with reduction of the anterior dislocation. In a minority of cases interposition of soft tissues makes closed reduction impossible and open reduction is required.

Open shoulder dislocation is rare but invariably results in severe disruption of the brachial plexus and vascular supply to the arm because the skin is the last structure to tear.

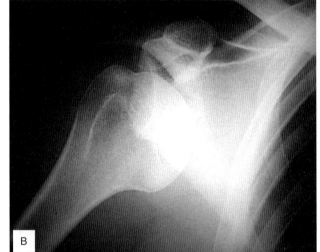

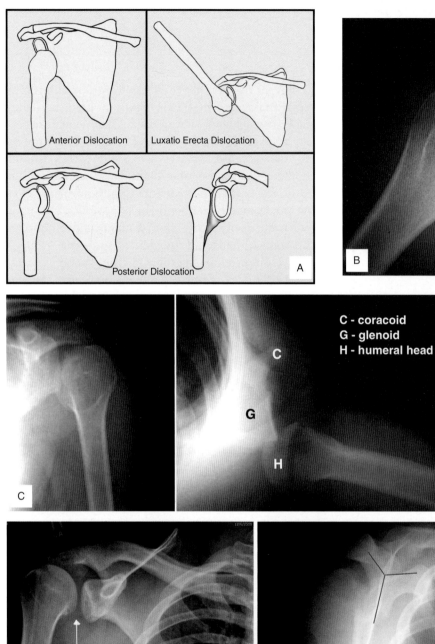

C - coracoid
G - glenoid
H - humeral head

Figure 6.26 (A) Illustration of types of shoulder dislocations. (B) Anteroposterior radiograph of an anterior shoulder dislocation with a large Hill–Sachs deformity. (C) Anteroposterior view of a posterior dislocation (left side) and axillary view of same patient (right side). (D) Posterior dislocation showing loss of ellipse sign (left) and scapular-Y view showing the humeral head lying posterior to the scapula (right). (E) Photograph of a patient with a luxatio erecta dislocation (left) and corresponding radiograph (right).

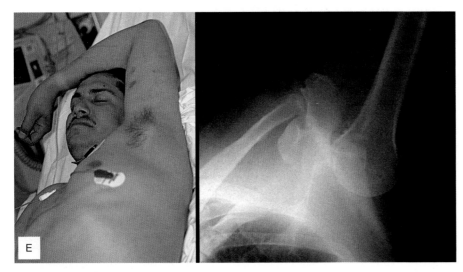

Figure 6.26 (*cont.*)

6.22 Clavicle Fracture

Clavicle fractures are common and can occur from a direct blow to the clavicle or from a fall on outstretched hand. Localized tenderness is found on examination, and radiography easily delineates the fracture. Complications are unusual but can include a host of serious injuries, including pneumothorax, subclavian vessel injury, tracheal injury, pacemaker malfunction, and thoracic outlet syndrome with brachial plexus injury.

Most clavicle fractures can be treated conservatively with a sling or a figure-of-eight bandage. Open reduction is usually not necessary and is reserved for patients with open fractures, irreducible fractures with soft tissue interposition, unstable fractures, associated acromioclavicular dislocation, associated brachial plexus injury, or nonunion.

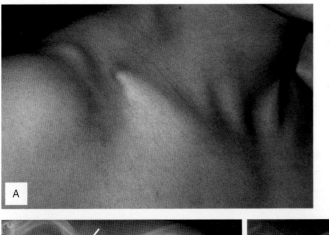

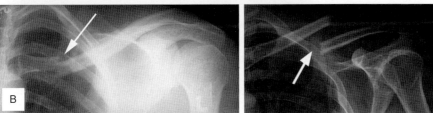

Figure 6.27 (A) Photograph of skin tenting seen with a displaced clavicle fracture. (B) Clavicular fractures. Slightly displaced medial clavicle fracture on plain radiography (left). Mid-shaft clavicle fracture with significant displacement. These types of fracture are sometimes associated with subclavian vascular injuries (right).

6.23 Sternoclavicular Dislocation

The sternoclavicular joint is the articulation of the medial aspect of the clavicle and the manubrium portion of the sternum. It is a "ball and socket" joint, and the dislocation may occur in any direction. The injury is rare, accounting for 1.5% of all dislocations, and is usually caused by high-energy mechanisms such as motor vehicle crashes or contact sports.

The injuries are classified as:

1. First degree: incomplete injury/stretching of the capsule.
2. Second degree: mild subluxation.
3. Third degree: complete dislocation.

The majority of these dislocations are anterior (>90%). The less commonly seen posterior dislocation is associated with life-threatening tracheal compression and airway compromise, vascular injury, and brachial plexus injury. First- and second-degree injuries are treated conservatively, but third-degree injuries may require reduction emergently if the airway is compressed. Reduction is accomplished by having the patient lie supine with the arm abducted while traction is applied to the arm by an assistant. A towel clamp may be used to lift the proximal clavicle anteriorly if necessary. Reductions are unstable and often need surgical reinforcement.

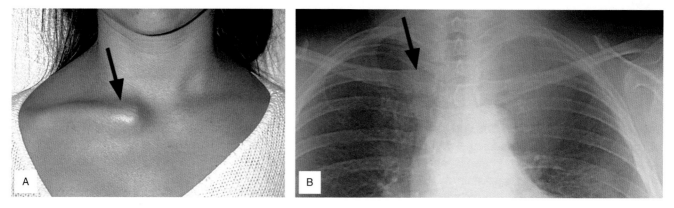

Figure 6.28 (A) Photograph of a woman with a right-sided anterior sternoclavicular dislocation. (B) The chest radiograph shows asymmetry of the clavicles with respect to the sternum, with the right sternoclavicular joint in an abnormal position (arrow).

6.24 Scapula Fracture

The scapula is integral to the normal function of the shoulder, and is rarely injured given its protection by thick surrounding musculature. Scapula fractures can be classified as the following:

- Body fracture
- Acromion fracture
- Scapula neck fracture
- Glenoid fracture
- Coracoid fracture.

Body fractures are the most serious of these types and form about 1% of all fractures. Mechanisms of injury include direct trauma, motor vehicle crashes, sports injuries, falls, and crush injuries. Examination reveals tenderness over the body of the scapula. Associated injuries are common, given the high energy required to fracture the scapula, and they need to be excluded. These injuries can include rib fractures, pneumothorax, hemothorax, pulmonary contusion, clavicle fracture, subclavian vessel injury, spine fracture, and skull fracture.

Anteroposterior and transscapular radiographic views are usually sufficient to delineate the injury. In general, these fractures are managed conservatively with sling and swathe, though some authors prefer operative therapy.

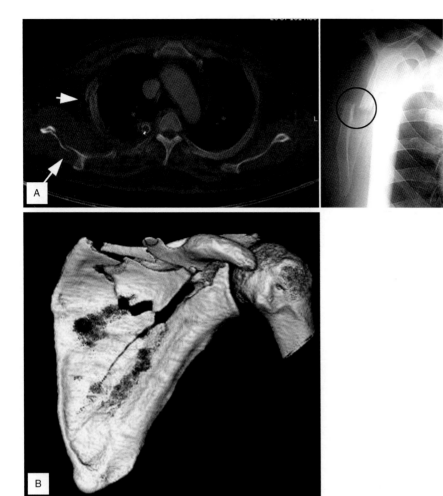

Figure 6.29 Scapula fractures. (A) CT scan of the chest showing a scapula fracture (large arrow) and rib fractures (small arrow) with a hemothorax (left). Scapular view radiograph illustrating a mid-body fracture with displacement (right). (B) CT scan with 3-D reconstruction of comminuted fracture of the scapula.

6.25 Pelvic Fractures

Pelvic fractures pose two major challenges for emergency physicians and surgeons. Firstly, there is a high incidence of associated intra-abdominal injuries (about 28% of all severe pelvic fractures). The clinical examination may be difficult and hollow viscus injuries, which occur in about 13% of all severe fractures, may be missed. Secondly, these fractures can bleed profusely and the bleeding is difficult to control.

A common classification of the pelvic fractures is based on the mechanism of injury and geography of the fracture, as follows:

Type A: Stable fractures. Isolated rami fractures, iliac wing fractures, or pubic symphysis diastasis less than 2.5 cm.

Type B: Partially unstable fractures (rotationally unstable, vertically stable).
B1: Pubic symphysis diastasis more than 2.5 cm and widening of sacroiliac joints (open book fractures), caused by external hemipelvis rotation forces.
B2: Pubic symphysis overriding, caused by internal hemipelvis rotation forces.

Type C: Disruption of the sacroiliac joint due to vertical shear forces. Unstable fractures (rotationally and vertically), often associated with severe bleeding.
C1: Unilateral.
C2: Bilateral.
C3: Involving acetabulum.

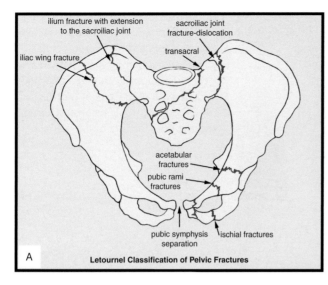

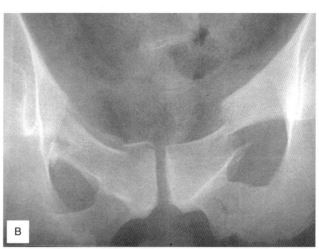

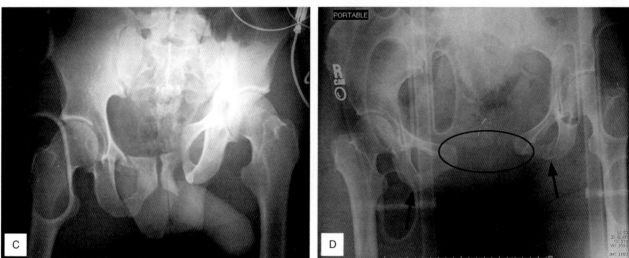

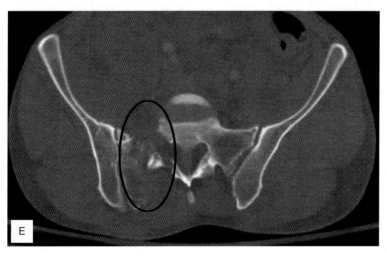

Figure 6.30 (A) Illustration of the different patterns of pelvic fractures. (B) Pelvic x-ray showing bilateral pubic and ischial rami fractures resulting in a "butterfly" fragment. This injury is often associated with significant bleeding. (C) Pelvic x-ray showing unstable Malgaigne fracture with widening of symphysis pubis, right acetabular fracture, left rami fracture, and left sacroiliac joint disruption. This type of fracture is always associated with severe bleeding. (D) Pelvic x-ray shows severe pubic symphysis diastasis. This is partially unstable and may be associated with significant bleeding. Arrows show bilateral inferior rami fractures. (E) CT scan shows fracture of the sacral bone with severe displacement. It is usually associated with severe bleeding from the presacral venous plexus or the iliac vessels.

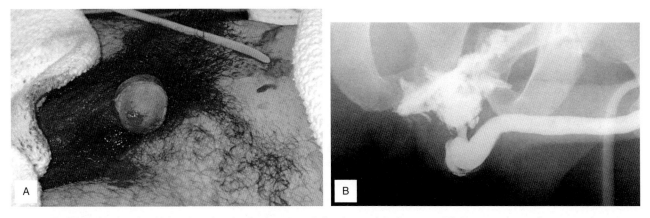

Figure 6.31 (A) Photograph of blood at the urethral meatus following pelvic fracture. (B) Retrograde urethrogram shows injury to the urethra.

Clinical Examination

The abdominal clinical examination is often difficult, because of the pain and abdominal wall hematoma associated with the fracture. The patient should be evaluated for instability by gentle compression over both iliac wings. This is a painful maneuver and should not be repeated by other physicians for confirmation or education. The clinical evaluation should include a rectal exam to rule out any rectal tears. In addition the prostate should be assessed for a high-riding position, which is indicative of posterior rupture of the urethra. The meatus of the urethra should be examined for any gross blood. A urethral catheter should be inserted without using any force. In the presence of any resistance the procedure should be abandoned and a urethrogram should be performed. In the appropriate cases a vaginal examination should be done to evaluate for vaginal tears.

Investigations

An anteroposterior portable pelvic x-ray is indicated in order to assess the type and severity of the fracture and the suitability of applying a pelvic binder. A trauma ultrasound (FAST) should be routinely performed to rule out any significant intraperitoneal bleeding. Retroperitoneal hematomas are usually missed by FAST. A diagnostic peritoneal aspirate (DPA) should be considered in the hemodynamically unstable patient with a negative FAST exam, who cannot safely be transported to the CT scan suite.

The most valuable investigation is an abdominal and pelvic CT scan with intravenous contrast. It provides reliable information about intraperitoneal injuries, the type and severity of pelvic fracture and can help in identifying those patients who may benefit from early angioembolization. Extravasation of contrast (blush) or a large hematoma are indications of significant bleeding and angiography should be considered.

Angiography with embolization of any bleeders should be considered early, before the patient becomes hypotensive and coagulopathic. Parameters which are predictive of the need of angioembolization include pubic symphysis diastasis >2.5 to 3 cm, sacroiliac joint disruption, older age, and female gender. In these cases early angiography should be considered.

Management

Immobilization of the fracture reduces pain and bleeding and should be done early. Rolling of the patient should be avoided and instead perform a straight lift using many helpers. Commercially available pelvic binders or sheet wrapping are practical and effective ways of pelvic fracture reduction and immobilization of open book fractures. Routine application of pelvic binder is not recommended and can be counterproductive in some types of fractures, such as in iliac wing or internal rotation fractures with pubic symphysis overriding. In these cases, application of pelvic binder may worsen the fracture displacement. An anteroposterior pelvic x-ray can easily select the cases that can benefit from a binder application. In highly unstable fractures, external pelvic fixation performed by the orthopedic team should be considered.

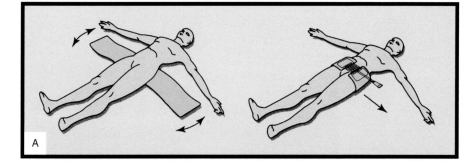

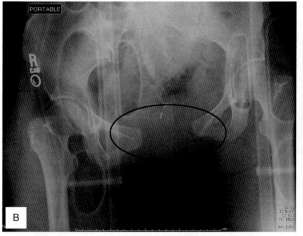

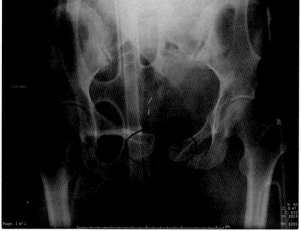

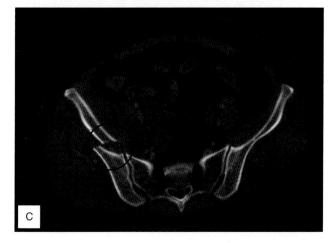

Figure 6.32 (A) Illustration of external pelvic binder device being placed (left). Patient with pelvic binder applied (right). (B) Radiographs of a patient with pubic symphysis diastasis before (left) and after (right) reduction and pelvic binder application. This type of immobilization is ideal for pubic symphysis diastasis but not other types of pelvic fractures. (C) CT scan showing fracture of the right iliac wing (circle). Application of a pelvic binder in this type of fracture is contraindicated because it worsens the fracture displacement.

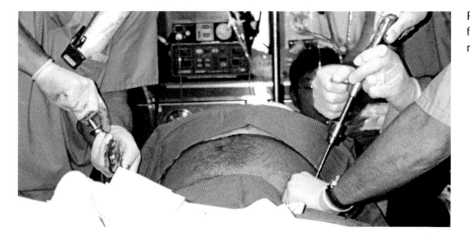

Figure 6.33 Photograph of external fixation applied in the emergency room, in an unstable pelvic fracture.

In the majority of pelvic fractures the bleeding can safely be managed with appropriate immobilization and blood transfusions. A small number of cases (about 5%) may need angioembolization. In rare occasions when the patient is too unstable for angiography or angioembolization fails, surgical intervention with damage control of the pelvic fracture bleeding can be life-saving. The management of these patients is a multidisciplinary team effort, including surgeons, emergency physicians, orthopedic surgeons, interventional radiologists, and anesthesiologists.

All patients with complex pelvic fractures should be admitted to the intensive care unit for close monitoring and timely therapeutic interventions. The intra-abdominal pressure should be monitored closely because some of these patients may develop abdominal compartment syndrome, which requires immediate surgical decompression. Definitive internal fixation should be considered a few days later (usually 4 or 5 days after admission) when the bleeding and hematoma are stabilized.

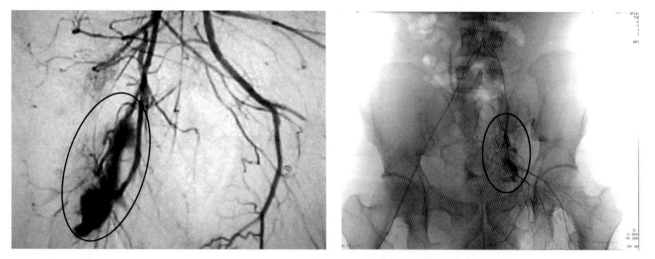

Figure 6.34 Angiograms of patients with complex pelvic fracture showing severe active bleeding.

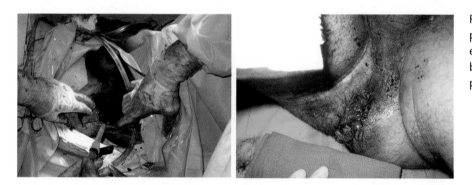

Figure 6.35 Photographs of open pelvic fractures. These patients require emergency operation for washout and bleeding control with tight gauze packing.

6.26 Hip Dislocation

Hip dislocations occur from high-energy trauma such as motor vehicle accidents and are true orthopedic emergencies because of the risk of ischemic necrosis of the femoral head. Because many patients present with severe associated trauma, other injuries may take priority, but the hip dislocation should be addressed before other orthopedic concerns. Ninety percent of all hip dislocations are posterior, with only about 10% being anterior dislocations. Rarely seen are central dislocations in which there is a concomitant fracture in the floor of the acetabulum. Given the energy involved, a femoral head fracture may also be present, and radiographs should provide good views of the femoral head and neck. In addition, the sciatic nerve is at risk with posterior dislocations and the femoral nerve and vessels may be damaged with anterior dislocations, thus the affected lower extremity requires a careful neurovascular examination.

Early closed reduction is paramount, as the femoral head has a limited blood supply. The average rate of avascular necrosis is 20%, and the risk rises to 50% in reductions performed 12 hours or more after the injury. Reduction can usually be accomplished using the Allis or Stimson techniques with appropriate deep sedation, though some patients will require operative reduction.

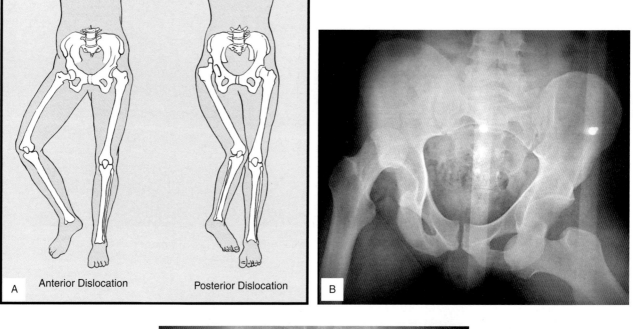

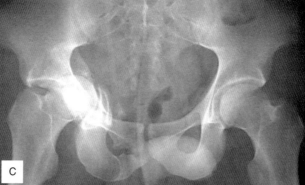

Figure 6.36 (A) Illustration of the classic position of adduction, flexion, and internal rotation seen in a posterior hip dislocation, and extension and external rotation seen in anterior hip dislocation. (B) Anteroposterior pelvis radiograph reveals both a posterior (right hip) and an anterior hip dislocation (left hip) occurring simultaneously in a patient involved in a motor vehicle crash. (C) Anteroposterior pelvis radiograph showing a right central hip dislocation with an acetabular fracture.

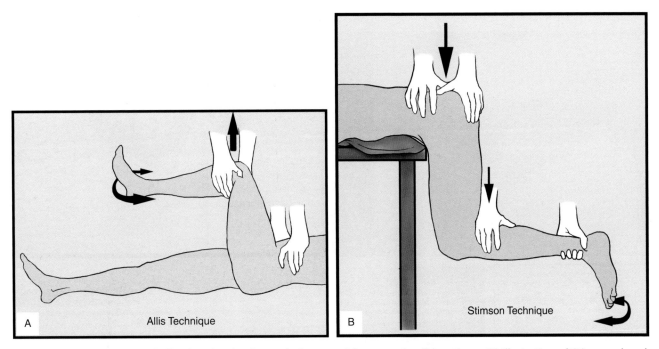

Figure 6.37 (A) Illustration of Allis closed reduction technique used for posterior dislocations. (B) Illustration of Stimson closed reduction technique used for posterior dislocation.

6.27 Hip Fractures

Hip fractures are commonly seen in the elderly, who are prone to osteoporosis and minor falls. Fractures in patients younger than 50 often require high-energy mechanisms or a pathological process affecting the hip. Most patients complain of pain in the medial thigh or groin, and there is significant discomfort with internal or external rotation. In addition, the affected leg is often shortened and externally rotated, though neurovascular status is usually intact.

Hip fractures can be classified as femoral head fractures, neck fractures, intertrochanteric fractures, and subtrochanteric fractures. Standard radiographic evaluation includes an anteroposterior pelvis view, along with coned views of the hip and a lateral view of the hip. On the anteroposterior pelvis view, it is important to examine the trabeculae carefully and to look for a disruption of Shenton's line (Figure 6.38C). Detection of minor fractures can be difficult, and plain radiographs can appear normal; thus, CT or MRI is indicated in patients with normal plain radiographs but persistent hip pain or inability to bear weight on the affected leg.

Femoral head and neck fractures are intracapsular fractures and have a limited blood supply, making avascular necrosis a serious concern. In contrast, both intertrochanteric and subtrochanteric fractures have an excellent blood supply. Prosthetic hip replacement or external fixation is used to manage most hip fractures. Early mobilization of elderly patients avoids numerous complications associated with prolonged immobilization, such as pulmonary embolus, pneumonia and sepsis. Femoral nerve block can provide excellent analgesia for these fractures in the emergency department.

Children differ from older adults in respect to this injury. Children's bones and periosteum are much stronger, and thus more severe trauma is required to produce hip fractures in this population. Communition is not seen as often, and the periosteum often remains intact, thus limiting displacement of the injury. The presence of the epiphyseal plate predisposes to late growth complications. And the incidence of avascular necrosis is also higher. In addition, children have a better tolerance to bedrest and immobilization, making these treatment options a possibility for some injuries.

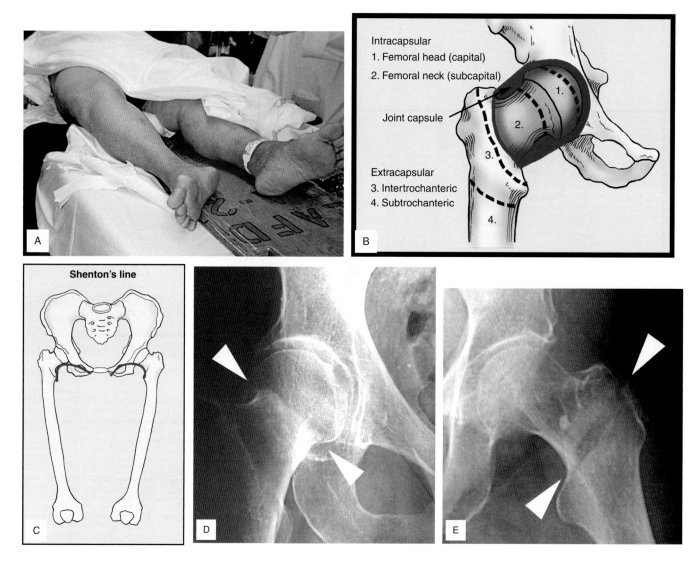

Figure 6.38 (A) Photograph of a shortened and externally rotated leg: the classic leg position after hip fracture. (B) Illustration of anatomic types of hip fracture. (C) Illustration of Shenton's line. (D) Hip radiograph of a femoral neck fracture. (E) Hip radiograph of an intertrochanteric hip fracture.

6.28 Femoral Shaft Fracture

The femur is the longest and strongest bone in the body, and thus fractures often require high-energy mechanisms such as major falls, motor vehicle accidents, or gunshot wounds. Physical examination reveals gross laxity of the femur, thigh swelling, and severe pain.

Significant blood loss can occur, and each fractured femur can easily lose three units of blood. Consequently, femur fractures are an important cause of hemorrhagic shock in the trauma victim. Gentle traction will reduce displaced fractures, and the limb should be splinted to maintain anatomic positioning to minimize soft tissue injury and blood loss. A careful physical examination is necessary to exclude neurovascular injury or compartment syndrome that may be present. Plain radiographs usually reveal the fracture clearly but should not delay the resuscitation of a critical patient, as they rarely will alter acute management. Emergency department treatment includes appropriate analgesia with limb traction. Orthopedic consultation is necessary, and most mid-shaft fractures will be treated operatively with an intramedulary rod.

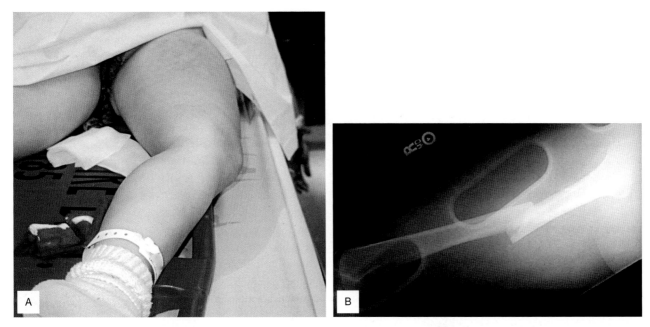

Figure 6.39 (A) Photograph of a swollen thigh and (B) plain radiograph in a patient with a femoral shaft fracture.

6.29 Patellar Fracture

Patellar fractures account for approximately 1% of skeletal fractures, and most are associated with direct trauma to the knee or resisted forceful extension of the knee. On examination, there is often point tenderness over the patella, with significant swelling and ecchymosis. A large hemarthrosis may occur with patellar fractures, and joint aspiration may be necessary for pain relief. The quadriceps extensor mechanism may be affected and thus should be tested for integrity by asking the patient to extend the knee against gravity and then against resistance. Radiographic assessment should include anteroposterior, lateral, and skyline views, although small undisplaced fractures can still be difficult to detect, and a bipartite patella can be a confusing normal variant. Three types of fractures are commonly seen: transverse, longitudinal, and stellate.

Most patellar fractures can be successfully treated by conservative therapy with cylindrical casting or a bulky Jones dressing for smaller fractures. Operative repair is done for open fractures, widely displaced fractures, severe articular disruption, osteochondral fractures, and longitudinal fractures.

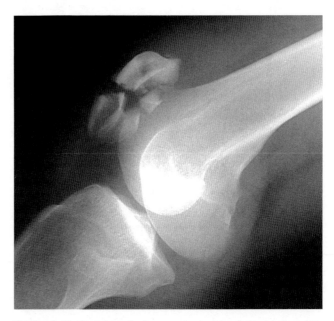

Figure 6.40 Radiograph shows a transverse fracture through the body of the patella.

6.30 Tibial Plateau Fracture

Tibial plateau fractures are often the result of direct shear forces. With most car bumpers being 20 inches high, the tibial plateau is at high risk in auto-versus-pedestrian accidents. Swelling, hemarthrosis, point tenderness, and pain with any motion of the knee make weight-bearing impossible. Ligamentous injury may coexist and thus should be sought out on the clinical examination. Standard anteroposterior and lateral radiographs with oblique views will make the diagnosis in most cases, but occasionally CT scanning may be needed to further define the injury. The medial plateau is stronger, and thus fractures usually involve the lateral plateau. Generally the fractures are of two varieties: split and/or depressed. Split fractures tend to occur in younger patients with stronger bone, and depressed fractures more often occur in the elderly patient with osteoporosis.

As tibial plateau fractures involve the articular surface of a major joint, they are at high risk for persistent pain and arthritis and thus should be managed by an orthopedic surgeon. In the past, the fractures have generally been casted, but because of the residual stiffness often associated with casting, surgical intervention and early mobilization are increasingly being used to achieve anatomic alignment and avoid complications.

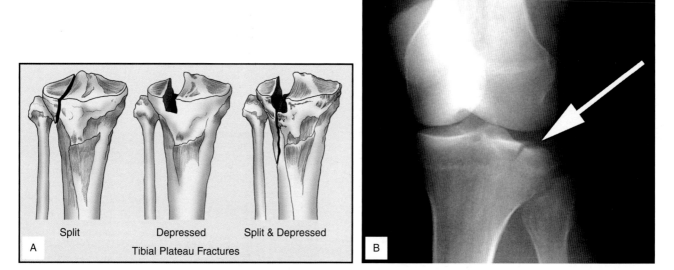

Figure 6.41 (A) Illustration of types of tibial plateau fractures. (B) This anteroposterior view of the knee reveals a lateral split plateau fracture.

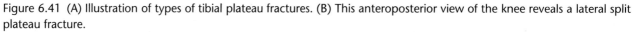

6.31 Knee Dislocation

Knee dislocation is rare but extremely important to recognize, as missed coexistent popliteal artery injury can lead to limb loss. This injury requires a high-energy mechanism and is often seen in the context of multiple trauma. Knee dislocation is classified according to the position of the tibia in relation to the femur. There are five major types of dislocation:

- Anterior: Anterior dislocation is often caused by severe knee hyperextension.
- Posterior: Posterior dislocation occurs with anterior to posterior force to the proximal tibia, such as a dashboard type of injury or a high-energy fall on a flexed knee.
- Medial, lateral, or rotator: Medial, lateral, and rotator dislocations require varus, valgus, or rotatory components of applied force.

Almost all dislocations are anterior or posterior, and both of these have a high incidence of popliteal artery injury. Physical exam of the affected limb will show gross deformity around the knee, with swelling and immobility. The finding of varus or valgus instability with the knee in full extension is suggestive of a complete ligamentous disruption and a spontaneously reduced knee dislocation.

A careful vascular examination is essential, as popliteal artery injury occurs in 35–45% of all knee dislocations, and the presence of normal pulses does not rule out a significant vascular injury. All patients should be initially evaluated using the ABI and CFD ultrasound. Patients with abnormal findings on these studies will need CT angiography or formal angiography. Patients with a cold, pale, pulseless distal extremity should undergo vascular repair directly without waiting for angiography if the 6-hour warm ischemia time limit is approaching. Coexistent peroneal nerve injury occurs in 25–35% of cases and manifests with decreased sensation at the first webspace with impaired dorsiflexion of the foot.

Emergency treatment consists of prompt reduction with gentle in-line traction. Definitive treatment includes identification and repair of the vascular injury. Limb loss occurs in about a third of all cases.

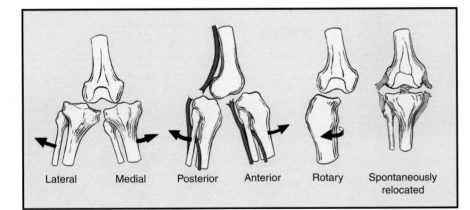

Figure 6.42 Illustration of types of knee dislocation.

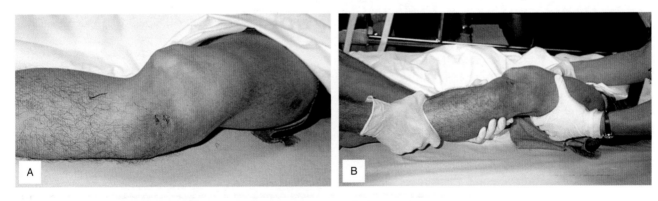

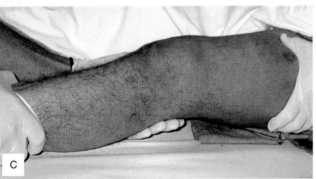

Figure 6.43 (A) Photograph of a lateral knee dislocation. (B) Reduction of the dislocation. (C) Postreduction showing knee in good position.

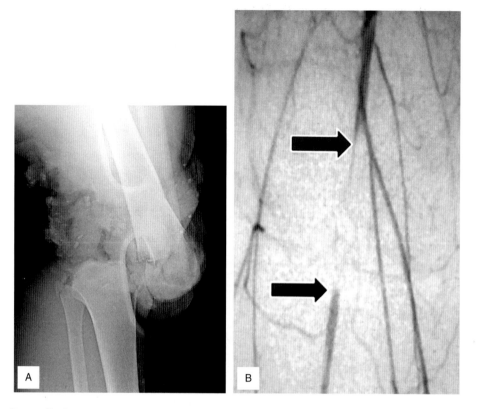

Figure 6.44 (A) Radiograph of a posterior knee dislocation and distal femur fracture. The patient had no peripheral pulses. (B) Angiogram shows popliteal artery injury.

6.32 Maisonneuve Fracture Complex

The Maisonneuve fracture complex represents 5–7% of all ankle fractures and can be easily missed if the treating physician is not familiar with this injury pattern. The mechanism typically involves external rotation of the inverted or adducted foot. The complex includes a combination of proximal oblique fibular fracture, disruption of the tibiofibular ligament distally, and a medial malleolar fracture or deltoid ligament tear. In addition, the interosseous membrane may be torn.

Typically the patient has severe ankle pain but with pain also through the entire lower leg. Careful examination reveals medial malleolar tenderness, and this fracture complex underscores the importance of noting coexistent tenderness at the proximal fibula. Plain radiographs reveal a medial malleolar fracture or widening of the medial mortise with an oblique proximal fibular fracture. Treatment is directed toward restoring integrity of the ankle mortise. Although some patients are treated conservatively with casting, most patients need operative repair.

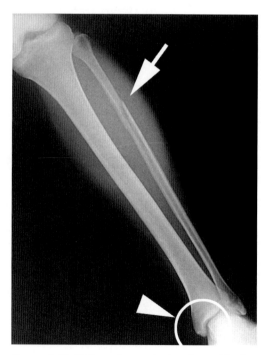

Figure 6.45 Plain radiograph showing widening of the medial ankle joint and a proximal fibular fracture.

6.33 Ankle Dislocation

Ankle joint dislocations are often secondary to sudden rotational forces, such as from sports injuries, falls, and motor vehicle accidents. Dislocations of the ankle are described according to the direction of displacement of the talus and foot in relation to the tibia and are most commonly lateral, although medial, posterior, and anterior dislocations are also seen. Dislocation without fracture is rare.

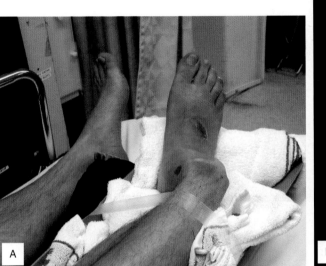

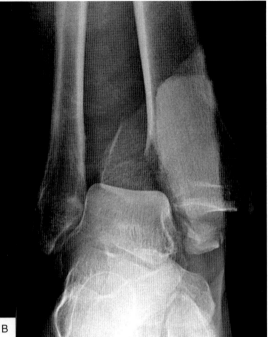

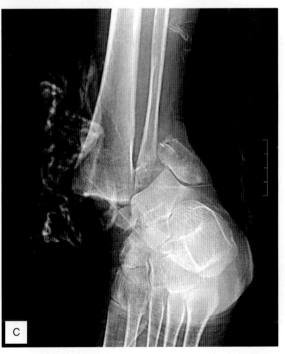

Figure 6.46 (A) Photograph of a medial ankle dislocation in a patient injured in a motor vehicle accident. (B) Radiograph of a medial ankle dislocation with distal tibia fracture. (C) Radiograph of lateral ankle dislocation with bimalleolar fracture.

Neurovascular status should be checked, although most often this remains intact. Reduction is relatively straightforward and accomplished by flexing the knee to 90 degrees, stabilizing the lower leg, plantar flexing the foot, and pulling forward and reversing the direction of the dislocation. Gross ligamentous disruption with or without fracture is consistently present, and thus surgical stabilization is necessary in this injury.

6.34 Subtalar Dislocation

Subtalar or peritalar dislocation requires the disruption of both the talocalcaneal and talonavicular joints without affecting the tibiotalar joint. This uncommon injury is usually the result of severe torsional forces, such as in falls or motor vehicle crashes. Dislocations can be anterior or posterior, although medial and

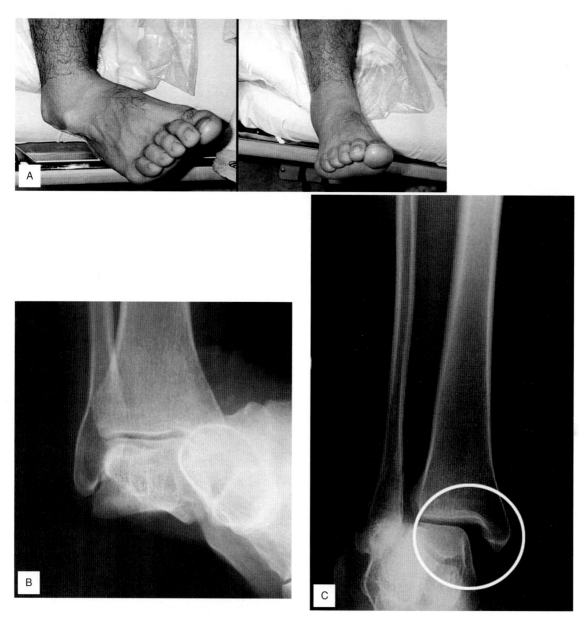

Figure 6.47 (A) Photograph of a medial subtalar dislocation (left) and post reduction (right). (B) Radiograph of a medial subtalar dislocation. (C) Radiograph of a widened ankle mortise signifying disruption of the deltoid ligament.

lateral are the most common. Obvious deformity is present, and the anteroposterior radiograph can be used to confirm the diagnosis.

Reduction should not be delayed and can usually be accomplished by in-line traction and reversal of the deformity. Most cases are managed conservatively with a below-knee cast with good results, although chronic limitation of motion at the subtalar joint may affect the gait.

6.35 Lisfranc Fracture

The tarsometatarsal joints are commonly called the Lisfranc joints, and dislocation or fracture/dislocation injury to this area is termed Lisfranc injury. The joint consists of articulations between the bases of the first three metatarsals and their respective cuneiforms and the fourth and fifth metatarsal with the cuboid. These joints are normally held in place by strong ligaments, and thus this injury is most commonly seen with high-energy mechanisms such as motor vehicle accidents.

Because of the strong ligamentous attachments, associated fractures of the metatarsals are often seen. Usually the injury to the foot is clinically evident,

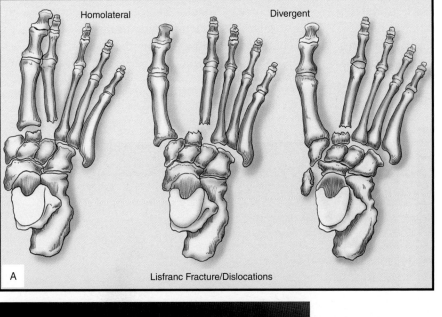

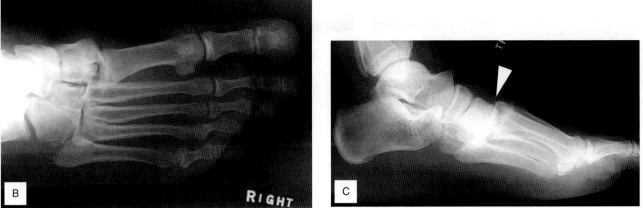

Figure 6.48 (A) Illustration of types of tarsometatarsal dislocations. (B) Homolateral tarsometatarsal dislocation seen on the anteroposterior foot x-ray. (C) Plain radiograph of divergent Lisfranc dislocation.

with significant swelling and tenderness of the forefoot. Occasional vascular injury may occur in a branch of the dorsalis pedis artery, which forms the plantar arch. Radiographically, the fracture dislocation may be grossly evident or quite subtle. The first four metatarsals should align with their respective tarsal articulations along the medial edges. Disruption in this area or widening around the bases of the first three metatarsals is suggestive of an injury. Therapy of Lisfranc fractures usually involves closed reduction with internal fixation using percutaneous Kirschner wires and casting.

6.36 Metatarsal Base Fractures

When assessing fractures at the base of the fifth metatarsal, it is important to distinguish isolated tuberosity fractures from diaphyseal fractures, as the treatment and incidence of complications varies significantly. Avulsion fractures usually occur with sudden inversion of the plantar flexed foot. The insertion of the peroneus brevis has been implicated in these fractures by causing avulsion of the styloid process. Fortunately, these fractures usually heal well without complication. Treatment of these isolated tuberosity fractures ("dancer's fractures") will be determined by the degree of pain and discomfort present, as these fractures may be treated with a compressive dressing, stiff shoe, or a short walking cast.

Diaphyseal fractures usually occur with running or jumping injuries, and transverse fractures within 15 mm of the proximal bone are often termed Jones fractures. Undisplaced fractures of this type are usually treated with non-weight-bearing casting for 6–8 weeks but may require longer immobilization or surgery. Displaced fractures are usually treated operatively. Complications of this diaphyseal fracture are common and include delayed union, nonunion, and recurrent fracture.

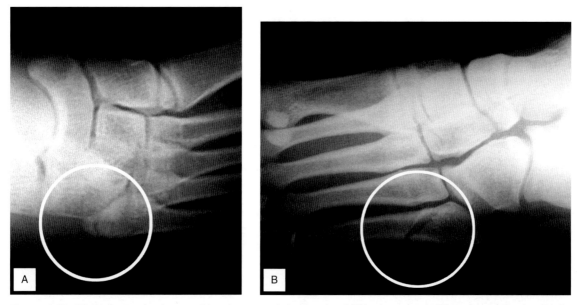

Figure 6.49 (A) Radiograph of an avulsion fracture of the proximal fifth metatarsal. (B) Radiograph of a diaphyseal fracture of the proximal fifth metatarsal.

6.37 Calcaneal Fractures

The calcaneus is the largest bone in the foot and requires high energy such as a major fall for fracture to occur. Associated injuries are also common and are important to detect. These include bilateral calcaneal injuries, lower leg injury, and vertebral fractures. Typically, significant pain and deformity around the heel is noted, and weight-bearing is impossible. Compartment syndrome can complicate this injury and must be considered.

Standard radiograph views include a lateral anteroposterior view shooting down the foot and an axial

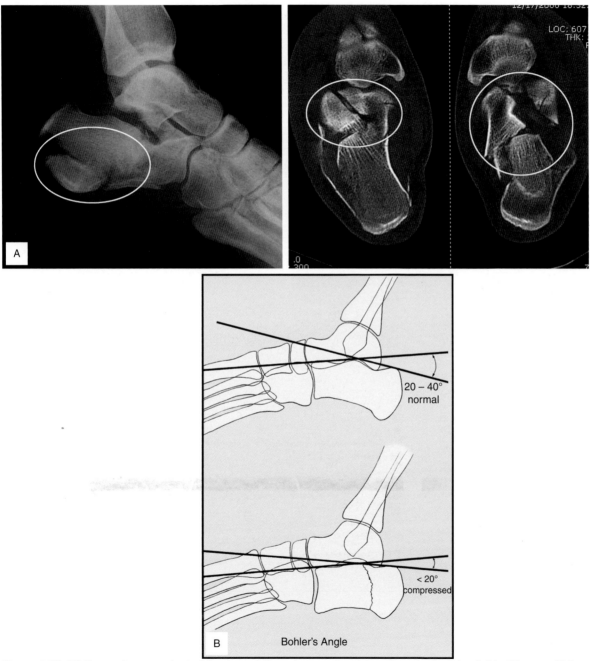

Figure 6.50 (A) X-ray of a comminuted fracture of the calcaneus involving the subtalar joint (left). CT scan of bilateral calcaneal fractures (right). (B) Illustration of Bohler's angle. This angle is seen on the lateral view and is the angle between lines connecting the three highest points of the calcaneus.

calcaneal view down the posterior half of the calcaneus (Harris view).

Comminution is commonly seen, as the bone is cancellous in nature. For examining the radiographs, Bohler's angle can assist in determining if compression has also occurred. This angle is normally 20–40 degrees, and loss of this angle suggests compression of the calcaneus. However, Bohler's angle is not always abnormal, even with comminuted calcaneal fractures, and it is more useful in determining prognosis than in diagnosis. In addition, subtalar joint involvement is important to recognize, as many of these patients are treated operatively. In contrast, nondisplaced extra-articular fractures will often be treated with casting for 6–8 weeks. Despite optimal therapy, chronic pain and joint dysfunction is seen in 50% of patients.

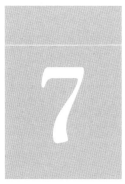

Spinal Injuries

Mark J. Spoonamore and Demetrios Demetriades

Introduction

One of the most devastating consequences of trauma is spinal cord injury. In the United States, approximately 10,000 spinal cord injuries yearly result in permanent disability. In the United States most spinal cord injuries are caused by motor vehicle accidents (40%), violence (30%), falls (20%), and sports accidents (6%). Although spinal fractures can occur in any age group, the peak incidence is in males from ages 18 to 25. Certain conditions predispose to spinal fracture or dislocation: old age, rheumatoid arthritis, osteoporosis, and spinal stenosis. Even relatively minor mechanisms can result in spinal fracture in these groups. Forces that injure the spinal column include flexion, extension, axial loading, shear force, and rotational acceleration.

About 90% of all spinal injuries due to blunt trauma are located at C-5–C-6, T-11–L-1, and T-4–T-6. The type and site of spine injuries depend on the mechanism of injury and the age of the victims. Motorcycle injuries usually cause thoracic spine trauma. High-level falls are associated with spinal trauma in about 24% of cases and usually involve the lower thoracic and lumbar spine.

Cervical spine injuries pose a special challenge because of the potential catastrophic consequences of any associated cord injury. The overall incidence of cervical spine injuries in blunt trauma is about 3% and increases with age. In the presence of severe head trauma the incidence of cervical spine trauma increases to about 9%. Very young or very old patients are more likely to suffer injuries of the upper cervical spine than younger adults who are more likely to have lower cervical injuries. In about 85% of blunt cervical spine injuries there is a fracture, in about 10% there is subluxation without fractures, and in about 4% there is isolated cord injury without fracture or dislocation.

Very young or very old patients are more likely to suffer cord injuries without skeletal trauma than young adults.

Clinical Examination

All trauma victims must be thoroughly evaluated for the possibility of a spinal injury. Blunt trauma patients should have the spine immobilized at first medical contact and remain in spinal immobilization until the integrity of the cord and spinal column can be verified. In patients with multiple severe injuries, the spinal clearance can be deferred until more critical injuries have been addressed, provided that immobilization of the spine and adequate precautions are maintained.

Patients with spinal fractures experience pain, and examination will reveal spinal tenderness on palpation and ecchymosis on inspection. Patients may also demonstrate a spinal deformity or step-off. However, patients who are unable to report pain because of concomitant head injury or intoxication may harbor occult spinal injuries and should remain immobilized until they can be accurately evaluated. Patients with spinal cord injury manifest symptoms according to the spinal cord level affected. With complete cord transection, all motor and sensory function below the level of the lesion is lost. The highest intact sensory level should be marked on the patient to determine whether the cord lesion is progressing proximally on subsequent examinations. A careful motor examination should corroborate the level of the cord lesion. Assessment of rectal tone and perianal sensation is important in detecting any sparing of lower cord segments which significantly improves the prognosis. Spinal shock is common in the immediate period after injury and consists of loss of all spinal reflexes and flaccid paralysis below the level of the lesion. During this phase the bulbocavernosus reflex (anal sphincter contraction with stimulation of the glans or urethra) is absent. In many cases, no definitive prognostication regarding the severity or level of the spinal cord lesion can be made while spinal shock is present. Once the bulbocavernosus reflex returns, spinal shock is resolved, reflexes become spastic, and the lesion is complete. Priapism is common in males after complete cord transection but resolves quickly in most cases.

Neurogenic shock is the hemodynamic effect of sympathetic denervation that results in vasodilation and hypotension. In high cervical cord injuries the hypotension is associated with severe bradycardia, because of disruption of the sympathetic innervation to the heart. Regardless of the presence of neurogenic shock, hypotension must be assumed to be due to hemorrhage and a diligent search for sources of blood loss must be made.

Incomplete cord syndromes may present with a confusing pattern of neurologic deficits. In central cord syndrome, the hands and arms sustain a much denser bilateral paralysis than the lower extremities. In Brown-Séquard syndrome, pain and temperature sensory loss occurs contralaterally, whereas motor loss and all other sensory loss are ipsilateral. With anterior spinal cord syndrome, there is preservation of posterior column function (position and vibration sense) bilaterally, but all other functions are lost. The syndrome of spinal cord injury without radiographic abnormality (SCIWORA) can occur in any age group but is particularly common in children. Neurologic deficits may be delayed many hours, and by definition, radiographs are normal. Consequently, it is difficult to make this diagnosis on initial evaluation. Patients who report persistent paresthesias should undergo computed tomography (CT) scan or magnetic resonance imaging (MRI) investigations.

Investigations

Trauma patients requiring cervical spine clearance can be classified into one of three categories: asymptomatic, symptomatic, or nonevaluable (obtunded/comatose).

Patients who are fully alert, not intoxicated, have no significant distracting injuries, and who are asymptomatic (no neurological symptoms, no neck pain) can be cleared safely based on clinical examination alone without imaging studies.

Trauma patients who present with neck pain, tenderness, spinal deformity, and/or neurologic symptoms or dysfunction require radiographic imaging. The standard radiological evaluation in a multiple trauma patient used to include a cervical spine series (anteroposterior, lateral, open mouth view). This approach has largely been replaced by routine CT scan evaluation. Most centers now utilize a multidetector CT scanner (MDCT) to rule out a cervical spine injury. A cervical CT scan with coronal and axial reconstructions has a sensitivity of 99% of detecting a cervical spine fracture or instability. This modality can also be rapidly accomplished as an extension of a primary CT of other body regions (head, thorax, abdomen, pelvis, etc.). Patients presenting with neurologic deficits and/or suspected ligamentous injuries should also be evaluated with a cervical MRI scan. The MRI can also provide accurate visualization of any cord lesion. Symptomatic trauma patients with suspected ligamentous injury may be evaluated with cervical flexion–extension radiographs. This investigation is rarely performed because of the superiority and safety of MRI. Flexion–extension radiological evaluation should be performed only in selected awake and alert patients, under the supervision of a physician.

The clearance of the cervical spine in obtunded and comatose trauma patients remains controversial. These patients should be evaluated with MDCT of the cervical spine. There is a less than 1% risk of a trauma patient having a purely ligamentous cervical spine injury that is not identified on MDCT. Some centers practice cervical spine clearance on the basis of normal MDCT. Others are more cautious and perform cervical spine MRI scan on all unevaluable patients with a normal CT scan. This is a controversial approach, and may be impractical and potentially risky to transfer a severe multitrauma patient for MRI scan. Many serious complications occur during transportation of the critically injured patients. In addition, although cervical MRI is very sensitive at detecting ligamentous injury, it has a lower predictive value and specificity, and may be over-read and lead to a high rate of false-positive findings that could potentially lead to unnecessary interventions. The use of dynamic flexion–extension radiographs or upright cervical radiographs in ruling out ligamentous injuries in obtunded trauma patients has not been clinically validated, and may be harmful.

Table 7.1 Clinical evaluation of the cervical spine

Asymptomatic
Awake/alert
No neck pain/tenderness
Normal neurologic exam
No intoxication or distracting injury
Minor/low-energy trauma
Symptomatic
Awake/alert
Neck pain/tenderness
Abnormal neurologic exam
Distracting injury
Major/high-energy trauma
Unevaluable
Obtunded/comatose
Intoxication
Abnormal cognitive function that interferes with clinical
   examination

Table 7.2 Algorithm for the evaluation of the cervical spine

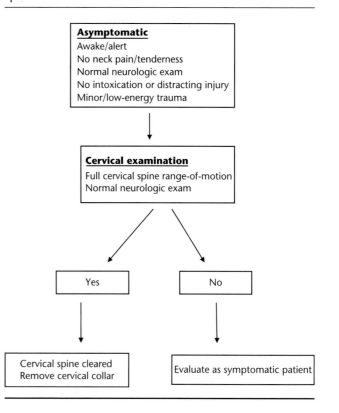

Table 7.3 Algorithm for the evaluation of the cervical spine in symptomatic patients

Table 7.4 Algorithm for the evaluation of the cervical spine in clinically unevaluable patients

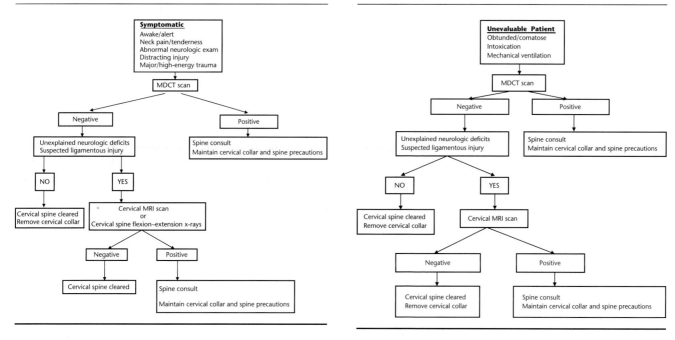

General Management

As with severe head injury, prevention of secondary injuries is the highest priority. Although cord lesions may progress in spite of proper medical care, avoidance of hypotension, hypoxia, seizure, hypoglycemia, hyponatremia, and mishandling of the patient are essential to avoid unnecessary deterioration.

Airway assessment occurs simultaneously with spinal immobilization. Patients with complete spinal cord injury above the level of C-4 will be apneic, as movement of the diaphragm and all other respiratory muscles is lost. Immediate assisted ventilation is required for the patient to survive, and the best means of accomplishing this is by endotracheal intubation and mechanical ventilation. In the past, concerns were expressed regarding the use of orotracheal intubation for fear that manipulation of the airway with a laryngoscope would cause movement of unstable spinal fractures and result in spinal cord injury. With the use of manual in-line stabilization by an assistant, orotracheal "rapid sequence intubation" using paralytic drugs has been shown to be safe. Alternatively, fiberoptic intubation should be considered in the appropriate cases.

Neurogenic shock usually responds to fluid administration, but pressor agents may be required to avoid hypotension and resultant hypoperfusion of the injured spinal cord. Severe bradycardia responds well to atropine administration. Patients with high spinal cord injury lose heat easily because of the peripheral vasodilation, and warming devices should be used to avoid hypothermia.

Once spinal cord injury is identified, administration of high-dose methylprednisolone may be considered, based on the National Acute Spinal Cord Injury Study (NASCIS) which demonstrated improved recovery in patients receiving steroids within 8 hours of injury. Methylprednisolone intravenously with a 30 mg/kg initial bolus followed by 5.4 mg/kg per hour for 24–48 hours is the recommended regimen. Administration of steroids beginning more than 8 hours after injury results in worse outcome and is not recommended. The therapeutic role of routine steroid administration in blunt spinal cord trauma is currently a controversial issue and many centers do not support their use. For medicolegal purposes it is recommended that each center has its own written protocol regarding the use of steroids in these patients. Steroids have not been studied in children or in penetrating injuries, and no recommendations regarding high-dose steroids can be made in these cases.

A Foley catheter should be placed as soon as the primary survey is completed. Nasogastric decompression is indicated if ileus develops.

Emergency surgical decompression of the cord and spinal fixation should be performed in patients with incomplete cord injuries, especially in cases with deteriorating neurological examination, and in the presence of significant epidural or subdural hematomas. The role of emergency spinal operation in complete cord transections is questionable and most neurosurgeons or spinal surgeons do not support it. However, an elective spinal fixation should be considered as early as possible in unstable fractures or dislocations in order to facilitate rehabilitation.

Common Mistakes and Pitfalls

1. Failure to assess the spine clinically or radiographically in high-risk patients who present with even relatively minor mechanisms of injury. Elderly patients who present with low-speed vehicular accidents or ground-level falls can suffer fractures because of their brittle or osteoporotic spines. A low threshold for obtaining radiographs or CT scan should be maintained in trauma involving high-risk patients.
2. Failure to intubate patients with fairly high cervical cord injury (above C-5) and quadriplegia, soon after admission. These patients often decompensate and develop severe respiratory failure a few hours after admission, requiring emergency intubation under suboptimal conditions, resulting in preventable morbidity.
3. Failure to recognize partial cord syndromes. In some series, the vast majority of patients with central cord syndrome were initially misdiagnosed because they were intoxicated or because they were thought to be malingering or have conversion disorder. Paralysis of both upper extremities without simultaneous paralysis of the lower extremities was thought by these clinicians to be anatomically impossible because they were unaware of the presentation of the central cord syndrome.
4. Mishandling of the patient with spinal fracture. Some patients who develop neurologic deficits do so after contact with medical personnel. Although some of these deficits would occur due to progressive edema or ischemia, others may be the result of inadequate care and poor spinal

immobilization during transfer of the patient from stretcher to x-ray table or CT scanner.

5. Intoxicated or head-injured patients should have spinal precautions maintained until they can reliably be evaluated by CT scan or clinical examination. Patients who report any symptoms require further investigation with CT scan or MRI, even if plain radiographs are normal.

6. There is often confusion between *spinal shock* (loss of reflexes and motor/sensory function for up to 24 hours after injury) and *neurogenic shock* (hemodynamic effects of sympathectomy due to high spinal cord lesions manifesting as hypotension with or without bradycardia, depending on the level of the cord injury). These terms are not interchangeable and should be used correctly to avoid miscommunication.

7. The inexperienced physician may incorrectly record normal or reduced rectal tone in the presence of a complete cord transection. This documentation may result in medicolegal complications because it can be claimed that a partial cord injury was allowed to progress to complete injury. If not sure, the physician should record "rectal tone difficult to evaluate."

8. The inexperienced healthcare provider may mistake reflexive minor extremity movements in complete cord injury as active movements. Such documentation may give the impression of partial cord injury and raises the expectations of the family. Only voluntary movements count!

9. Chance fracture of the lumbar spine is frequently associated with a small-intestinal injury that may be initially occult.

10. Patients who present with calcaneal fracture(s) after jumping from a height should be screened for coexistent lumbar compression fractures because these fractures are commonly associated.

11. Approximately 10% of spinal fractures are associated with another noncontiguous spine fracture, thus the finding of any spinal fracture should initiate a search for other fractures elsewhere in the spine.

Spinal Cord Injuries

7.1 Complete Spinal Cord Transection

Complete transection of the spinal cord is a devastating injury. Transection above the level of C-4 results in acute respiratory failure as the nerve supply to both the diaphragm (C-3–5) and intercostal muscles (T-1–12) is lost. Such patients frequently expire in the field unless immediate ventilation is provided.

At more distal levels, acute spinal cord transection results in complete flaccid motor paralysis and anesthesia below the level of the injury. Deep tendon reflexes are absent distal to the lesion. Examination will reveal urinary retention and diminished or absent rectal sphincter tone. In males, transient priapism is very common and indicates complete cord transection although it often resolves by the time the patient arrives in the emergency department (ED).

Loss of sympathetic innervation results in loss of vasomotor tone and hypotension. In cervical cord injuries, loss of sympathetic innervation to the heart prevents the normal response of reflex tachycardia. Consequently, the hemodynamic picture of hypotension, inappropriate bradycardia, and warm, flushed skin constitutes the classic syndrome of neurogenic shock secondary to high cord transection. Transection of the upper thoracic cord usually results in hypotension associated with tachycardia. Inability to vasoconstrict also prevents the normal response to cold stress, and these patients are at risk for hypothermia. Treatment is initially directed at restoring intravascular volume and ensuring that hypotension is not due to occult blood loss. If volume infusion does not restore adequate blood pressure, pressor agents such as dopamine are indicated to improve perfusion and consequently the survival of the spinal cord proximal to the transection.

During the acute phase of spinal cord injury, all distal reflexes are absent, and the patient is said to be in "spinal shock" (not to be confused with neurogenic shock with its hemodynamic manifestations). To confirm that all reflexes are absent, the most distal reflex arc or bulbocavernosus reflex is examined. Stimulation of the glans or clitoris or tugging on a Foley catheter normally produces a reflex anal sphincter contraction. During spinal shock, no response will occur. During this phase, it is possible that spinal cord dysfunction is due to concussion or contusion of the cord, and dramatic recovery of function can occur. Over the ensuing 24–48 hours, spastic reflexes that are typical of an established spinal cord injury begin to appear. The first such reflex to return is the bulbocavernosus reflex. Once this reflex reappears, the period of spinal shock has ended, and significant recovery is unlikely. Sparing of sensation in the perianal area should be elicited, as this represents a positive prognostic sign of potential recovery of spinal function.

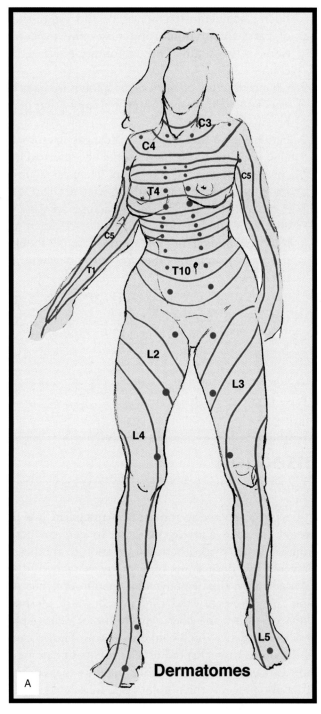

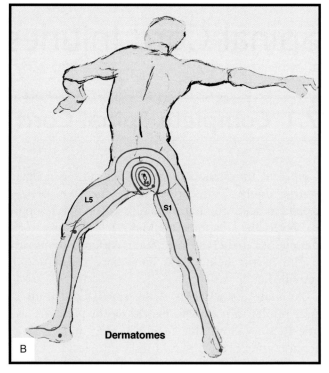

Figure 7.1 (A) Illustration showing anterior dermatomes. (B) Illustration showing posterior dermatomes. (C) Illustration of the bulbocavernosus reflex arc. Stimulation of the glans or the urethra causes contraction of the anal sphincter. (D) Photograph showing priapism in a child with complete transaction of the spinal cord. The presence of priapism is a bad prognostic sign. (E) Autopsy photograph of severe distraction of the spinal column and extrusion of the spinal cord.

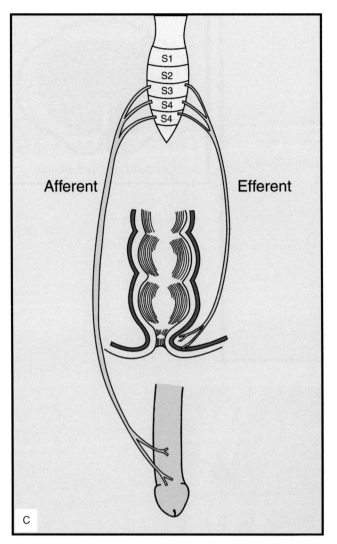

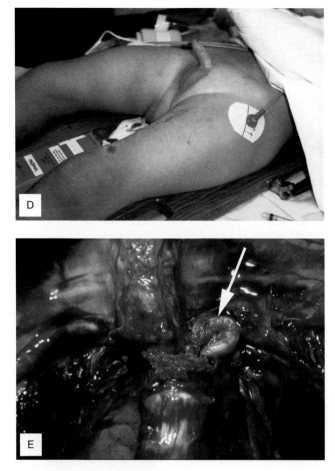

Figure 7.1 (*cont.*)

7.2 Central Cord Syndrome

Central cord syndrome represents 3% of all cervical spine injuries and occurs mainly in older patients with osteoarthritic changes of the cervical vertebrae. It typically results from hyperextension of the neck with resultant inward buckling of the ligamentum flavum. This produces compression of the central portion of the cord, with subsequent edema and variable amounts of hemorrhage. Because of the stereotopic organization of the lateral corticospinal tract, the hands (lying closest to the center of the cord) are

more affected than the arms, which in turn are more affected than the lower extremities. Clinically the syndrome consists of motor weakness that is most profound in the hands and arms, patchy sensory deficits, and variable dysfunction of bowel and bladder. Plain radiographs of the cervical spine are often normal because the condition may occur without a fracture or dislocation. CT scan may reveal central cord edema, but MRI is the most sensitive imaging modality in diagnosing this condition.

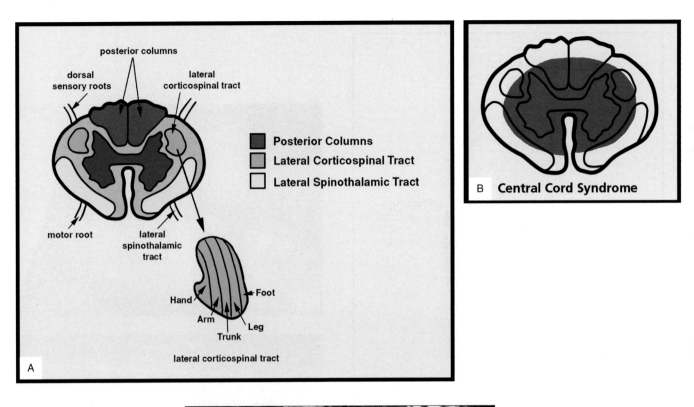

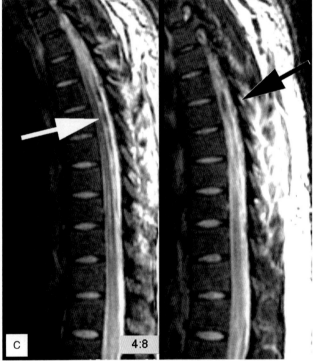

Figure 7.2 (A) Illustration of the cross-section of cervical spinal cord showing ascending sensory and descending motor tracts and stereotypic organization of the lateral corticospinal tract. (B) Illustration of cross-section of cervical spinal cord. The red area shows section of the spinal cord affected in central cord syndrome. (C) T2-weighted cervicothoracic MRI showing hemorrhagic contusion of the central cervical cord (black arrow) and edema of the adjacent spinal cord (white arrow).

Because of the apparent incongruity of the clinical presentation, the condition is often misdiagnosed initially in the ED, especially if the patient is concurrently intoxicated. Misdiagnosis of the condition as "malingering" or "conversion disorder" is common.

Treatment is immobilization of the neck and administration of high-dose corticosteroids. Surgical decompression may be indicated if there is significant spinal stenosis or instability. Recovery of bowel and bladder function and ambulation is the rule, although recovery of full manual dexterity is rare.

7.3 Brown-Séquard Syndrome

Brown-Séquard syndrome is due to an incomplete transection or hemisection of the spinal cord, usually caused by penetrating trauma. It consists of a characteristic constellation of findings with loss of pain and temperature contralateral to the side of the injury and

loss of motor function (corticospinal tract), light touch (spinothalamic tract), position, and vibration sensation (posterior columns) ipsilateral to the injury. Although true Brown-Séquard injury is due to an exact hemisection of the spinal cord, the clinical findings may vary if more or less of the cord is transected.

As with other penetrating injuries, the use of high doses of corticosteroids has not been found to be beneficial in prospective series, although it is still sometimes used in individual cases. Broad-spectrum antibiotic coverage is indicated, and surgical debridement may be required. Impaled objects should always be removed in the operating room. Functional recovery is often surprisingly good in spite of the permanent cord lesions.

Table 7.5 Neurologic deficits distal to site of hemisection of spinal cord in Brown-Séquard syndrome

Light touch	Ipsilateral
Position/vibration	Ipsilateral
Motor function	Ipsilateral
Pain sensation	Contralateral
Temperature sensation	Contralateral

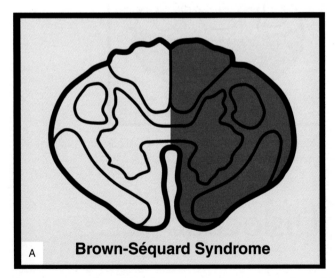

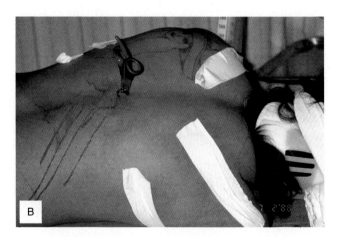

Figure 7.3 (A) Illustration showing spinal cord tracts affected in Brown-Séquard syndrome (red area). (B) Photograph of a patient with scissors embedded in the mid-thoracic spine who manifested classic Brown-Séquard syndrome. (C) CT scan of the cervical spine showing a gunshot wound (black arrow) with bone fragments impinging on the lateral spinal cord (white arrow), resulting in a Brown-Séquard type lesion.

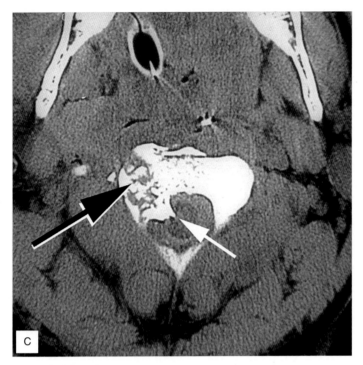

Figure 7.3 (*cont.*)

7.4 Anterior Cord Syndrome

Anterior cord syndrome results from damage to the anterior spinal artery, producing infarction of the anterior spinal tracts, or by direct laceration of the anterior part of the cord by retropulsed bony fragments. Posterior column function (position and vibration sense) is preserved. Clinically, there is bilateral loss of motor function, light touch, pain, and temperature sensation below the level of the injury.

Anterior cord syndrome is usually seen in elderly patients in conjunction with medical conditions, particularly arterial embolization from the heart. However, it may also result from prolonged cross clamping of the aorta, prolonged hypotension, or direct injury from bone fragments or foreign bodies.

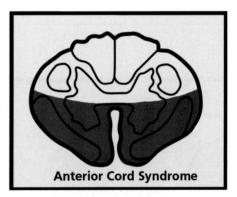

Figure 7.4 Schematic drawing of spinal cord tracts affected in anterior cord syndrome.

Upper Cervical Spine Dislocations

There are multiple strong ligamentous attachments from the cervical spine to the base of the skull. These include the anterior and posterior longitudinal ligaments, the anterior and posterior atlanto-occipital membranes, the apical ligament from the odontoid, and the capsular ligaments of the atlanto-occipital joint.

Separation of the cervical spine from the base of the skull is almost invariably fatal at the scene of the trauma. Fatalities occur from disruption of the spinal cord above the level of C-4 which results in complete paralysis of respiratory effort and asphyxial death or from injury to the brainstem or vertebral arteries. In patients who survive to reach a hospital, mortality is high due to brainstem injury, associated head and systemic trauma, and prolonged coma with its attendant complications. Nevertheless, survivors have been reported, and a full resuscitative effort should be made.

7.5 Atlanto-Occipital Dislocation

Atlanto-occipital dislocation occurs from the application of massive shearing force to the head in an anteroposterior direction as seen in high-speed motor vehicle crashes. The injury is primarily ligamentous, although associated fractures of the face and skull are common.

There are several radiologic methods of detecting subluxation or dislocation of the atlanto-occipital joint, although the ratio of Powers is the most commonly used and is described as follows:

The length of the line BC is compared to the length of line OA (see Figure 7.5D):

Normal :   BC/OA = 0.77
Upper limit of normal :   BC/OA = 1.0
Abnormal :   BC/OA > 1.0

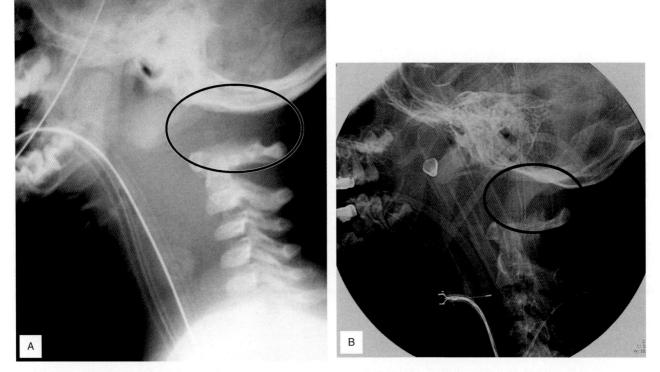

Figure 7.5 (A–B) Lateral radiographs of the cervical spine in young children showing severe atlanto-occipital dislocation and massive soft tissue swelling anterior to the spinal column.

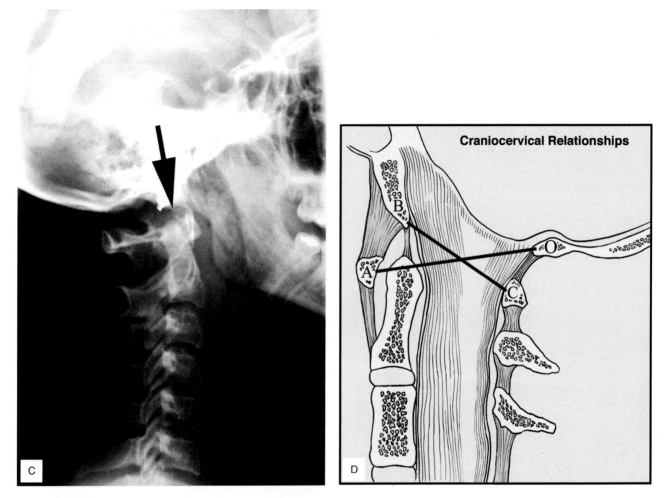

Figure 7.5 (*cont.*) (C) Lateral radiograph of the cervical spine in an adult showing a subtler atlanto-occipital dislocation (arrow) with significant soft tissue swelling anterior to the spinal column. (D) Schematic drawing illustrating the measurements used in calculating the "ratio of Powers" to detect atlanto-occipital dislocation.

7.6 Atlantoaxial Dislocation

Atlantoaxial dislocation is a rare injury of unclear mechanism. There is disruption of the transverse and alar ligaments that connect the odontoid process to the ring of C-1, which displaces superiorly (see Figure 7.9A). Neurologic deficits are uncommon with superior dislocation (as shown) or when associated with fracture of the odontoid, although the condition is unstable due to disruption of the ligaments. Anterior dislocation is usually fatal as the spinal cord is compressed against the intact odontoid.

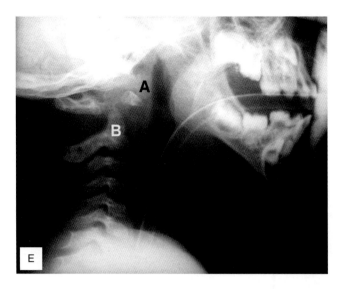

Figure 7.5 (*cont.*) (E) Lateral radiograph of the cervical spine in a child showing atlantoaxial disclocation. The ring of C-1 (A) is seen lying completely above the tip of the odontoid process (B).

7.7 Rotatory Subluxation of C-1 on C-2

Another form of ligamentous injury in this area is rotatory subluxation of C-1 on C-2 which results from torsional forces applied to the head and neck. Neurologic deficits are rare because the space for the spinal cord is not encroached upon.

The plain radiographic appearance of this injury is subtle and may be confused with a burst fracture of C-1. In the case of rotatory subluxation, one lateral mass rotates anteriorly and the other posteriorly. The anteriorly subluxed lateral mass appears larger and

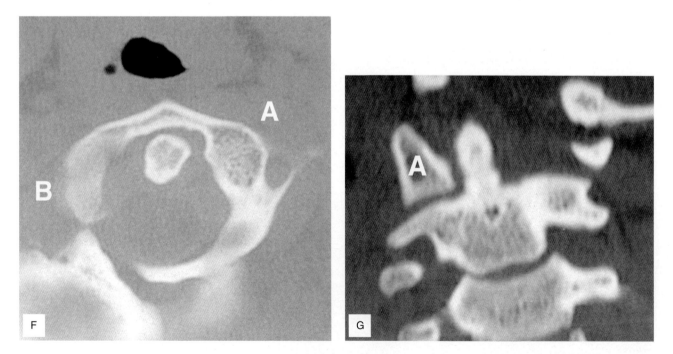

Figure 7.5 (*cont.*) (F) CT scan of C-1 and C-2 showing the left lateral mass of C-1 (A) rotated anteriorly and the right lateral mass (B) rotated posteriorly. On a plain radiograph anteroposterior view, the left lateral mass will appear larger (because it is farther from the x-ray film) and closer to the odontoid because of the rotation. Conversely, the right lateral mass will appear smaller and farther from the odontoid process. (G) CT scan of C-1 and C-2 in the anteroposterior orientation. The right lateral mass is seen clearly but the left lateral mass of C-1 has rotated posteriorly out of view.

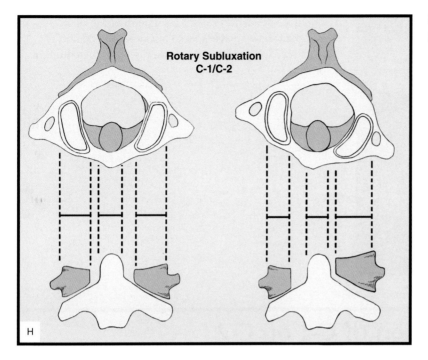

Figure 7.5 (*cont.*) (H) Schematic drawing of rotator subluxation of C-1 on C-2.

closer to the odontoid process, whereas the other lateral mass appears smaller and farther from the odontoid. On the plain radiographic open-mouth odontoid view, the distance from the odontoid to the lateral mass is increased on one side and decreased on the other, in contrast to a burst fracture of C-1, in which both lateral masses are displaced laterally. In burst fractures that occur on only one side of the ring of C-1, that lateral mass will be displaced laterally, whereas the unaffected side will show a normal relationship of the lateral mass of C-1 to the articular plate of C-2.

7.8 Ligamentous Injuries

Flexion and extension views of the C-spine are supplementary radiographs that are indicated in patients with increased soft tissue swelling anterior to the vertebral bodies or suspicion of misalignment on the lateral C-spine film. They are contraindicated in patients with apparent neurologic injury or in those whose diagnosis is clear.

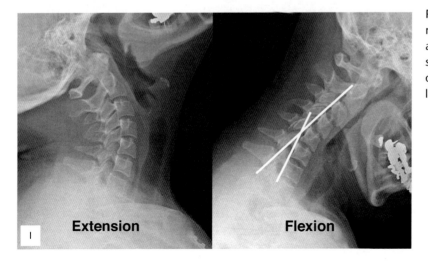

Extension **Flexion**

Figure 7.5 (*cont.*) (I) Flexion–extension lateral radiographic series. The extension view appears normal, but the flexion view shows significant angulation and anterior subluxation of C-4 on C-5, indicating posterior ligamentous disruption.

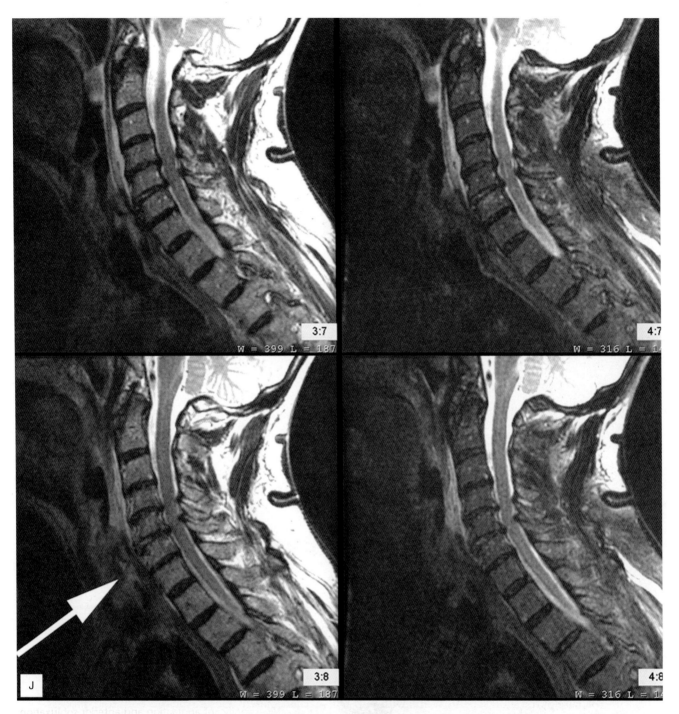

Figure 7.5 (*cont.*) (J) T2-weighted MRI showing ligamentous injury and soft tissue edema to the vertebral bodies of C-5 through C-7. (K) Lateral radiograph showing C-4 on C-5 subluxation.

The patient must be awake and able to cooperate. He or she should be instructed to actively flex and then extend the neck up to the point of experiencing pain and no further. At the point of maximal voluntary flexion and extension, a lateral radiograph is obtained. The patient's neck should never be passively flexed or extended by the physician during this examination.

Positive findings are increased subluxation of the vertebrae in either flexion (posterior ligaments disrupted) or extension (anterior ligaments disrupted). CT scan is relatively insensitive in detecting ligamentous injuries or misalignment of the spine. MRI may be required to fully delineate the extent of ligamentous injury and in many centers it has become the investigation of choice in these cases.

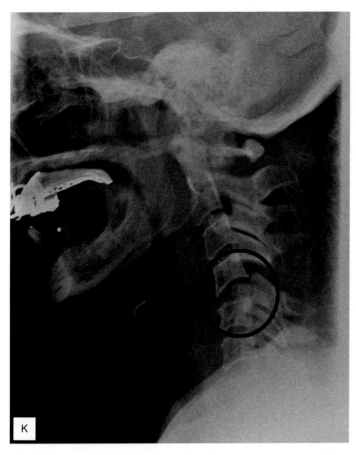

Figure 7.5 (*cont.*)

Cervical Spine Fractures

7.9 C-1 Burst Fracture (Jefferson Fracture)

C-1 or the "atlas" is a ring-shaped vertebra that articulates with the base of the skull superiorly and with C-2 inferiorly. Fractures usually result from axial compression of the head and spinal column (e.g., from diving into a shallow pool or when a passenger's head strikes the inside of the roof of a car in a motor vehicle accident). Because of the angles at which C-1 articulates with the occiput and C-2, the axial force is translated into a lateral force at C-1, causing the fragments to burst outward. Consequently, neurologic deficits are relatively uncommon with C-1 fracture because the space for the spinal cord within the spinal canal is actually increased. A Jefferson fracture is unstable,

however, and must be adequately immobilized. An associated fracture of the odontoid process may occur.

On plain films, the open-mouth view is essential to diagnose C-1 fracture. Although some studies question the utility of including an open-mouth view in the standard initial series of x-rays in trauma patients, it is difficult to reliably diagnose a Jefferson fracture on a single lateral view.

CT scan is very accurate in detecting C-1 fractures and is indicated for any suspicious abnormalities or for inadequate visualization on plain radiographs.

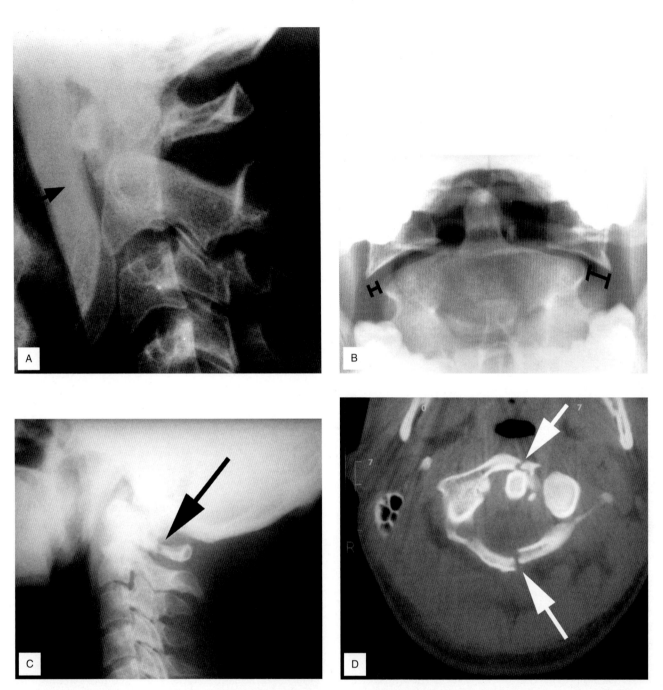

Figure 7.6 (A) Lateral C-spine radiograph showing increased preodontoid space and prevertebral soft tissue swelling suggestive of a C-1 fracture. Normal measurements of the preodontoid space are 3 mm in adults and 5 mm in children. A greater space is allowed in children because the odontoid process is incompletely calcified until adolescence. Normal measurements for the prevertebral space anterior to C-3 are 5 mm in adults and 7 mm in children, due to a higher position of the esophagus in children which increases the prevertebral space. (B) Open-mouth radiograph of C-1 and C-2. Lateral displacement of the articular portion of the ring of CT is the typical finding, as the ring of C-1 generally bursts outward. The distance between the ring and the odontoid process is increased. Displacement of the lateral masses of C-1 on C-2 may be unilateral or bilateral as shown here. (C) Lateral radiograph showing fracture of posterior arch of C-1 (arrow). (D) CT scan of C-1 showing outwardly displaced fracture fragments. Because C-1 is a ring-shaped structure, at least two fracture sites inevitably exist (arrows). CT scan is particularly useful in a child, whose small mouth and inability to cooperate make the open-mouth view difficult to obtain. (E) CT scan of C-1 showing fracture of the anterior arch of C-1.

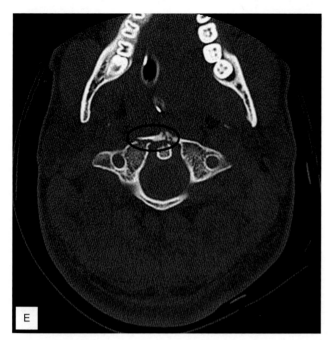

Figure 7.6 (*cont.*)

7.10 Odontoid (Dens) Fractures (C-2)

There are three types of odontoid fracture. Type I odontoid fracture occurs at the tip of the odontoid process, above the level of the alar ligaments. This is a rare fracture, caused by avulsion of the tip of the odontoid by apical ligaments attached to the base of the skull. It is a stable fracture because the alignment of C-1 on C-2 is maintained by the alar and transverse ligaments (see Figure 7.9A). Neurologic deficit is uncommon.

Type II odontoid fracture occurs at the "neck" of the odontoid process, below the level of the transverse ligaments. It usually results from shear forces that cause anterior-to-posterior displacement of the entire C-1–C-2 complex from the body of C-2. It is a highly unstable fracture, more frequently associated with neurologic deficits, and often complicated by nonunion.

Type III odontoid fracture runs through the vertebral body of C-2. It may be comminuted and unstable. There is usually no associated spinal cord injury unless the fracture is significantly displaced or fragments of C-2 are retropulsed into the canal.

Treatment of odontoid fractures begins with immobilization in a halo vest if there is no evidence of neurologic deficit. Operative reduction may be required for fractures with impingement on the spinal cord or for persistent instability due to nonunion of the fracture fragments.

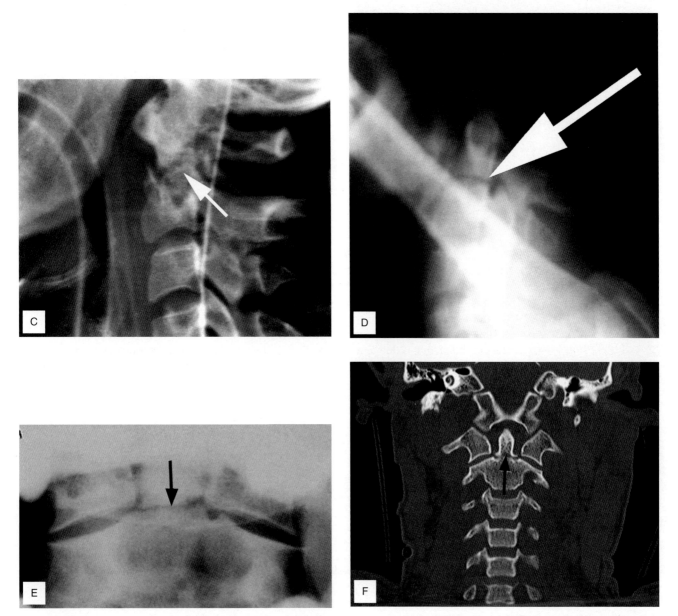

Figure 7.7 (A) Schematic showing the ligamentous attachments of C-1 and C-2. (B) Schematic showing the three types of odontoid fracture. (C) Lateral plain radiograph of type II odontoid fracture. Arrow shows fracture line at the base of the odontoid process. (D) Swimmer's view of the cervical spine showing type II odontoid fracture. (E) Open-mouth radiograph showing type II odontoid fracture. (F) CT scan showing type II odontoid fracture (arrow).

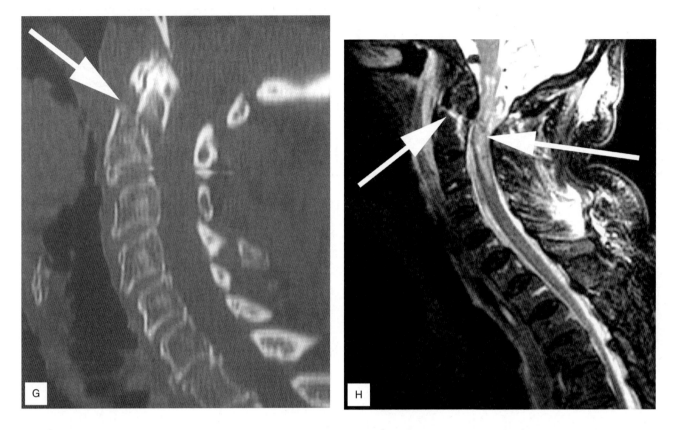

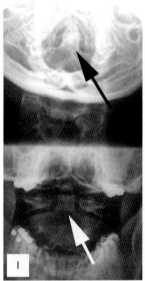

Figure 7.7 (*cont.*) (G) Lateral CT showing displaced type II odontoid fracture (arrow).
(H) T2-weighted MRI of the cervicothoracic spine of an elderly female who fell downstairs and
presented with quadriplegia. MRI shows displaced type II fracture of the odontoid (short arrow)
with injury to the spinal cord from C-1 to C-3 (long arrow). (I) Pseudofracture of the odontoid.
The upper image appears to show a type II odontoid fracture (white arrow), whereas
the lower image (modified open-mouth view) shows a normal odontoid (black arrow).
The pseudofracture is due to a "Mach effect," which is a lucency created by the overlap
of two bones.

7.11 Hangman's Fracture (C-2)

Hangman's fracture is traumatic spondylolisthesis of the pars interarticularis of C-2. In common usage, however, the term is applied to bilateral pedicle fractures of C-2 as well. The fracture results from hyperextension of the neck with compression of the posterior elements of C-2 by the hyperextending occiput. This is the type of injury produced by a judicial hanging, hence the name. Displaced hangman's

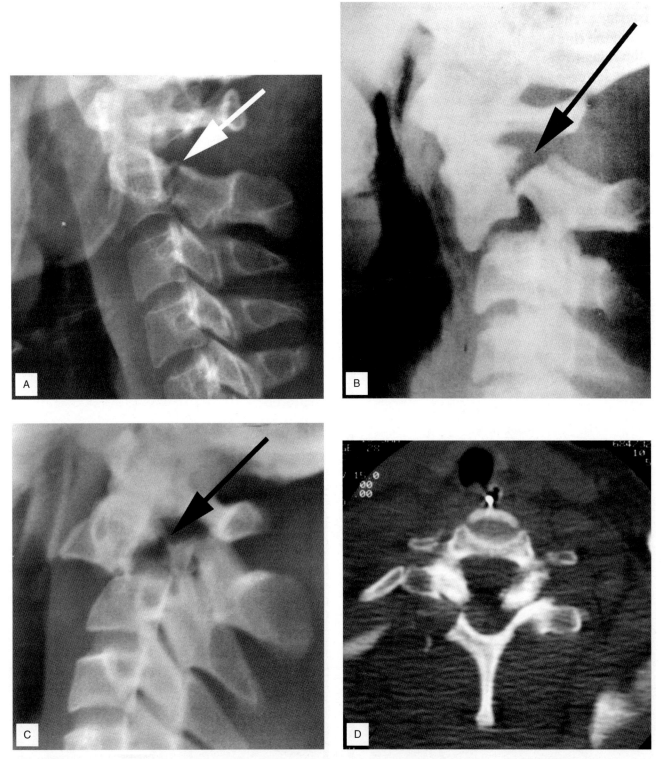

Figure 7.8 (A) Lateral C-spine radiograph showing bilateral pedicle fracture (hangman's fracture) of C-2: undisplaced hangman's fracture. (B) Moderately displaced hangman's fracture. (C) Severely displaced hangman's fracture. (D) CT scan of a hangman's type of fracture, extending through the laminae rather than the pedicles of C-2.

fractures are commonly associated with severe neurologic deficits. Cord lesions at this level result in paralysis of respiratory muscles and therefore apnea, as well as complete paralysis and sensory loss distal to the lesion.

Nevertheless, patients may sustain this injury without any injury to the spinal cord. These patients should be immobilized in a halo vest and often require operative fixation.

7.12 Fractures of the Lower Cervical Spine (C-3–C-7)

Fracture Types

Vertebral body fractures are common and usually occur as a result of hyperflexion. The severity of the fracture ranges from minor to critical, depending on the degree of comminution and displacement of fragments posteriorly into the spinal canal. Unstable fractures require operative fixation and ultimately spinal fusion.

Table 7.6 Classification of vertebral body fractures

Type I	Anterior inferior fragment (flexion or extension "teardrop" fracture)
Type II	Anterior wedge compression fracture
Type III	Fracture of the anterior half of the vertebral body with minimal or no displacement of the fragments posteriorly
Type IV	Comminuted "burst" fracture of the vertebral body with retropulsion of the fragments into the spinal canal

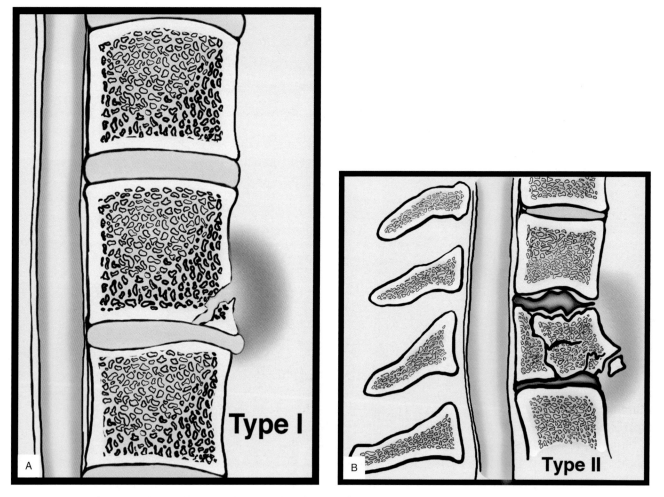

Figure 7.9 (A) Schematic of type I fracture of vertebral body. (B) Schematic of type II fracture of vertebral body. (C) Schematic of type III fracture of vertebral body. (D) Schematic of type IV fracture of vertical body.

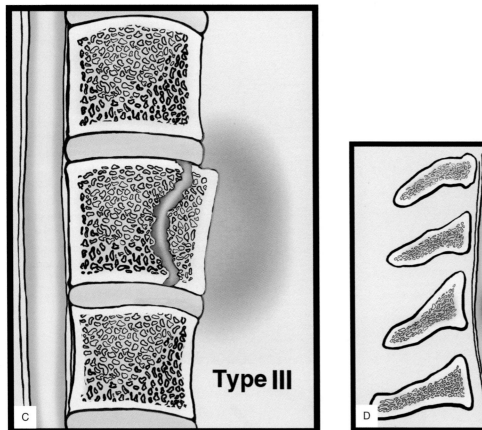

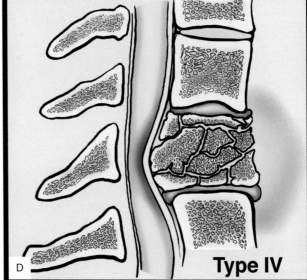

Figure 7.9 (cont.)

7.13 Flexion and Extension Teardrop Fracture

The flexion teardrop fracture is seen as a small triangular fragment at the anterior–inferior border of the vertebral body. Although the flexion teardrop fracture appears radiographically innocuous, it is a highly unstable fracture that is associated with spinal cord injury in up to 50% of cases. The injury is caused by hyperflexion of the neck, resulting in disruption of the posterior ligaments. As the flexion continues, the anterior inferior fragment of a vertebral body is fractured off by contact with the subjacent vertebral body. This disrupts the anterior longitudinal spinal ligament, rendering the cervical spine unstable as both anterior and posterior ligamentous support is disrupted. This fracture occurs most commonly at the C-5 level. Often there is associated slight posterior subluxation of the affected vertebral body or of the vertebral column above it.

The extension teardrop fracture appears radiographically similar to the flexion teardrop in that a small anterior fragment is avulsed from either the inferior or superior aspect of the vertebral body. The anterior longitudinal ligament is stretched during hyperextension of the neck and eventually tears, avulsing a small fragment of bone from the anterior aspect of the vertebral body. Because the posterior ligaments remain intact, the fracture is stable with the neck flexed. It may be necessary to perform flexion–extension radiographic views to demonstrate this fracture and determine its stability.

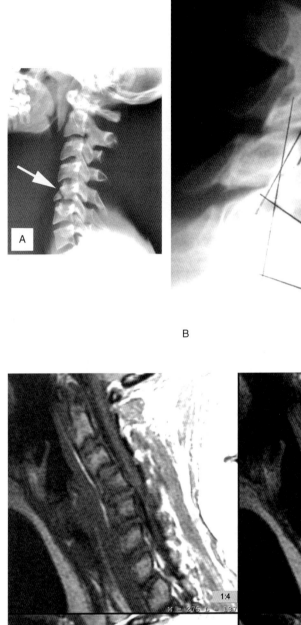

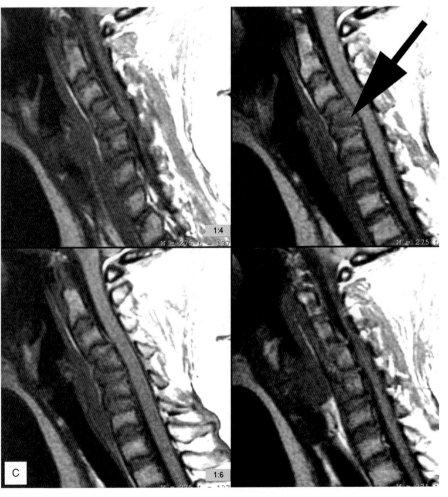

Figure 7.10 (A) Lateral radiograph of a flexion "teardrop" fracture at the base of C-5. Arrow indicates the typical triangular anterior–inferior fragment. (B) Lateral radiograph of the cervical spine showing a flexion teardrop fracture of C-4 with lines showing the posterior displacement and angulation of C-4 on C-5. (C) T1-weighted MRI of flexion teardrop fracture of C-4 and C-5, with retropulsion of the vertebral bodies into the spinal canal producing slight spinal cord compression.

7.14 Compression or Burst Fracture of the Vertebral Body

Axial compression or hyperflexion can produce variable degrees of injury to the vertebral body, ranging from a minor anterior compression "wedge" fracture to complete bursting of the vertebral body with retropulsion of fragments into the spinal canal, causing spinal cord injury.

Anterior compression is apparent on anteroposterior radiographs of the spine as loss of height of the anterior vertebral body compared with its posterior height or compared with the adjacent vertebrae. In comparing the normally parallel vertebral endplates, angulation of greater than 11 degrees suggests either ligamentous disruption, facet dislocation, or anterior

compression fracture. On the anteroposterior radiograph, compression fracture is seen as a loss of height of the vertebral body compared with the adjacent ones, loss of space between adjacent spinous processes, or loss of distance between the pedicles above and below the fracture. Separation of the pedicles laterally compared with those above or below suggests a burst fracture of the vertebral body.

Higher-grade fractures involve comminuted fragments displaced centrifugally. Consequently, plain radiographs reveal loss of vertebral height, increased anteroposterior and lateral diameters, and loss of the normal lordotic lines of alignment. A step-off of

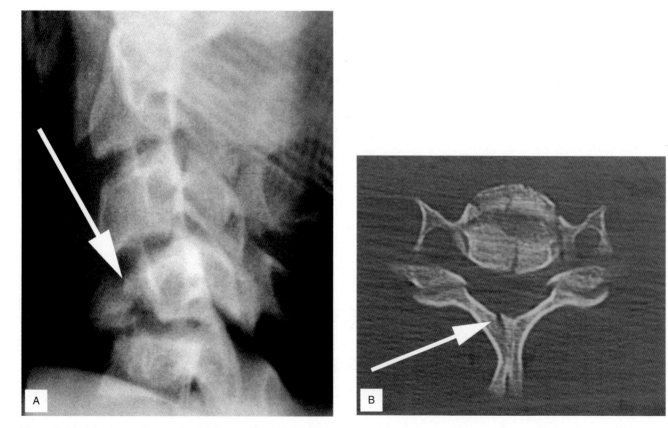

Figure 7.11 (A) Plain radiograph of a flexion-burst fracture (type IV) of C-4 with a large displaced anterior fragment (arrow), slight posterior displacement of the remainder of C-4, and severe angulation at the C-4/C-5 level. (B) CT scan showing a comminuted fracture of the vertebral body with an undisplaced posterior arch fracture (arrow). (C) Lateral radiograph of a comminuted type III fracture of C-5 (arrow).

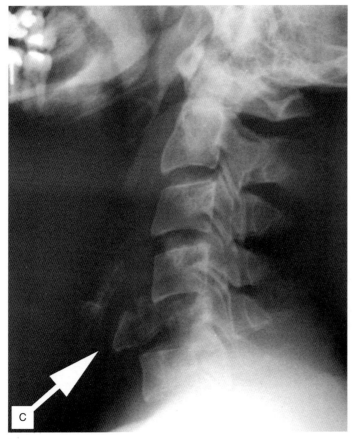

Figure 7.11 (*cont.*)

more than 3.5 mm in the anterior or posterior vertebral lines suggests ligamentous disruption with subluxation, facet dislocation, or burst fracture of the vertebral body. The presence of both anterior and posterior step-offs is diagnostic for burst fracture.

CT scan often reveals more severe comminution of fractures that appear as simple anterior wedge compressions on plain radiographs, and it should be performed when compression fractures are detected on plain films.

All suspicious findings on the initial three-view C-spine series must be delineated further. Use of flexion–extension views for questions of alignment or ligamentous injury can reveal instability that was unsuspected on the initial lateral radiograph. CT scan of the cervical spine can examine regions of the spine that were poorly visualized on plain radiographs and delineate not only the exact extent of the fracture but also its effect on the spinal cord. However, CT scan is not reliable in looking for misalignment and purely ligamentous injuries. MRI is more valuable in visualizing soft tissue disruption in these situations.

7.15 Clay Shoveler's Fracture

Clay shoveler's fracture is a painful but stable fracture of the spinous process of C-7. It is caused by forced flexion of the neck against resistance. The spinous process is avulsed by the pull of the posterior ligaments. Treatment is immobilization of the neck for comfort with either a soft or hard cervical collar, as well as appropriate analgesia. Admission is not required unless indicated for other injuries.

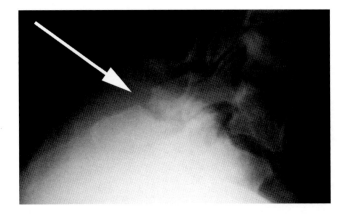

Figure 7.12 Lateral radiograph showing a displaced fracture of the spinous process of C-7, also known as a clay shoveler's fracture.

7.16 Fractures of the Pedicles, Laminae, and Lateral Masses

The pedicles and laminae form a diamond-shaped bony encasement of the spinal cord. Isolated fractures of a single pedicle or lamina are usually due to penetrating injury, most commonly a gunshot wound. With blunt trauma, any combination of pedicle and laminar fractures can occur, depending on

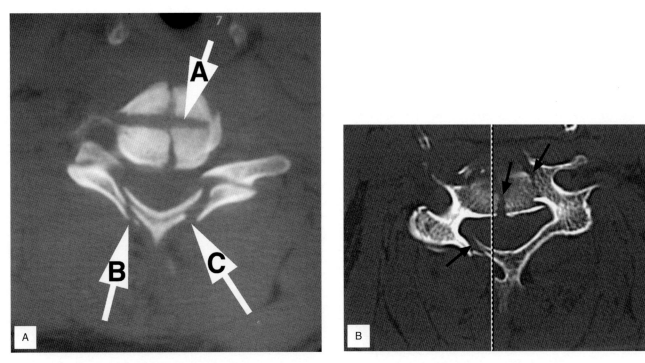

Figure 7.13 (A) CT scan showing a comminuted fracture of the vertebral body (arrow A) with fractures of both laminae (arrows B and C) in a patient who sustained an injury after diving into a swimming pool. (B) CT scan showing a very unstable cervical spine fracture, involving the body and anterior and posterior arches of the vertebra. (C) CT scan showing fracture of the left lamina of T-1 (arrow). (D) CT scan of a patient with a gunshot wound showing fracture and bullet fragments at the right lamina of T-1 (arrow).

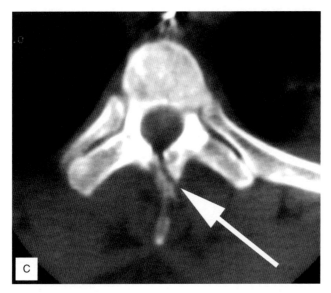

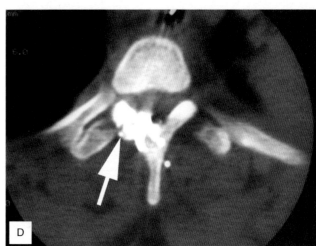

Figure 7.13 (*cont.*)

the angular or rotational forces applied in addition to hyperextension or, less commonly, hyperflexion. Displacement of pedicle or laminar fragments medially can result in direct spinal cord injury. Bilateral pedicle or laminar fractures render the spinal column unstable.

The lateral masses represent the lateral articulations of the spinal column and contain the facet joints. They also form the bony margins of the neural foramina through which nerve roots enter and exit the spinal cord. Consequently, fractures of the lateral masses are often associated with nerve root injury.

7.17 Facet Dislocation

Unilateral facet dislocation results from forced flexion of the neck with a rotational component to one side or the other. If sufficient flexion or rotation occurs, one superior facet will become locked anterior to the inferior facet on that side. The opposite side will show normal alignment of the facets. Oblique radiographs of the spine will often more clearly demonstrate the dislocation. Subluxation of the vertebral bodies is less than 50%, and approximately 25% will have associated spinal cord injury. Reduction is accomplished by sedation and simple traction in most cases.

Bilateral facet dislocation results from forced flexion of the neck, causing the superior facets to glide anteriorly on their inferior counterparts. Once the facet joints reach the peak of the inferior facet, they are said to be "perched" atop the inferior facet. If the superior facet continues anteriorly, it becomes locked in the dislocated position. Bilateral facet dislocation results in greater than 50% subluxation of the superior vertebral body on the inferior one and almost inevitably results in complete spinal cord injury.

Plain radiographs are usually sufficient to demonstrate facet dislocation, but CT scan will also demonstrate this injury and may reveal unsuspected fractures of the facets, lateral masses, pedicles, or laminae.

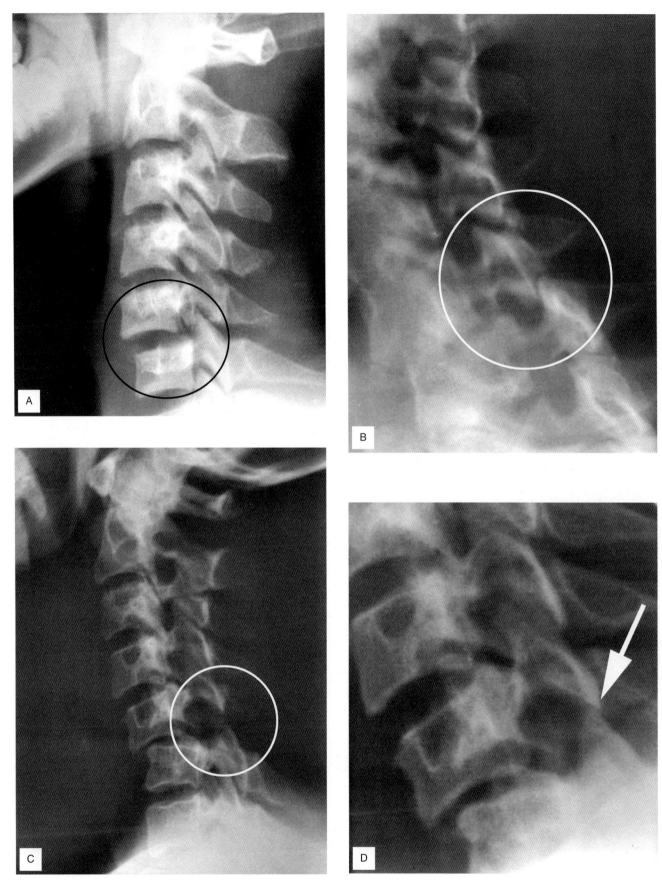

Figure 7.14

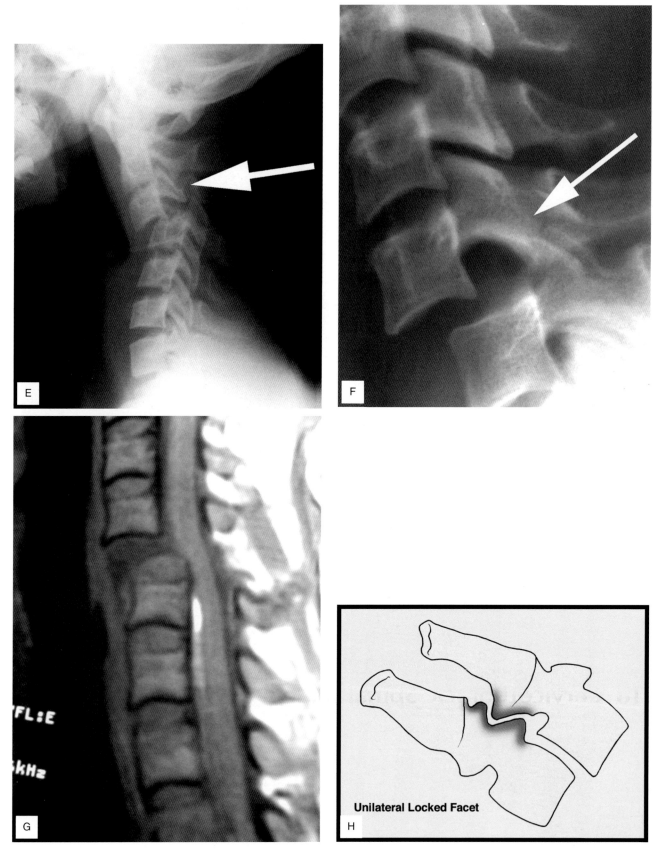

Figure 7.14 (cont.)

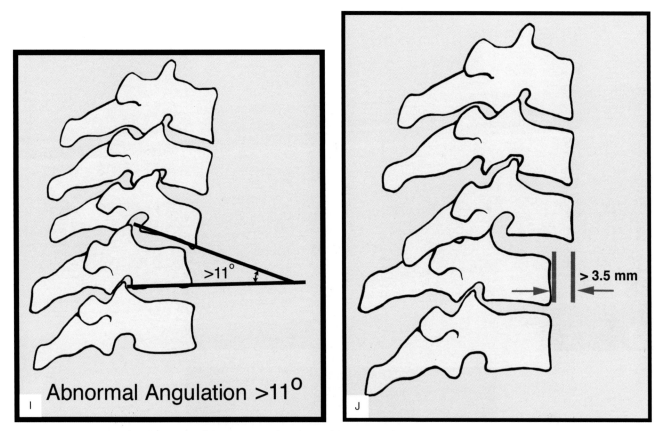

Figure 7.14 (A) Lateral radiograph of the C-spine showing subluxation of C-5 on C-6 due to unilateral facet dislocation of C-5 (circle). (B) Oblique view of unilateral facet dislocation. (C) Lateral radiograph of the C-spine showing subluxation and angulation of C-5 on C-6. Both superior facets (C-5) are seen resting atop the lower facets (C-6), a condition known as perched facets. (D) Close-up view of perched facets (arrow). (E) Lateral radiograph of a 15-year-old girl, injured while jumping on a trampoline, who arrived with quadriplegia. X-ray shows complete bilateral facet dislocation of C-3 on C-4 with significant anterior subluxation and angulation of C-3 (superior facets are lying anterior to the lower facets; see arrow). (F) Close-up of bilateral facet dislocation. (G) T1-weighted MRI of C-5 on C-6 bilateral facet dislocation. (H) Schematic illustrating unilateral facet dislocation. (I) Schematic illustrating abnormal angulation measurements with perched facets. (J) Schematic illustrating anterior subluxation with perched facets.

7.18 Cervicothoracic Spinal Injury

The junction of C-7 and T-1 is a relatively common location for spinal injury, up to 20% of spinal fractures in some series. Consequently, it is essential to visualize this area with plain radiographs on the initial examination prior to clearing the cervical spine. Visualization of this area is difficult to accomplish in children, patients with large, muscular shoulders, and those with upper extremity injuries that make it difficult to pull on the arms for a lateral x-ray. Unless the lateral x-ray extends to the top of T-1, a swimmer's view is often required to verify alignment in this area. Detection of fractures with the swimmer's view is difficult because of superimposed bones and soft tissues, and CT scan should be used when visualization of the cervicothoracic junction is not possible with conventional radiography or when suspicious areas are identified on the swimmer's view.

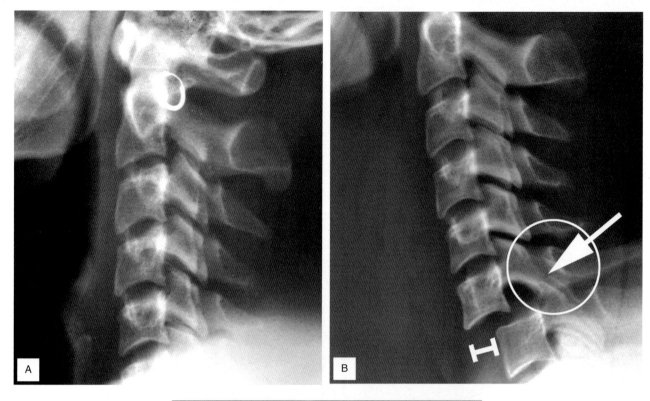

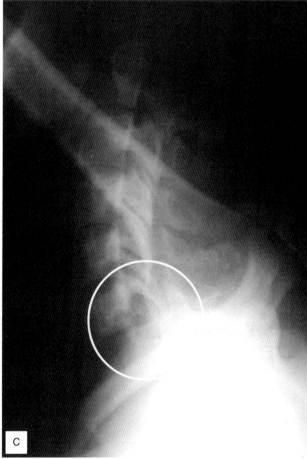

Figure 7.15 (A) Lateral cervical spine radiograph appearing normal to the top of C-6 level. (B) Repeat lateral view of the same patient with a clearly apparent bilateral facet dislocation of C-6 on C-7 (arrow) and significant subluxation of C-6 on C-7. (C) Swimmer's view showing bilateral facet dislocation at the cervicothoracic junction.

Thoracic Spine Injuries

Fracture of the thoracic spine is relatively rare because of the stabilizing influence of the ribs and their liga- mentous attachments and protection by the large para- spinous musculature posteriorly and by the thorax itself

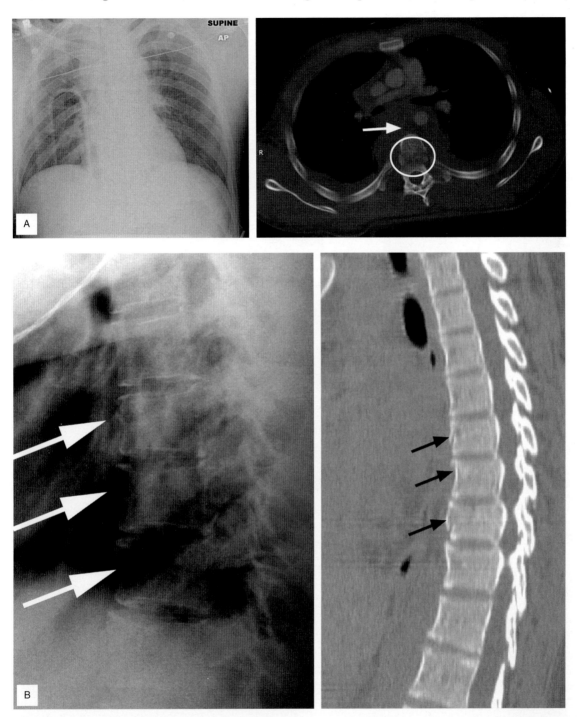

Figure 7.16 (A) Chest radiograph of a patient involved in a motorcycle accident shows a widened mediastinum (left). The differential diagnosis, besides thoracic aortic injury and fracture of the sternum, should include fracture of the thoracic spine. A CT scan of the same patient (right) shows a fracture of the thoracic spine (circle). Note the large hematoma around the fracture site (arrow). (B) Lateral radiograph of the thoracic spine showing three contiguous vertebral compression fractures (arrows) in a young woman who was in a motor vehicle accident (left). Lateral CT scan of the thoracic spine showing anterior compression fractures in the previous patient (right).

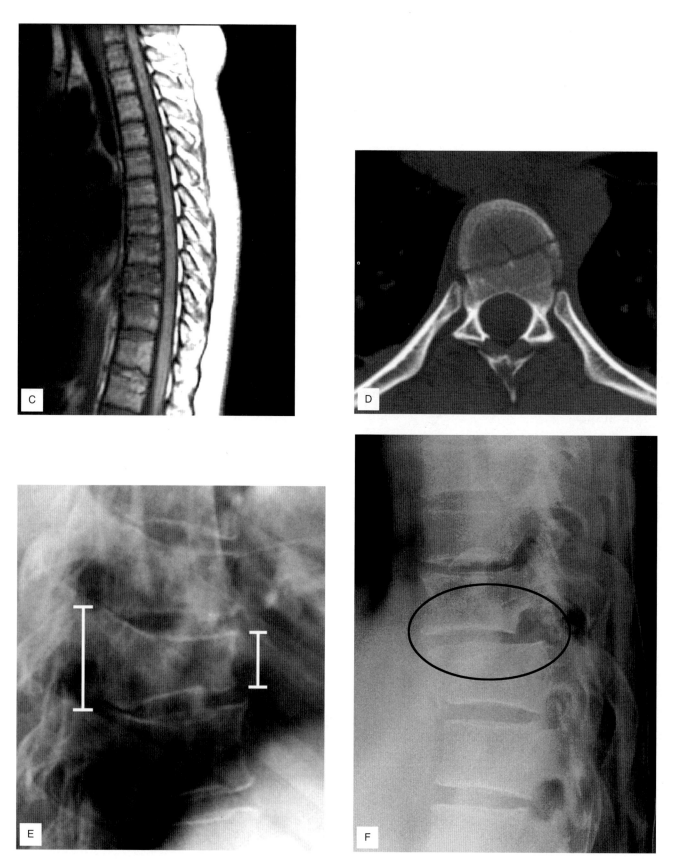

Figure 7.16 (*cont.*) (C) TI-weighted MRI of the spine showing the same compression fractures without damage to the spinal cord. (D) CT scan showing a comminuted thoracic vertebral body fracture. (E) Lateral radiograph of the thoracic spine showing anterior wedge compression fracture of T-6. (F) Fall from height presenting with paraplegia at T-9. Plain radiograph showing compression fracture of T-10 with anterior subluxation of T-9 on T-10 and a small fracture of the anterosuperior aspect of T-10 body.

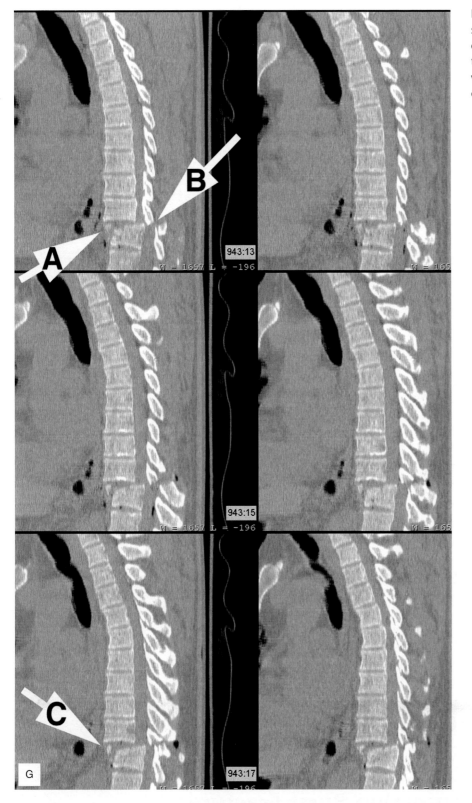

Figure 7.16 (*cont.*) (G) Lateral CT scan series reveals posterior displacement and impingement on the spinal cord (arrows A and C), as well as fracture of the posterior elements of T-9 (arrow B).

anteriorly. In addition, the anatomy of the thoracic vertebrae inherently limits lateral movement and extension. Motorcycle accidents often result in thoracic spine injuries. Fractures in this segment of the spine are commonly associated with spinal cord injury because of the limited amount of space for the cord within the spinal canal in this area. The most common mechanism is hyperflexion from deceleration injuries or falls. Penetrating injury in this area is another relatively common etiology for thoracic cord injury.

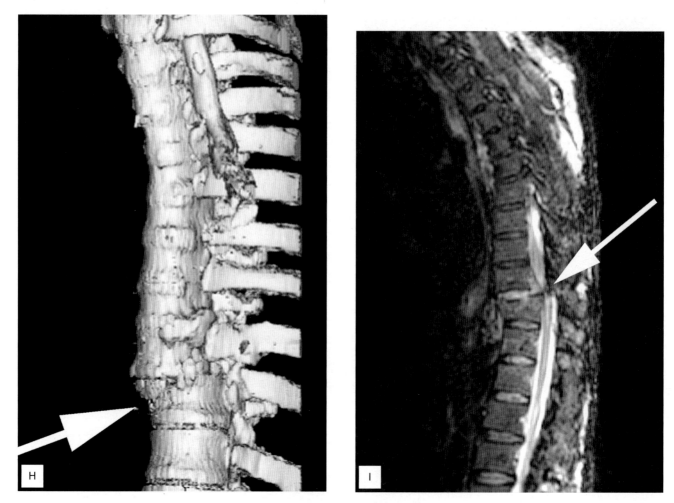

Figure 7.16 (*cont.*) (H) 3-D CT scan reconstruction of the previous fracture. (I) T2-weighted MRI of the same patient showing severe compression of the spinal cord at the T-9–T-10 level (arrow).

Associated thoracoabdominal injuries may take precedence for stabilization, so it is important not to overlook the possibility of concurrent spinal injury.

The chest x-ray often shows a widened upper mediastinum because of the presence of hematoma around the fracture. The radiological appearance is very similar to that in blunt trauma to the thoracic aorta.

Visualization of the thoracic spine by plain radiographs is difficult on account of numerous overlying structures. Consequently, CT scan is often necessary to clearly delineate the nature and extent of the injury, as well as the impact on the spinal cord.

Lumbar Spine Injuries

7.19 Lumbar Compression Burst Fractures

Compression fracture of a lumbar vertebra is one of the most common spinal fractures. It occurs in two distinct age groups. The first group is the elderly, in whom anterior vertebral body collapse can occur with relatively minor trauma and often signals underlying bone pathology, such as advanced osteoporosis or

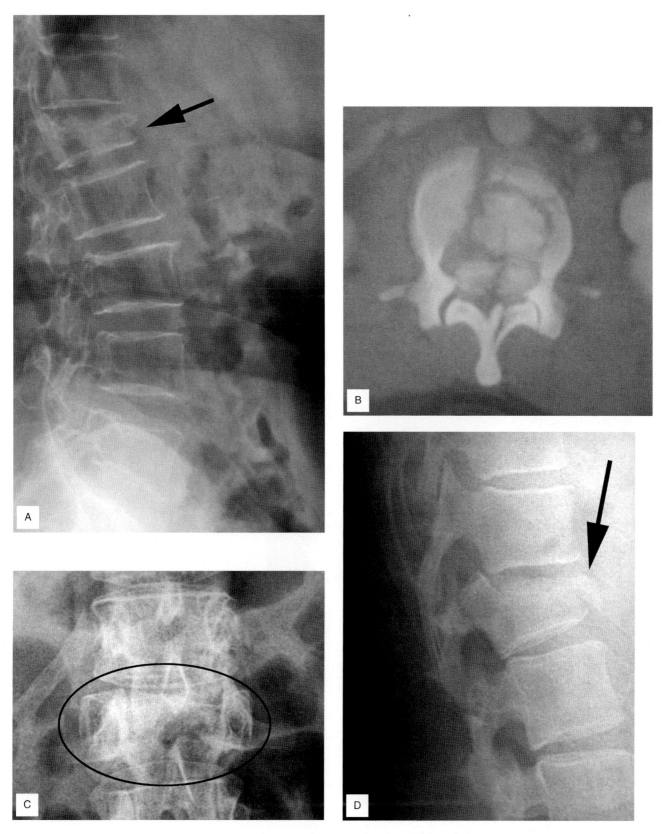

Figure 7.17 (A) Lateral radiograph of the lumbar spine of a suicidal patient who jumped out of a hospital window. It shows an anterior wedge compression fracture of L-1 (arrow). (B) CT scan of the same patient. The L-1 vertebral body shows a comminuted fracture with intrusion of bony fragments into the spinal canal. (C) Plain radiograph showing close-up view of the L-1 burst fracture with lateral displacement of both pedicles of L-1 compared with T-12. (D) Radiograph showing severe compression fracture of L-1 (arrow) with retropulsion of a large fragment into the spinal canal.

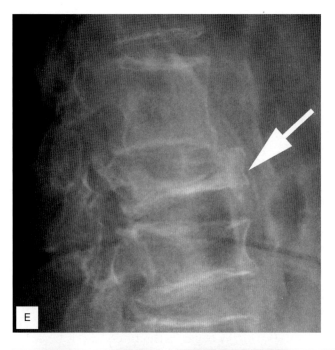

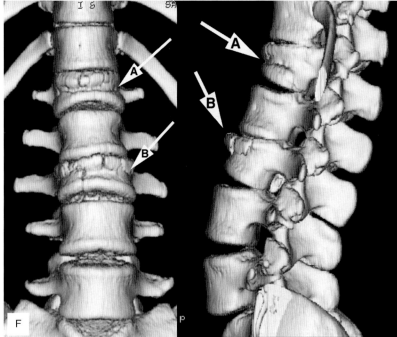

Figure 7.17 (*cont.*) (E) Lateral radiograph of the lumbar spine showing severe compression fracture of L-1 (arrow) and less severe fracture of L-2. (F) 3-D CT scan reconstruction showing anterior wedge compression fractures of L-1 (arrow A) and L-3 (arrow B) on the anterior and lateral views.

metastatic lesions. The second group is made up of younger patients who sustain severe hyperflexion of the lumbar spine, usually during a fall from height. In these patients, associated injuries, such as calcaneal, acetabular, and other lower extremity fractures, mesenteric or renal arterial injury, aortic avulsion, and additional spinal column injuries, are common.

Lumbar compression fracture occurs as a result of acute hyperflexion at the waist, resulting in an anteriorly wedge-shaped vertebral body. The posterior wall of the vertebra is intact, and spinal cord injury is very rare. Collapse of more than 30% of the anterior height may result in progressive collapse of the vertebral body and increasingly severe kyphosis. Consequently, fractures with greater than 30% anterior compression are treated more aggressively. Associated adynamic ileus is commonly associated with these fractures. Radiographically, these fractures appear wedge-shaped with loss of anterior vertebral height on the lateral view. The presence of a burst fracture should be suspected if the anteroposterior view shows separation of the pedicles. This finding indicates a burst fracture rather than a wedge compression fracture.

The extent of fracture comminution may be underestimated on plain radiographs, and a CT scan of the affected vertebra often shows a more extensive fracture. Fractures of the transverse process, lateral mass, or vertebral body in the lumbar spine from L-2 to L-4 may be associated with renal injury. Assessment for the presence of abdominal or retroperitoneal organ injury is indicated by either CT scan or IVP.

7.20 Chance Fractures

Chance fracture typically occurs to a rear seat passenger wearing a lap belt, when the car is involved in a front-end collision. The patient sustains acute hyperflexion at the waist around the axis of the lap belt. The normal flexion point of the spine is located in the center of the vertebral body. An improperly worn lap belt shifts the flexion point anteriorly and acts as a fulcrum that pries apart the vertebral elements from back to front. There are several variations of Chance fracture, depending on the course of the fracture line. For example, the fracture line may begin in the interspinous ligament

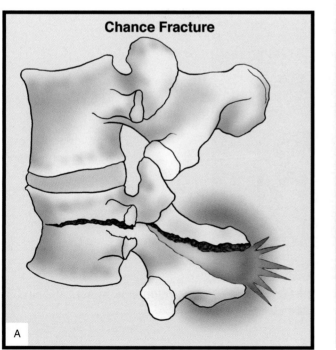

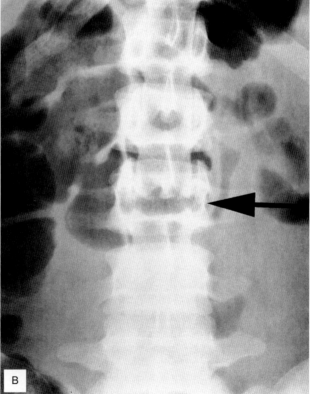

Figure 7.18 (A) Schematic drawing demonstrating classic Chance fracture. (B) Lumbar spine radiograph showing a fracture line (arrow) coursing through the entire vertebral complex, including the spinous process, laminae, pedicles, and vertebral body. Anteroposterior radiograph view shown.

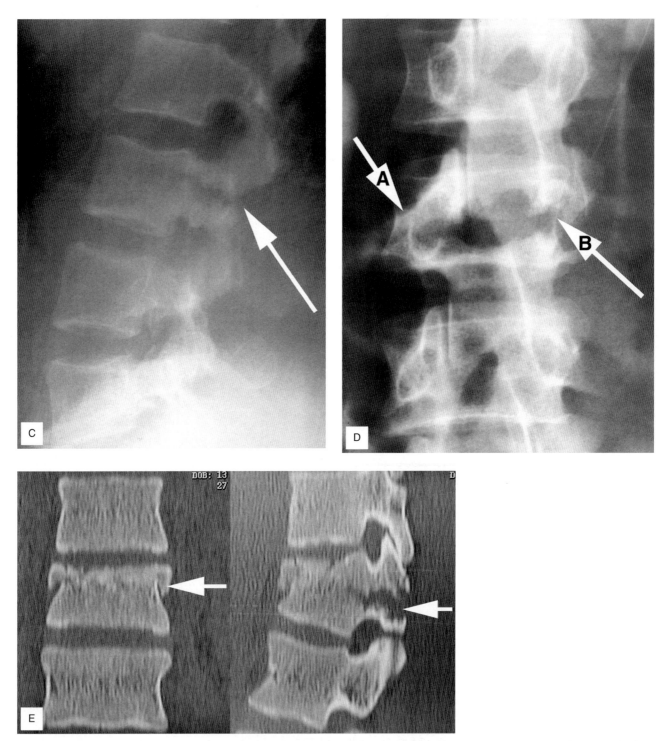

Figure 7.18 (*cont.*) (C) Lateral view of Chance fracture (arrow). (D) Oblique showing pedicle fracture (arrow A) and vertebral body fractures (arrow B). (E) CT scan showing Chance fracture on anteroposterior and lateral view.

and then enter bony elements, only to terminate in a disruption of the disk space. The impact on spinal stability is identical regardless of the exact course of the fracture because both posterior and anterior elements are disrupted. Consequently, this is an unstable fracture.

Because hollow viscera are compressed between the lap belt and the spinal column, Chance

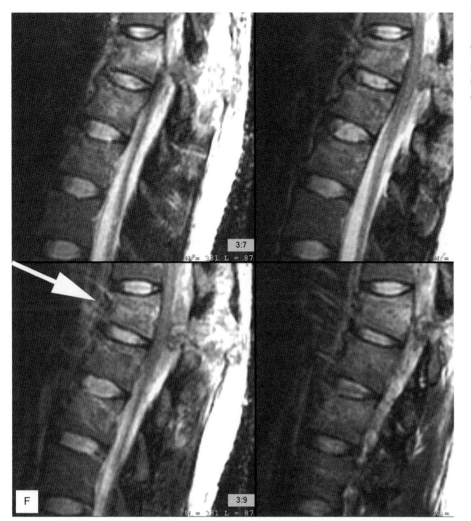

Figure 7.18 (*cont.*) (F) T2-weighted MRI lateral view showing Chance fracture with severe disruption of the posterior elements and soft tissues (arrow), as well as complete spinal cord compression and edema.

fractures are commonly associated with blunt intestinal injury, and patients should be investigated for this possibility.

The presence of a seatbelt sign on the lower abdomen should alert the clinician to the possibility of Chance fracture as well as intestinal injury.

7.21 Fracture-Dislocation of the Lumbar Spine

The spinal cord ends at the level of L-1 or L-2 as the conus medullaris. Nerve fibers supplying the pelvis and lower extremities continue distally as the cauda equina. Injuries to the lower lumbar vertebrae may produce injury to this structure, resulting in the cauda equina syndrome. This syndrome is characterized by the presence of asymmetric weakness and numbness of the lower extremities, often with saddle anesthesia of the perineum, as well as sphincter dysfunction of bowel and bladder. As with compression fractures, injury to the kidneys, ureters, and other retroperitoneal structures must be considered with lumbar fracture-dislocations.

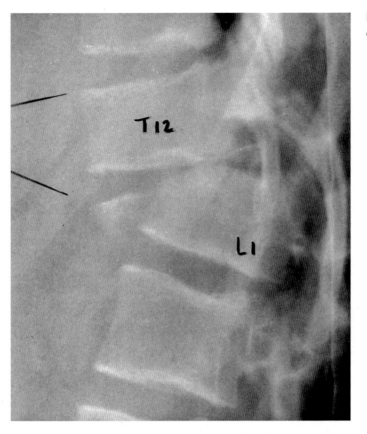

Figure 7.19 Lateral radiograph showing fracture–dislocation of T-12 on L-1.

Pediatric Spinal Injury

Cervical spine fractures are relatively rare in children because of the inherent flexibility of the pediatric spine. When spinal fractures do occur, the upper cervical vertebrae (C-1–C-3) are most commonly involved.

The interpretation of spinal radiographs in children is difficult. Soft tissue thickness may vary considerably depending on the phase of respiration. The presence of epiphyses makes the detection of fracture lines difficult. Incompletely calcified vertebrae cause vertebral bodies to appear wedge-shaped, suggesting possible compression fracture. Physiologic anterior subluxation of C-2 on C-3 or C-3 on C-4 occurs in up to 50% of children and persists until mid adolescence in 10% of patients. In the presence of apparent subluxation, drawing a line between the posterior spinolaminal line of C-2 through C-3 will demonstrate normal alignment if the spinolaminal line of C-2 lies within 2 mm of this line (Swischuk's line). Greater distances of C-2 from this line suggest true subluxation.

It is often difficult to obtain adequate open-mouth views of C-1 and C-2 in children because of their small mouths and inability to cooperate. Consequently, it is often necessary to obtain a CT scan of the upper vertebrae in children when the mechanisms of injury or physical findings suggest the possibility of spinal injury.

Although it may occur at any age, the syndrome of spinal cord injury without radiographic abnormality (SCIWORA) accounts for approximately one-third of spinal cord injuries in children younger than age 8 years. Symptoms may be delayed for 24 hours in a significant proportion of these cases. Consequently, obtaining normal radiographs of the spine and a normal neurologic examination at the time of injury does not necessarily exclude delayed spinal cord injury. The presence of any neurologic symptoms such as transient paresthesias at the time of injury requires investigation with either CT scan or MRI. Administration of high-dose steroids for spinal cord injury has not been well studied in children but may be helpful when abnormalities are detected on CT or MRI and when neurologic deficits are present.

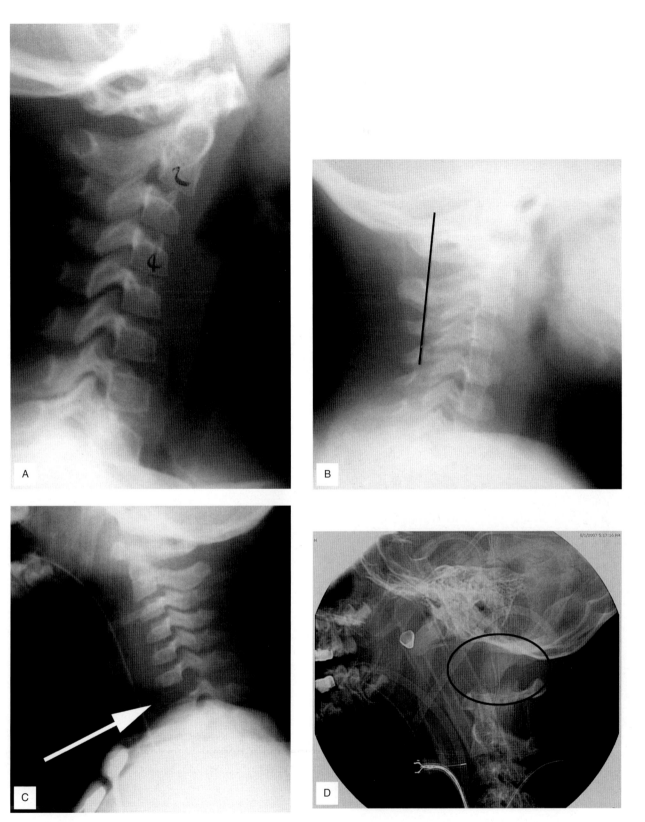

Figure 7.20 (A) Lateral C-spine radiograph showing physiologic subluxation of C-2 on C-3. (B) Lateral C-spine radiograph showing alignment within Swischuk's line confirming that the subluxation is physiologic rather than pathologic.
(C) Lateral C-spine view of bilateral facet dislocation of C-6 on C-7 and massive anterior soft tissue swelling in a young child.
(D) Lateral C-spine of a 5-year old child shows atlanto-occipital dislocation.

Penetrating Injuries to the Spinal Cord

Penetrating injuries account for about 14% of all spinal cord injuries in the United States. Most penetrating spinal injuries, including gunshot wounds, are stable. It is highly unlikely that victims of gunshot injuries, who are neurologically intact, have unstable fractures.

Stab wounds usually result in partial cord injuries and the prognosis is fairly good. However, the majority of gunshot wounds produce extensive cord damage and the prognosis is poor.

Many patients with penetrating cord injuries have associated serious injuries to the surrounding structures in the neck, chest, or abdomen. The clinical evaluation of the abdomen in a paralyzed patient is very difficult and unreliable. These patients should be evaluated with contrast CT scan. Patients with penetrating cervical or thoracic spinal cord injuries may need further investigation by means of endoscopy or swallow studies to rule out associated aerodigestive injuries. All penetrating injuries to the abdomen in paralyzed patients should undergo exploratory laparotomy, because the abdomen is clinically unevaluable.

The management of penetrating cord injuries is usually supportive and operative intervention has little or no role. In most cases, surgery to remove the bullet does not improve outcome and may increase the risk of complications, such as infection, cerebrospinal fluid leak, and bleeding. However, some cases with incomplete cord injury due to gunshot wounds, especially if there is deterioration of the neurological function, may require surgical decompression. Similarly, victims with incomplete cord injuries and a missile lodged in the spinal canal may benefit from operative removal.

Steroids have no role for routine use in penetrating spinal cord trauma and there is some evidence that they increase the risk of complications. In selected cases with extensive surrounding edema or shock wave injury due to high velocity missiles, some physicians might give steroids.

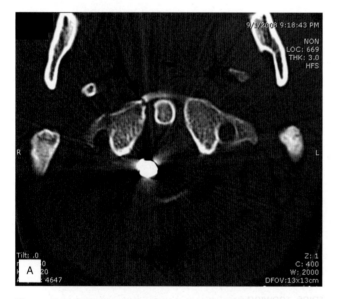

Figure 7.21 (A) Gunshot wound with fracture of the anterior arch of C-1. The bullet is lodged in the spinal canal. Patients with complete spinal cord transection at this level die within a few minutes because of complete respiratory muscle paralysis. This patient, in addition to the quadriplegia, suffered severe hypoxic brain damage.

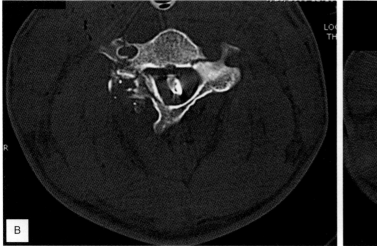

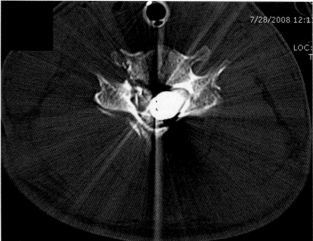

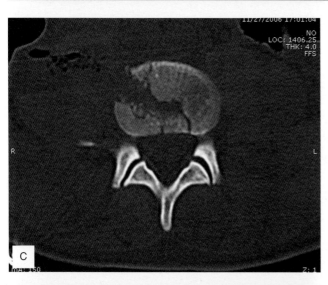

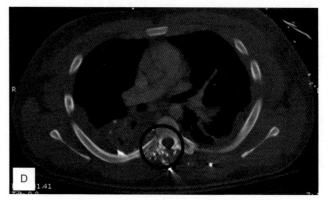

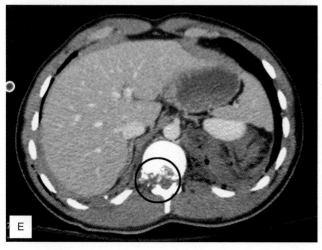

Figure 7.21 (*cont.*) (B) Patients with gunshot injury to the cervical spine, with extensive bone damage and the bullet lodged in the spinal canal. These patients survived with permanent quadriplegia. (C) Gunshot wound to the spine with extensive vertebral body damage but intact spinal cord. (D) CT scan of patient with gunshot wound to the thoracic spine, showing extensive bony damage posteriorly but incomplete cord injury. (E) CT scan of patient with gunshot wound to the thoracic spine with complete cord transection and paraplegia.

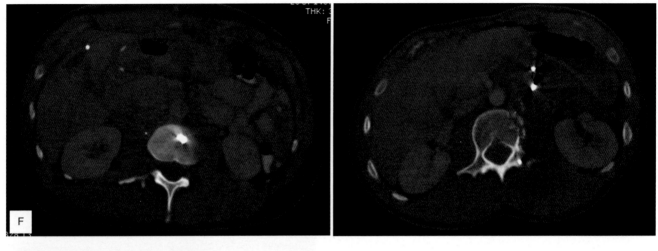

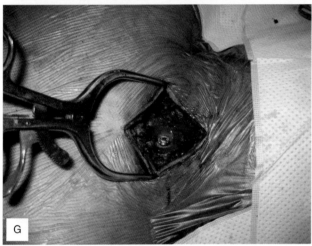

Figure 7.21 (*cont.*) (F) Gunshot wound to the lumbar spine with no cord injury. The bullet is lodged in the vertebral body and does not need to be removed (left). CT scan of a victim showing a fracture of the vertebral body (right). This fracture does not need any specific treatment. (G) Intraoperative appearance of a bullet lodged in the intervertebral space causing partial cord injury.

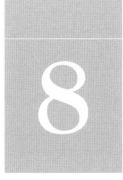

8 Burn Injuries

Andrew Tang, Charity Wip, Warren Garner, and Demetrios Demetriades

Introduction

The skin serves as an effective barrier to external agents such as pathogens, loss of internal constituents like water, electrolytes, and proteins, and provides protection from mechanical trauma. Cutaneous burns range from inconsequential superficial injuries that can heal without medical intervention to overwhelming skin loss and patient death. The extent of the burn depth and size is directly related to the degree of fluid loss and the extent of the systemic inflammatory response. Patients require careful fluid resuscitation for this mixed hypovolemic and hyperdynamic state.

In the United States, burns account for approximately 40–50,000 admissions per year with 80% of patients being candidates for outpatient treatment. The American Burn Association has devised specific referral criteria for transfer to specialized burn centers, which have been shown to decrease mortality and improve functional outcome of patients. Burn mortality has decreased drastically over the past three decades as a result of early excision and grafting, control of sepsis, advances in ventilatory and nutritional support, and wound care adjuncts such as synthetic skin substitutes.

Clinical Examination

The initial assessment of a burn patient is similar to any trauma patient based on the priorities established by Advanced Trauma Life Support (ATLS). After quickly securing the airway–breathing–circulation (ABCs), ongoing tissue damage should be prevented by carefully removing hot or chemically saturated clothing and jewelry. There are additional concerns related to the burn injury:

1. Early assessment for airway compromise from inhalation injury.
2. The inhaled products of combustion can induce pulmonary parenchymal damage and further worsen the patient's respiratory status.
3. Patients with greater than 20% total body surface area (TBSA) burns are hypovolemic from the predictable wound evaporative fluid loss and transudation of fluids into the extracellular space.
4. Approximately 10% of burn patients suffer concomitant injuries. Therefore a focused examination is important to determine the possibility of neurologic or musculoskeletal injury.
5. The patient should be completely exposed to assess for the extent of burn, and for evidence of any associated trauma.

Proper initial resuscitation is dependent on accurate assessment of both the extent and depth of burn. Percentage of body surface area involved may be estimated by applying the "Rule of Nines" or the Lund–Browder chart for second-degree or higher burns. In this calculation, the head and each upper extremity is 9%, while the lower extremities, the anterior and posterior trunks are each 18% of the body surface area. The perineum accounts for the remaining 1%. For children, a modified rule of nine is used to account for the larger heads, which is 18% of the TBSA. The lower extremities are 14% each with the remaining distribution the same as adults. Smaller burns may be estimated based on the patient's palm, which is approximately 1% TBSA.

In the first 24–48 hours the extent of burn size and depth may not be clear as the injury progresses. Inadequate resuscitation or acute infection can impede the healing process. Deeply burned skin looses elasticity and manifests as a loss of compliance in response to underlying tissue swelling. Large chest burns can

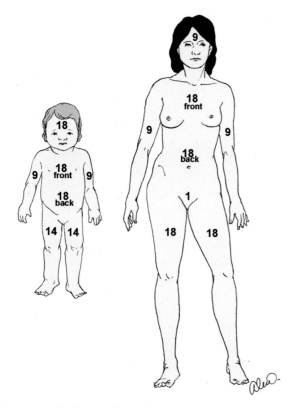

Figure 8.1 The "Rule of Nines" in determining body surface area burns in adults and children.

3. Chest radiography. Though the initial chest radiographs may be normal in early inhalation injury, it may demonstrate parenchymal abnormalities such as pulmonary edema.

4. Flexible laryyngoscopy/bronchoscopy. These procedures can be done at the bedside to further evaluate the airways of patients with suspected inhalation injury. Visualization of airway erythema, edema, carbonaceous sputum, and singed nose hair all signify inhalation injury.

5. Doppler stethoscope. Extensive burns of the extremities and subsequent edema make peripheral pulses difficult to palpate, and Doppler stethoscope may help detect weak pulses.

6. Compartment pressure measurement. A high index of suspicion should exist for compartment syndrome. Whenever suspected, objective measurements can assist in further clinical management.

7. Serum glucose. Glycemic control can reduce osmotic diuresis and infectious complications, and may improve survival. Although, the precise target range is yet to be defined, most practitioners attempt to keep glucose below 180 mg/dL.

present with loss of chest wall excursion and high ventilatory pressures. Similarly, circumferential burns of the extremities can impede blood flow and induce limb ischemia. Clinical vigilance and early escharotomy are imperative to prevent respiratory compromise or further tissue ischemia.

Investigations

History and physical examination clarifies the circumstances surrounding the burn and may reveal any associated injuries. Additional important investigations include:

1. Arterial blood gas and pulse oximetry. Early detection of hypoxia and/or hypercapnia in patients with inhalation injury is documented by these tests.

2. Carboxyhemoglobin levels. Patients in closed-space fires are at risk for carbon monoxide (CO) poisoning. CO has an affinity for hemoglobin 40 times that of oxygen and may falsely elevate pulse oximetry readings. A carboxyhemoglobin level up to 10 may be normal for chronic smokers.

General Management

Similar to any traumatized patients the initial management of the thermally injured patient consists of securing the ABCs. All burn patients with history, signs, or symptoms of smoke inhalation should be promptly assessed by direct laryngoscopy and be placed on 100% supplemental oxygen to facilitate CO dispersion. Patients showing any signs of acute inhalational injury should undergo immediate endotracheal intubation either as a prophylactic or therapeutic measure. Remaining clothing may continue to harbor the burning process, and thus the patient should be completely undressed and all jewelry removed. Dry chemical powders should be brushed off the skin while liquid chemicals should be removed with copious water irrigation. Once the skin has been completely cleansed and fully evaluated, the patient should be promptly dried and covered with warm blankets to prevent hypothermia. Small partial or full-thickness burns may be treated at the local hospitals. However, specific transfer criteria have been established by the American Burn Association to achieve the optimal care at specialized burn centers. The guidelines are:

- Partial thickness burns greater than 10% TBSA
- Burns that involve the face, hands, feet, genitalia, perineum, or major joints
- Third-degree burns in any age group
- Electrical burns, including lightning injury
- Chemical burns
- Inhalation injury
- Burn injury in patients with preexisting medical disorders that could complicate management, prolong recovery, or affect mortality
- Any patients with burns and concomitant trauma (such as fractures) in which the burn injury poses the greatest risk of morbidity or mortality
- Burned children in hospitals without qualified personnel or equipment for the care of children
- Burn injury in patients who will require special social, emotional, or long-term rehabilitative intervention.

Silver sulfadiazine is the most commonly used topical antimicrobial in burn wound care. After its application, sterile dressings should be used to cover the wound. Sometimes proteinacous exudate, silver sulfadiazine, and fibrin combine to produce a pseudoeschar which should be removed during daily dressing changes. Otherwise, its presence delays wound healing and increases the risk of infection. Burns over cartilaginous areas such as the nose and ear can be covered by mafenide acetate, which has superior eschar penetration to silver sulfadiazine. Tetanus vaccination status should be obtained and prophylaxis administered when necessary. Careful serial neurovascular examination of circumferential burn is critical. Patients demonstrating signs of compartment syndrome should undergo emergent escharotomy. In addition to providing pain relief, adequate analgesia has been shown to decrease the incidence of post-traumatic stress disorder, particularly in the pediatric population. Titrated doses of intravenous narcotics and anxiolytics should be liberally used. Burn patients are in a hypermetabolic state and may require greater than normal doses of medications to achieve the desired effect.

Aggressive crystalloid hydration is necessary to maintain adequate circulating blood volume due to the evaporative loss and third space fluid shifts. It is generally agreed that burns exceeding 20% TBSA cause systemic physiologic derangements through various proinflammatory mediators. Early aggressive fluid resuscitation should be initiated to achieve a urine output of at least 0.5 cc/kg per hour for adults and 1 cc/kg per hour for children. Although various formulas exist to guide the initial resuscitation of the burned patient, the most commonly applied is the Parkland formula. This resuscitation strategy is based on Ringer's lactate administered at 4 cc/kg per % TBSA. Half of this volume is given in the first 8 hours post burn, and the remaining given over the next 16 hours. Mental status, vital signs, and central venous pressure also serve as useful adjuncts to guide resuscitation. However, urine output remains the most reliable indicator of adequate end organ perfusion. Adequate urine output is particularly important for patients who suffer from burn-associated rhabdomyolysis.

Common Mistakes and Pitfalls

1. Missed or delayed diagnosis of inhalation injury. These patients can develop progressive airway edema that can quickly change a safe elective intubation to an airway emergency.
2. Incorrect estimation of burn size. The entire body surface must be examined to assess for injury. First-degree burns with intact epidermal barrier are not included in the TBSA calculations. Another pitfall that results in TBSA overestimation is using the entire body region percentage as designated by the Rule of Nines rather than counting only the burned areas.
3. Missed coexisting major blunt trauma. Ten percent of burn patients suffer from concomitant trauma, and liberal imaging modalities should be used to clarify the injury burden.
4. Missed or delayed diagnosis of compartment syndrome. Circumferential burns should raise the suspicion of compartment syndrome. Serial examination and compartment pressure measurements should be performed.
5. Inadequate fluid resuscitation. The evaporative loss, third space fluid shift, and the proinflammatory hypermetabolic state cause tremendous fluid loss. Aggressive crystalloid resuscitation is required to maintain hemodynamic stability and adequate end organ perfusion.
6. Inadequate analgesia and sedation. Large amounts of intravenous analgesic are often needed to achieve adequate relief.
7. Inadequate wound evaluation. Partial thickness burns may convert to full thickness either due to

the extent of injury or inadequate resuscitation. The same team of clinicians should serially examine the wound in order to appreciate the wound progression and plan management.

Extent of Burn Injury

Second-degree and higher burns are characterized into three zones of injury. The central irreversibly damaged tissue is the zone of coagulation. It transitions to the zone of stasis where the moderately injured tissue experiences decreased perfusion secondary to injury-induced vasoconstriction. Depending on the extent of tissue damage and the adequacy of resuscitation, this tenuous zone may progress to necrosis or may recover. The zone of hyperemia consists of a clearly viable, but inflamed rim of tissue.

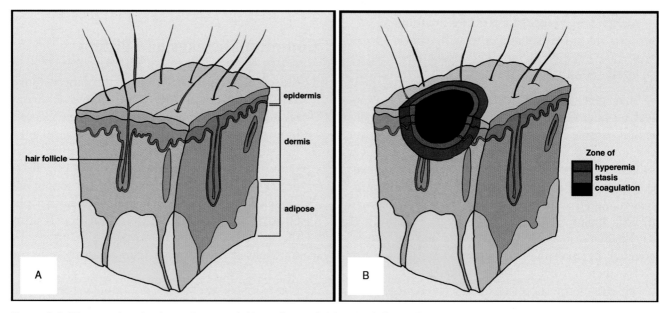

Figure 8.2 Diagram showing layers in normal skin and superficial second-degree burn. (A) Normal skin layers. (B) Zones of injury with a superficial second-degree burn. The central coagulation zone is irreversibly damaged tissue. The zone of stasis may progress to necrosis or may recover, depending on good resuscitation and prevention of infection.

8.1 First-Degree Burn

First-degree burn is equivalent to sunburn in terms of tissue injury depth and prognosis. The extent of thermal penetration is limited to the epidermis while the dermis and all elements of the dermal appendages remain intact. The burned skin is erythematous, painful, blanches with touch, but does not blister. Skin regeneration typically happens within a few days as the damaged epidermal layer desiccates and sloughs off. Treatment is aimed at providing comfort with moisture cream to create a supportive environment for healing and nonsteroidal anti-inflammatory drugs or acetaminophen for pain.

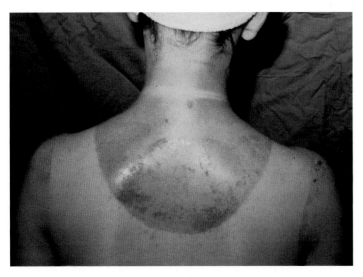

Figure 8.3 Sunburn is a typical first-degree burn. The skin is erythematous and painful, but without blistering.

8.2 Second-Degree Burn

Second-degree burns result when thermal injury penetrates into the dermis. Its division into two classifications, superficial and deep, is based on depth of injury, but more importantly has treatment and prognostic significance.

Superficial Second-Degree Burn

The wound in a superficial second-degree burn is erythematous, moist, blanches with touch, blisters, and tends to be more painful than deep second-degree

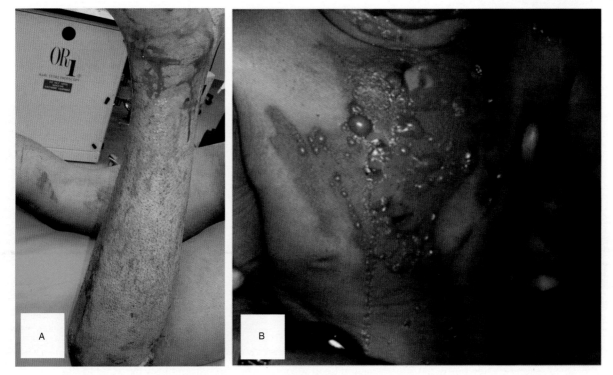

Figure 8.4 Superficial second-degree burns. (A) Lower extremity circumferential second-degree burn from hot-water scald. (B) Superficial second-degree burn from hot-water scald. Notice the classic blistering appearance. (C) Superficial second-degree burn from radiator fluid scald on the forearm. The ruptured blister had been debrided.

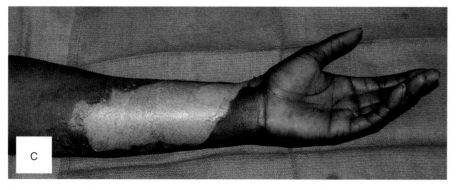

C

Figure 8.4 (*cont.*)

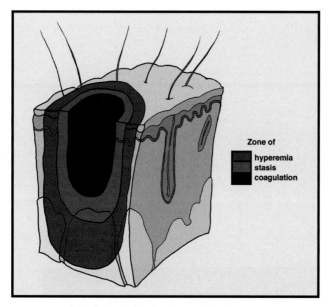

Zone of
hyperemia
stasis
coagulation

Figure 8.5 Deep second-degree burn cross-section. Note the zone of necrosis extending into the deep dermal layer.

burns due to the intact dermal appendages and sensory nerve endings. Tissue response to injury is a dynamic process, particularly in the first 24–48 hours post injury. Appropriate fluid resuscitation and wound care that establish a moist antibacterial environment may arrest conversion of a superficial to deep second-degree burn and facilitate healing. Spontaneous re-epithelialization takes place from the rete ridges, hair follicles, and sweat glands and is typically complete by 14 days. Discoloration and scarring can occur.

Deep Second-Degree Burn

A deep second-degree burn extends to the deep dermal layer. For this reason, these wounds tend to

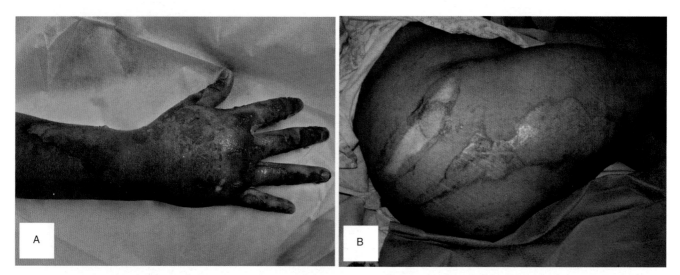

A

B

Figure 8.6 Deep second-degree burns. (A) Superficial and deep second-degree burn from hot-water scald to the hand. (B) Deep second-degree burn with central third-degree burn. Notice the classic color differentiation. (C) Foot scald injury consisting of largely nonblanching pale appearing third-degree burn and erythematous deep second-degree burn over the medial forefoot.

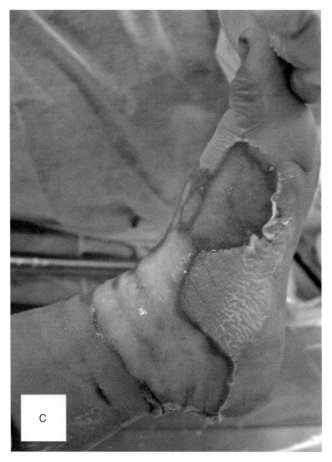

C

Figure 8.6 (*cont.*)

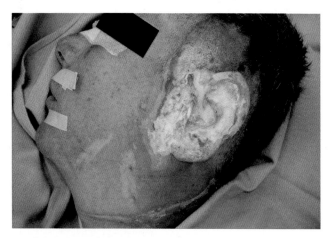

Figure 8.8 Gasoline burn over the face resulting in loss of soft tissue coverage over the ear with exposed cartilage. Mafenide acetate efficiently penetrates cartilage and should be used for burns over the ear and nose.

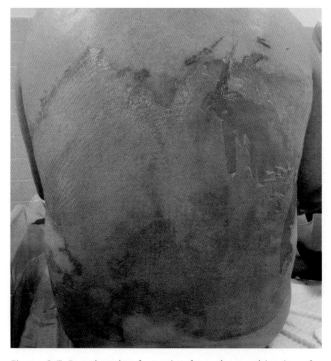

Figure 8.7 Pseudoeschar formation from the combination of silver sulfadiazine, proteinaceous exudate, and fibrin. It should be removed during daily dressing to promote wound healing.

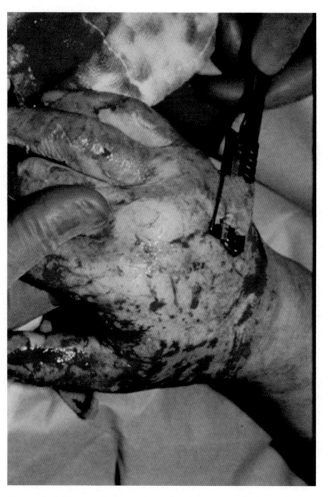

Figure 8.9 Tangential excision of a deep second-degree burn with a Weck knife.

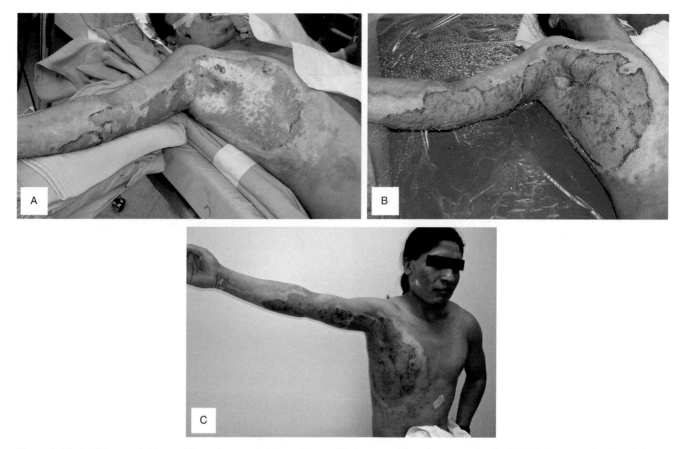

Figure 8.10 Excision and skin grafting of second-degree burns. (A) Preoperative photograph of a 14% TBSA superficial and deep second-degree burn resulting from a car fire. (B) The same wound after tangential excision and split-thickness skin grafting. (C) The functional and cosmetic appearance of the wound 10 days after the operation.

be less sensate due to damage of the sensory elements. While deep second-degree burns may heal spontaneously, the rate and quality of that healing is often poor and there is a higher propensity to convert to full-thickness burns, develop infections, and form contractures. Depending on the size of injury and the status of the surrounding tissues, a small deep second-degree burn may be treated expectantly with local wound care and antimicrobial dressings. However, large affected areas or those in close proximity to third-degree burns are best treated by early tangential excision and grafting. This approach has been shown to decrease septic wound complications, decrease hospitalization and associated morbidity and mortality, and improve functional outcome. Supportive measures include early enteral nutrition, anabolic agents, and appropriate antibiotic usage. Silver sulfadiazine is the most commonly used burn topical agent. It has a broad spectrum of activity against both gram-

positive and gram-negative organisms, including *Staphylococcus aureus* and certain species of *Pseudomonas* and *Candida*. It has limited eschar penetrating and side effects include neutropenia and thrombocytopenia. Mafenide acetate provides the best eschar penetration with the broadest antimicrobial coverage against *Pseudomonas* and gram-negative rods. However, it is painful on application and can cause metabolic acidosis due to its carbonic anhydrase activity.

Treatment of deep second-degree or deeper burns begins with tangential removal of the necrotic tissue followed by closure. Burn wound coverage usually consists of autografts and temporary synthetic alternatives. In patients with extensive burns, the donor graft harvested at a depth of 8–14/1000th of an inch can be meshed to provide expanded wound coverage. Meshed grafts are also less susceptible to seroma accumulation and have better conformance to contoured areas such as the knee or ankle. For cosmetically

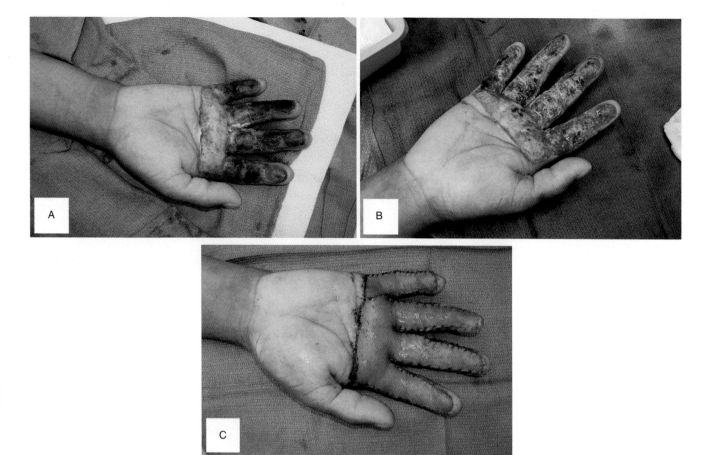

Figure 8.11 Excision and skin grafting of second-degree burns of the hand. (A) Heat press deep second-degree burn to the hand. (B) The hand after tangential excision of the devitalized tissue. (C) Intraoperative photograph of the wound covered with a sheet graft. Sheet grafts are used for cosmetically sensitive areas such as the face and hand.

sensitive areas such as the face or hands, a sheet graft is best used to avoid the weave-like appearance of mesh grafts. However, seroma formation beneath the sheet graft is more common, and this needs to be carefully drained to avoid graft loss.

8.3 Third-Degree Burn

When thermal injury extends to the subcutaneous fat with destruction of the overlying epidermal and dermal elements, the third-degree burn uniformly needs early excision and grafting. The wound is insensate and appears leathery and dry. There is notable absence of tissue edema compared to surrounding second-degree burns. If left untreated, third-degree burns will form a classic burn eschar that will separate from the surrounding viable tissue over the ensuing days to weeks. Spontaneous wound closure takes place by contracture formation from the wound edges as all regenerative elements within the wound bed are destroyed. The mainstay of therapy is early excision with grafting.

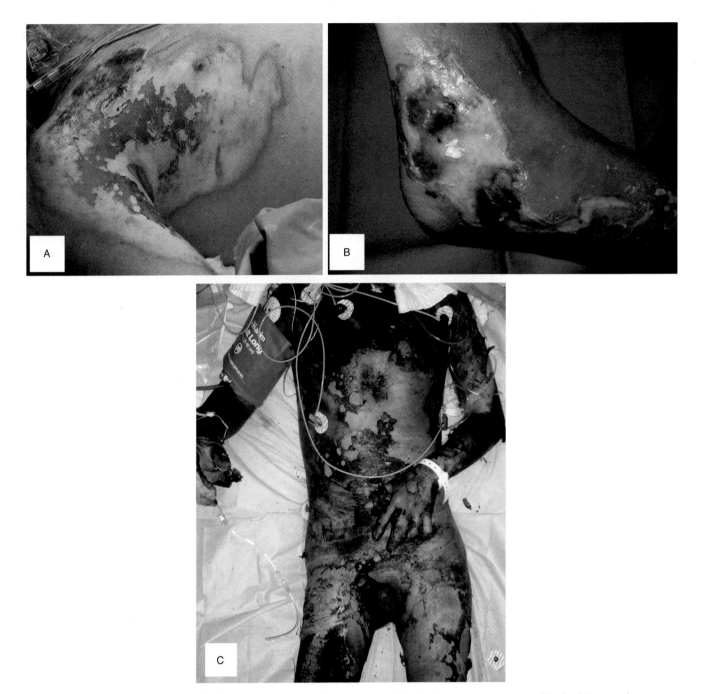

Figure 8.12 Third-degree burns. (A) Third-degree burn with its characteristic leathery appearance and lack of tissue edema. (B) Third-degree burn of the foot from hot cooking-oil splash. (C) Fatal 95% TBSA fourth-degree burn from a houschold fire.

8.4 Fourth-Degree Burn

Fourth-degree burns involve extensive thermal destruction of subcutaneous tissue, fascia, muscles, and bone. It is charred in appearance and requires extensive debridement, complex reconstruction, and in certain cases, amputation.

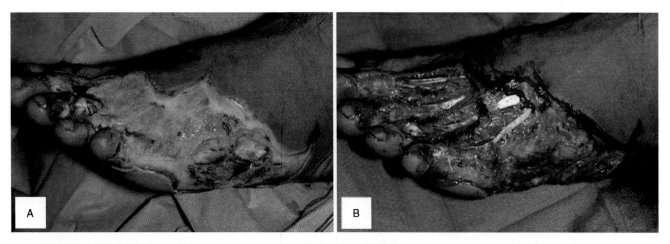

Figure 8.13 Fourth-degree burn. (A) Fourth-degree burn of the foot. (B) Same patient after surgical excision. Note the exposed tendons and bone.

Special Considerations of Burn Injury

8.5 Inhalation Injury

Inhalation injuries typically happen in the setting of explosions or fires in enclosed quarters. Although inhalation injury is present in 6.5% of burn patients and carries mortality up to 50%, its initial manifestation may be deceivingly mild. The upper airway suffers from direct thermal damage up to the level of the glottis. The closure of the glottis and the moist airway environment limits the extent of thermal transmission distally. However, toxic compounds of combustion including hydrogen cyanide, ammonia, and aldehydes propagate to the level of the alveoli and induce further chemical injuries that underlie the development of acute lung injury (ALI) and acute respiratory distress syndrome (ARDS).

Clinical suspicion should be high in cases of fire within an enclosed space. Clues on physical examination include facial burns, singed nasal hair, carbonaceous sputum, and hoarse voice. Direct laryngoscopy demonstrating mucosal erythema, edema accompanied by carbonaceous sputum, is diagnostic of inhalation injury. There should be a low threshold for intubation, even in cases of what appears to be mild inhalation injury, due to the progression of airway edema that can turn an elective situation into an airway emergency.

Currently there is no reliable method to quantify the extent of inhalation injury. Serum carboxyhemoglobin, extrapolated to the time of injury, provides a crude estimation of severity. Treatment is largely supportive with 100% oxygen which shortens the half-life of carboxyhemoglobin from 4.5 hours to 50 minutes, mechanical ventilation, and aggressive respiratory care. High-frequency oscillatory ventilation, based on the principles of delivering small stacked tidal volumes through an uncuffed endotracheal tube, thus reducing barotraumas and facilitating airway clearance, has been shown to improve oxygenation, decrease the incidence of ARDS, and improve mortality against historical controls.

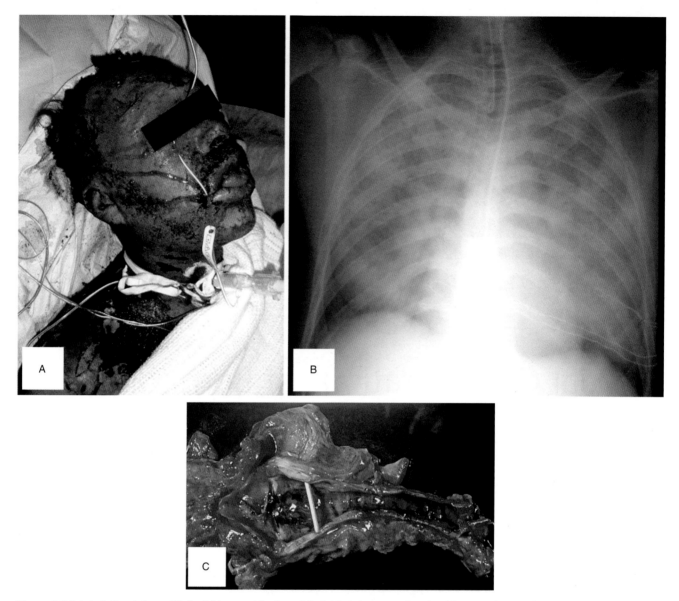

Figure 8.14 Inhalation injury. (A) Facial burn with singed facial hair in a man involved in a car fire. High suspicion for inhalation injury. This patient should undergo bronchoscopy. (B) Chest x-ray demonstrating noncardiogenic pulmonary edema in a patient with severe inhalation injury. (C) The laryngotracheal view of inhalation injury at autopsy. Note the extensive erythema and carbonaceous materials throughout the airway.

8.6 Abdominal Compartment Syndrome

Abdominal compartment syndrome (ACS) develops in 5% of hospitalized burn patients as a result of fluid resuscitation, injury-induced capillary permeability, and bowel edema. This entity progresses to multisystem organ failure and is uniformly fatal if left untreated. Alarming signs of ACS include a tense abdomen, increased ventilatory pressures from loss of diaphragmatic excursion against increased intra-abdominal pressure, decreased urine output from renal vascular compression, and hypotension secondary to preload compromise from inferior vena cava compression. An elevated bladder pressure coupled with clinical signs prompt early intervention. An abdominal ultrasound can reliably identify free fluid within the abdominal space. In selected cases, percutaneous catheter decompression with a flexible drainage catheter directed toward the pelvis is effective in achieving adequate abdominal decompression. However, decompressive laparotomy may serve as the primary therapy or may be reserved for cases unresponsive to catheter decompression.

8.7 Circumferential Burn

A high index of suspicion for the development of compartment syndrome is key when taking care of patients with deep second-degree or third-degree circumferential burns of the extremity, thorax, or abdomen. Tissue edema that accumulates under a constrictive burn eschar can ultimately lead to compromise in the perfusion gradient resulting in pressure and ischemia induced neuromuscular damage, limb loss, and life-threatening compartment syndrome.

It is important to perform frequent serial examinations for capillary refill, sensation, compartment pressures, and digital artery Doppler signal to detect the development of compartment syndrome. Clinical suspicion may be confirmed by objective measurements of compartment pressure. An absolute compartment pressure >30 mm Hg or a $\Delta P <30$ mm Hg (MAP − compartment pressure) mandates escharotomy.

Escharotomies are performed with electrocautery to limit blood loss. Incisions are made over the limb on both the medial and lateral aspects to achieve complete eschar release. The underlying osteofascial compartments should be examined for compartment syndrome, and if suspected, standard fasciotomies are performed.

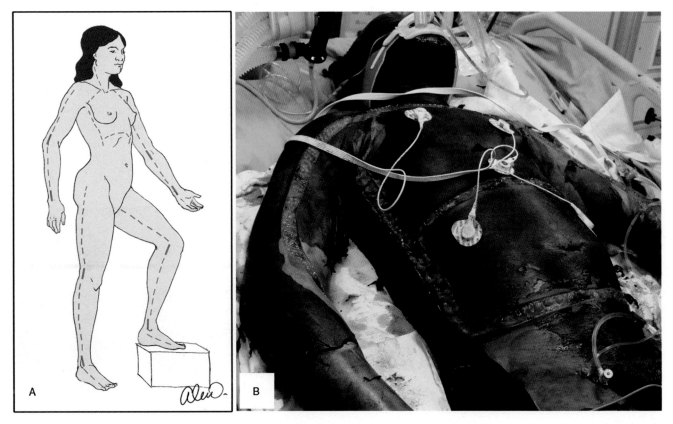

Figure 8.15 Escharotomy for circumferential burn. (A) Illustration of the recommended escharotomy incisions. (B) Truncal and extremity escharotomies in a household fire victim.

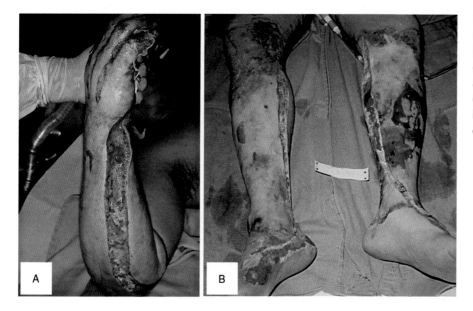

Figure 8.16 Escharotomy for circumferential extremity burn. (A) Circumferential deep second-degree burn requiring forearm and hand escharotomies. (B) Circumferential burns of the lower extremities requiring escharotomies.

Circumferential burns of the thorax may present with decreased chest wall compliance resulting in oxygenation and ventilation compromise. Thoracic compartment syndrome should be suspected if increased peak airway pressures, hypercarbia, and hypoxia are encountered. Properly performed escharotomies result in immediate improvements in chest wall compliance and improved arterial blood gas.

8.8 Scald Burns

Scald burns commonly result from hot water and mostly involve the elderly or children under 5 years old. Water at 60 degrees Celsius can cause full-thickness burns in 3 seconds, and governmental regulations to lower hot water tank temperatures have led to a decrease in such injuries. Scalds on skin with light clothing tend to be worse than on exposed skin areas, as the clothing tends to retain heat. Similarly, thick soup and sauce also tend to cause deep thermal injury. Cooking oil and grease can reach 200 degrees Celsius and is another common cause of scald injury. Tar burns are unique with similarly high temperatures

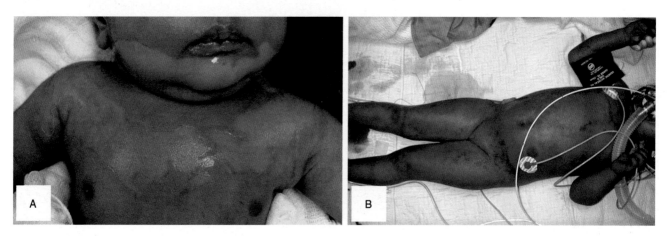

Figure 8.17 Scald burns. (A) Hot-water scald in a child. (B) A victim of child abuse by immersion into hot water.

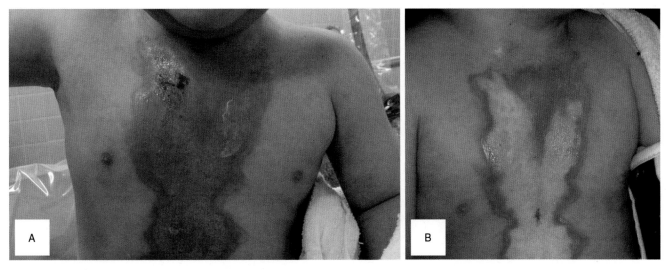

Figure 8.18 Scald burns. (A) Hot-milk scald in a child upon presentation. (B) The same child 2 days after presentation. Notice the conversion of superficial to deep second-degree burn.

and adherence to the skin. Removal of tar is facilitated with petroleum-based ointment. Deliberate scald burns account for 10% of child abuse cases.

Characteristic "immersion" patterns should promptly alarm the clinician of such possibility.

8.9 Chemical Burns

As a general rule, chemical burns should be copiously irrigated with water to limit further corrosion. The degree of tissue destruction is dependent on several factors including the concentration, form, and pH of the offending agent, duration and volume of contact, and the extent of irrigation.

In comparison to acids, alkaline agents typically produce more extensive damage by liquefactive

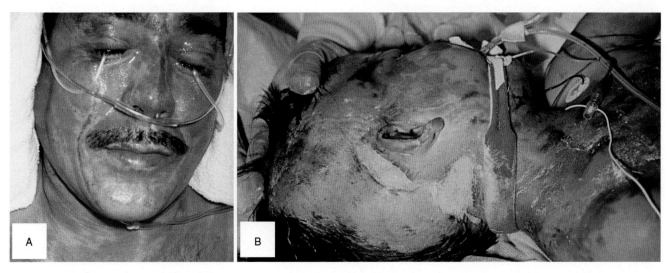

Figure 8.19 Chemical burns. (A) Muriatic acid burns to the face and eyes. Morgan lens eye irrigation is being performed. (B) Large second- and third-degree burns from 90% hydrosulfuric acid. This child accidentally reached for an open container that fell on his face.

necrosis in which the process continues through protein denaturation and fat saponification until all alkaline substances have been neutralized by the host tissue. On the other hand, the coagulative necrosis caused by acids is a self-limiting process once the denatured proteins and damaged tissue form a coagulum, thus limiting further acid penetration and tissue damage.

Hydrofluoric acid, typically found in household rust removal and cleaning products, is a special circumstance in that the acid produces liquefactive necrosis. With extensive exposure to biologic tissues, the fluoride ion precipitates calcium and can cause severe systemic hypocalcemia. In addition to copious wound irrigation, 2.5% calcium gluconate gel should be applied to the affected areas to create a CaF_2 precipitate which limits the spread of fluoride ion and also relieves pain. Patients should be monitored for signs of hypocalcemia, particularly cardiac manifestations such as prolongation of the QT interval, torsade de pointes, or ventricular fibrillation. Intravenous 10% calcium gluconate may be used in severe cases of hypocalcemia.

8.10 Electrical Burns

Electrical burns are differentiated into low voltage (<1000 V) and high voltage (>1000 V). Four mechanisms of injury exist: direct contact, electrical arc, flame, and flash burn. Current passing through the body from the point of entry to the grounding exit subjects the skin and underlying tissues to direct electrothermal injury. Electrical arc happens when current sparks between two objects of different electrical potentials that are not in physical contact with each other. These are high-voltage burns that may cause electrothermal injury as well as flame burns by igniting flammable items on the person such as

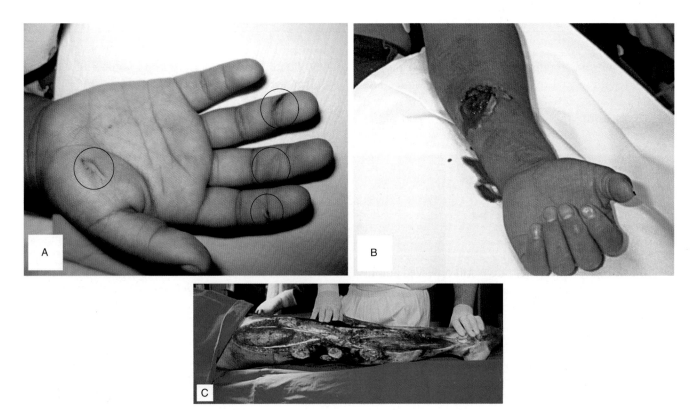

Figure 8.20 Electrical burns. (A) Low-voltage electrical burns to the hand from holding a defective electrical cord. (B) High-voltage electrical injury to the forearm of an electrician. (C) High-voltage electrical burn requiring lower extremity fasciotomies.

clothing. Flash burns are usually partial thickness and result from heat generated by nearby current arcs that cause thermal injury but do not actually enter the body.

Electrical burns are a unique entity in that the external signs of injury are deceptively benign in comparison to the extent of soft tissue damage. Electrical currents cause different amounts of tissue damage based on distinct tissue resistive properties. Nerves, vessels, and muscles are more susceptible to electrothermal damages while bone and skin are less so. Extensive myonecrosis may develop with resultant myoglobin-induced renal failure. Treatment is based on aggressive fluid resuscitation to achieve a urine output of 1 cc/kg per hour. Other unproven but commonly practiced treatments include the use of mannitol to induce an osmotic diuresis, and urine alkalinization with bicarbonate to prevent myoglobin precipitation in the renal tubules. Patients should be monitored for a minimum of 6 hours, and often up to 24 hours, for cardiac arrhythmias and the development of extremity compartment syndrome. When suspected, decompressive fasciotomy should be promptly performed to minimize ischemic and pressure-induced myonecrosis. Nerves and the lens are particularly susceptible to electrical insult. Long-term sequelae include permanent debilitating peripheral neuropathy and cataracts.

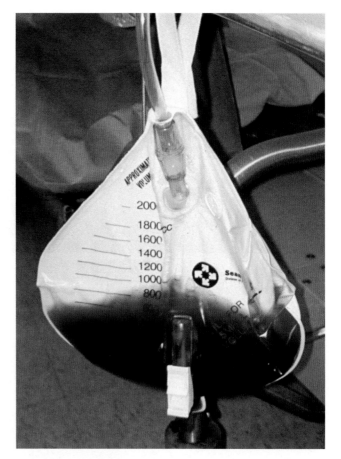

Figure 8.21 Myoglobinuria from electrical-burn-induced rhabdomyolysis.

8.11 Outcome of Burn Injury

Advances in burn wound management and critical care have improved mortality from 6.5% in 1995 to 4.7% in 2005. The highest mortality rate is still observed among inhalation injury. Among the 6.5% of admissions with inhalation injury, the mortality rate increased to 26.3%. Most of the mortalities occur at the ends of the age spectrum with 38% due to multisystem organ failure and only 4.1% due to wound sepsis.

Increased burn survival over the past several decades raises important quality of life issues. Studies have shown that the most significant predictors of improved quality of life include the size of full-thickness burn, age, degree of functional recovery of the hands, and perceived social support. Sixty-six percent of burn patients return to work, the likelihood and timing of which are directly related to the size and severity of the injury.

Cosmetic outcomes range from minor skin discoloration or hypertrophic scars, to debilitating contractures in untreated wounds.

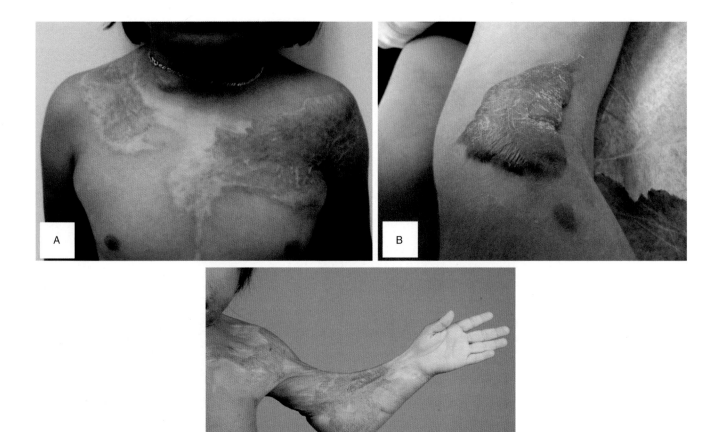

Figure 8.22 Late burn complications. (A) Healed appearance of split-thickness skin graft in a child who suffered scald burn. There is also noticeable skin discoloration in areas of superficial second-degree burn that healed without surgery. (B) Hypertrophic scar resulting from minor superficial second-degree burn over the lateral knee. (C) Debilitating contractures in a child with deep second- and third-degree burns that were not treated.

9 Soft Tissue Injuries

Demetrios Demetriades and Marko Bukur

Introduction

Extensive blunt soft tissue trauma may occur after traffic accidents, falls from significant heights, and crush injuries. They are common after major earthquakes (see Chapter 11, Disaster Medicine). They can be closed, open, or both.

Extensive soft tissue trauma following penetrating injuries may occur after high-velocity bullet wounds, closed-range shotgun injuries, and explosions (see Chapter 10, Ballistics).

Meticulous systematic and local examination should be performed to rule out other associated injuries. Locally, the physician should evaluate for underlying vascular, nerve, tendon, and bone injuries

Avulsion type injuries occur when a flap of tissue is separated from underlying tissue structures. The most extreme form of this injury is a degloving injury, which occurs when all the skin and subcutaneous tissues are separated from the underlying fascia. Tissue

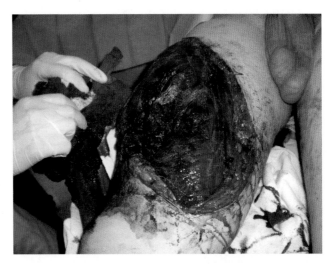

Figure 9.1 Auto-versus-pedestrian injury with significant tissue loss and an open femur fracture. The wound needs pressure irrigation and intravenous antibiotics to reduce the risk of osteomyelitis.

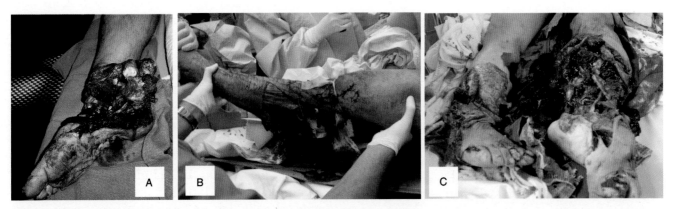

Figure 9.2 Mangled extremities: bleeding control by direct pressure or tourniquet application is the first priority. All these cases required amputations. Attempts to salvage these limbs are almost always unsuccessful and result in serious complications and prolonged hospitalization.

ischemia of the flap segment is the greatest concern and may lead to areas of large soft tissue defects.

Mangled extremity injuries often involve soft tissues, neurovascular structures, and bones. These injuries require a multidisciplinary approach because of their complexity and high risk of serious complications, including death, amputation, renal failure, and infection.

Complications

The following systemic complications may occur after extensive soft tissue trauma:

1. Hypovolemic shock, due to extravasation of blood and fluid externally or into the tissues.
2. Renal failure due to myoglobinemia and myoglobinuria.
3. Electrolytic abnormalities: Hyperkalemia (release of potassium from damaged cells), hypocalcemia (deposition of calcium in the injured tissues), or hyperphosphatemia. This combination of electrolytic abnormalities is highly cardiotoxic.
4. Hematological changes: Disseminated intravascular coagulopathy (DIC) due to release of tissue thromboplastin from the injured tissues.

Local complications
1. Compartment syndrome.
2. Infection of open wounds, closed hematomas, or damaged tissue.
3. Necrotizing soft tissue infection.

Investigations and Monitoring

All patients with extensive soft tissue trauma should have serial monitoring of the hemoglobin levels, platelet count, coagulation parameters, electrolytes, creative phosphokinase (CPK), and hourly urine output. In extremity injuries close monitoring for compartment syndrome is indicated. Vascular studies (CT scan angio, color flow Doppler, formal angiogram) should be performed as indicated to evaluate for associated vascular injuries. Compartment pressures should be considered in suspicious extremity injuries to rule out compartment syndrome.

Management

The treatment should address local and systemic problems. The local care of large open wounds should be provided in the operating room, often under general anesthesia. Only minor or closed wounds should be managed in the emergency room. Antibiotic prophylaxis should be administered routinely and tetanus prophylaxis should be considered in the appropriate cases.

Initial priorities should include hemorrhage control, a quick neurological exam, and photo documentation. Hemorrhage control is best achieved with digital compression when possible. Blind clamping of bleeding in the emergency department is not advised as this can lead to further neurovascular injury. If digital pressure is unable to control bleeding a commercial tourniquet or inflated blood pressure cuff may provide temporary hemostasis. Documentation of neurologic function and extent of tissue damage is important in cases where the extremity is unsalvageable and primary amputation necessary. In amputations, early involvement of a replant team, if available, is important to determine the likelihood of extremity salvage but should not delay addressing other life-threatening injuries.

Primary repair should be considered only in selected cases with clean incising wounds. In the majority of cases of extensive soft tissue trauma the wound should be debrided and left open to heal by secondary intention. Negative pressure dressings may be helpful in removing effectively any infected exudates and prevent the retraction of the wound edges.

Good hydration with intravenous fluids and aggressive diuresis to maintain the urine output at about 100 mL/hour for the first 24 hours may prevent acute renal failure in cases with severe myoglobinemia (CPK >5000 U/L). The urine pH should be neutral or slightly alkaline. This can be achieved by good hydration and intravenous $NaHCO_3$. Mannitol administration might be helpful as well.

In extremity injuries the muscle compartments should be monitored clinically and pressure measurements and timely decompressive fasciotomy should be performed in the appropriate cases (see Section 9.6, Extremity Compartment Syndrome).

9.1 Dog Bite Injury

About 2 million mammalian bite injuries occur yearly in the United States, 60–80% of which are attributed to dogs. Most of these bites occur in children and young adults and are usually secondary to unintentional provocation or perceived threatening behavior exhibited by the victim. In approximately 90% of cases the animal is known to the victim. Canine bites most commonly affect the extremities, followed by the head and neck, and trunk. However, children are more likely to suffer injuries to the head and neck due to their smaller stature. Injuries in this age group can be devastating as dogs can create depressed skull fractures, large scalp avulsions, intracranial bleeding, or major vascular injury in the neck or thoracic inlet. Similarly, large breeds can inflict serious wounds in adults as well with bite forces exceeding 450 pounds per square inch.

Dog bites may cause a variety of injury patterns including punctures, avulsions, tears, abrasions, and severe crush injury. Additionally, a high degree of suspicion for occult vascular injury should be maintained in attacks from larger dog breeds or law enforcement animals. Tenets of wound care include initial cleansing and irrigation which serves to remove debris and bacteria, and has been shown to decrease the transmission of the rabies virus. For large wounds, x-rays are important to rule out retained foreign bodies and underlying fractures. Grossly devitalized tissue and visible debris should be removed.

Liberal consultation of an orthopedic specialist should be obtained when the bite involves the hand. The hand contains a number of bones, nerves, and joints enclosed within a small space and relatively superficial location. Additionally, infection can rapidly progress along the fascial planes and tendon sheaths in the hand resulting in permanent disability if not rapidly treated. Primary closure of bite wounds remains a controversial issue. After appropriate wound care, simple lacerations can be repaired, especially on the face and neck, where cosmesis is a concern and wound infection less likely due to abundant vascular supply. Wounds that involve deep punctures, present more than 24 hours after injury, or have signs of infection should not be closed. Tetanus history should also be obtained from the patient and boosters and/or immunoglobulin administered where appropriate.

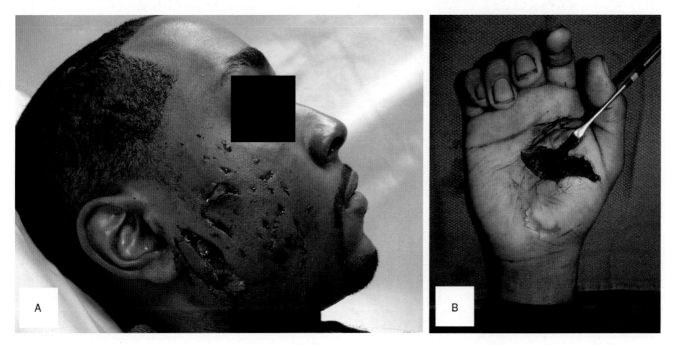

Figure 9.3 (A) Multiple facial lacerations caused by a pit bull bite attack, resulting in a parotid gland injury. The puncture wounds should be cleaned and left open. However, incising wounds like the one over the parotid should be repaired primarily. (B) Laceration of the hand with partial degloving of tissue from a pit bull bite. Hand injuries should be evaluated clinically for underlying tendon injuries and radiologically for associated fractures.

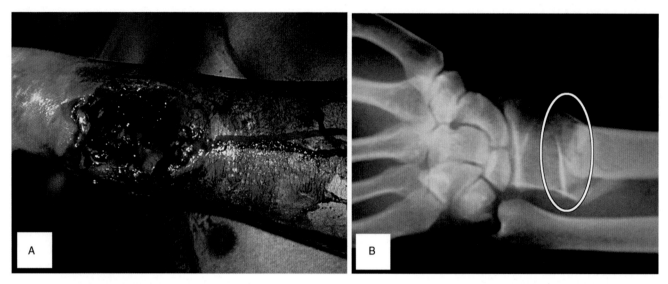

Figure 9.4 Severe dog bite of the forearm with tissue loss (A) and underlying radius fracture (B). The tendons and nerves should be evaluated clinically.

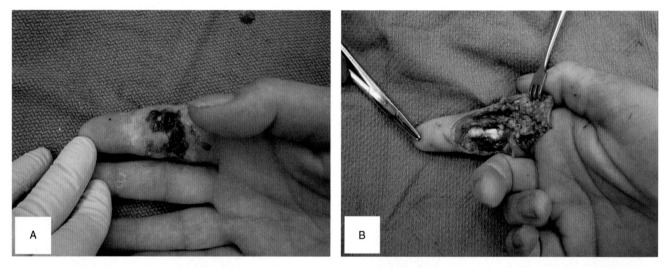

Figure 9.5 Dog bite injury with delayed presentation and severe finger infection (A). Surgical exploration shows spreading of the infection along the tendon sheath (B).

Infection after dog bite injury is a concern and dependent on multiple factors including bite location, type of bite, and delay in treatment, patient age, and comorbid factors. Infections are often polymicrobial and involve one or more of the following micro-organisms: *Pasteurella* spp., *Streptococcus* spp., *Staphylococcus* spp., *Morexella* spp., *Fusobacterium* spp., and *Bacteroides* spp. *Pasteurella* is sensitive to penicillin, tetracycline, and cephalosporins but resistant to erythromycin and aminoglycosides. Antibiotic prophylaxis after simple dog bite injuries is not indicated and should be reserved for complex wounds, injuries to the hand, delayed presentations, and the immunocompromised. Outpatient oral antibiotic

prophylaxis for a 3–5 day period is acceptable in those patients without clinical signs of local or systemic infection. Empiric coverage should be aimed at the aforementioned pathogens that colonize the offending animal's mouth. Amoxicillin–clavulanic acid is an excellent single agent choice for prophylaxis in those patients that are not allergic to penicillin. Alternative choices include doxycycline with metronizadole, fluoroquinolones with clindamycin, or trimethoprim–sulfamethoxazole. Established infections should be treated with intravenous antibiotics in the inpatient setting as these wounds are likely to require surgical debridement. Initial empiric therapy should cover the canine oral flora and potential skin flora of the patient. Ideally cultures of draining purulent fluid should be obtained prior to initiating therapy, but this should not delay care. Acceptable choices for initial therapy include β-lactam/β-lactamase inhibitor combinations (e.g., piperacillin–tazobactam, ampicillin–sulbactam), carbapenems, or cephalosporins and fluoroquinolones with metronizadole. Urgent surgical evaluation should also be obtained for source control particularly for injuries to the hand.

Infection with rabies is the most serious potential complication associated with canine bites, and is a rare entity in the United States due to effective animal control and vaccination. However, the high mortality rate with established infection demands vigilance for screening and prophylaxis as immunotherapy is ineffective once clinical symptoms have manifested. When the offending animal is unavailable for observation, has unknown vaccination status, or suspected to be a stray, local public health consultation should be contacted to obtain the local prevalence of rabies in the assaulting species. Rabies prophylaxis should be given based upon the exposure risk and epidemiological data for the area.

9.2 Cat Bite Injury

Cat bites are the second most common mammalian injury and account for 5–15% of all bite injuries in the United States. Almost two-thirds of bites involve the upper extremities followed by the head/neck, and lower extremities. Due to the small size of domestic cats in North America these injuries are less destructive and life-threatening compared with dog bites.

Many of these injuries are not initially evaluated by medical personnel because of their innocuous appearance, thus delaying presentation. However, the sharp, slender teeth of cats cause puncture wounds which inoculate organisms deep into the soft tissues, predisposing cat bites to a higher risk of infection. Additionally, if bites occur near joints there is a risk of subsequent osteomyelitis or septic arthritis.

Liberal imaging and orthopedic consultation should be obtained when injuries occur in these areas to prevent debilitating complications associated with uncontrolled infection. Because of the high risk of infection, prophylactic antibiotics and close follow-up are necessary to detect complications. The oral flora of cats is almost identical to that found in dogs and thus antibiotic therapy is similar. Rabies transmission, though less common than in dogs, is possible and should be screened for adequately. These bites are almost always punctures and they should never be sutured because of the high risk of infection. Tetanus history should be obtained from the patient and prophylaxis should be administered where appropriate.

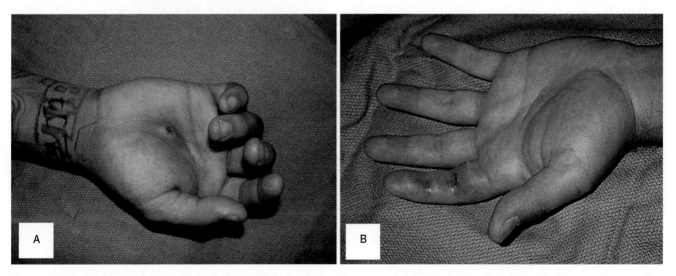

Figure 9.6 Examples of typical cat bite injuries. (A) Note the small puncture wound of the palm surrounded by erythema and edema from resultant infection. (B) Infected cat bite resulting in flexor tenosynovitis of the index finger.

9.3 Human Bite Injury

Most commonly these bites are the result of assault with injuries frequently involving the hands and upper extremity. A crushing and tearing mechanism causes tissue destruction and devitalization. Additionally, the human mouth contains a high concentration of about 100 different virulent bacteria. This combination results in a high incidence of infections. The most common pathogens are *Streptococcus* and *Staphylococcus* species.

A special category of human bites is the clenched-fist injuries, otherwise known as the "fight bite." These injuries occur from one individual punching another in the mouth with considerable force at impact. The wounds classically appear over the dorsal aspect of the third, fourth, or fifth metacarpophalangeal joints and appear benign due their small size. Careful examination of the dorsum of the hand in the "clenched-fist" position should be carried out after a history of fist fighting. In over 50% of clenched fist injuries there is penetration of the metacarpophalangeal joint with subsequent tendon and cartilage injury. The bone may be involved in many cases. Patients typically extend their hands after injury which allows deeper penetration of bacteria into the joint space or tendon sheath allowing proximal extension into hand or wrist causing tenosynovitis, septic arthritis, or osteomyelitis. Infections may spread aggressively due to the complex tendon sheath anatomy of the hand as well as the relative avascularity of these structures. Plain film investigation should also be done to rule out occult fractures or retained teeth. All clenched-fist injuries should be examined by an experienced hand surgeon due to the limited options of reconstruction once established infection has set in. Only 10% of patients with septic arthritis will regain function and amputation may be necessary in many cases.

Most human bites can safely be managed on an outpatient basis. However, infected bites and those with joint or tendon sheath penetration should be admitted for intravenous antibiotics, debridement, and close observation.

The early management of these bites should include wound irrigation to facilitate examination and removal of any visible foreign bodies. Immobilization in the point of function of the extremity and elevation are essential. Surgical exploration may be indicated for those bites where tendon or joint damage is suspected.

Most bites can safely be sutured primarily, especially in cases with lacerations or loss of tissue in the face and neck. However, puncture bites, any type of bites on the hands, or cases with delayed presentation at the hospital the wound should never be sutured because of the high risk of infection. Close follow-up should be done in the 48–72 hours after wound closure to ensure that no delayed infection has occurred. In addition, prophylactic antibiotics and tetanus therapy is necessary in these high-risk wounds. Acceptable agents for prophylaxis include amoxicillin–clavulanic acid, fluoroquinolones with clindamycin or trimethoprim–sulfamethoxazole, or doxycycline in those that are allergic to penicillin. Prophylaxis is generally carried out for a period of 3–5 days. Established infections such as cellulitis, abscess formation, and septic arthritis will require longer durations of therapy and treatment should be tailored based upon available cultures.

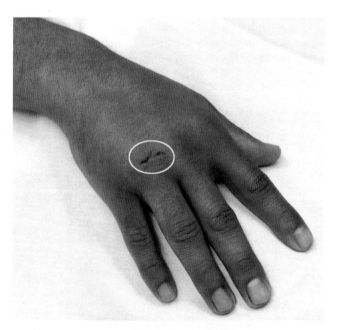

Figure 9.7 Classic appearance of the "fight bite" injury. It is imperative to rule out underlying tendinous and osseous injuries. This type of injury is associated with a high risk for serious infection.

It is also important to consider infectious disease transmission after human bite exposure. Transmission of herpes, syphilis, hepatitis B and C, as well as other infectious pathogens has been reported. Additionally, the human immunodeficiency virus (HIV) has been detected in the saliva of infected patients and case reports of possible infection have been reported. However, given the low level of the virus in saliva routine post-exposure prophylaxis for HIV is not needed. Consideration for prophylaxis should be reserved for those patients assaulted by a known HIV-positive individual with a high viral load. Baseline and 6-month serological tests should also be offered to the patient. Similarly, routine prophylaxis for hepatitis B is unwarranted. For those individuals bitten by an individual known to harbor the virus, immunoglobulin and accelerated vaccination should be offered to unimmunized individuals.

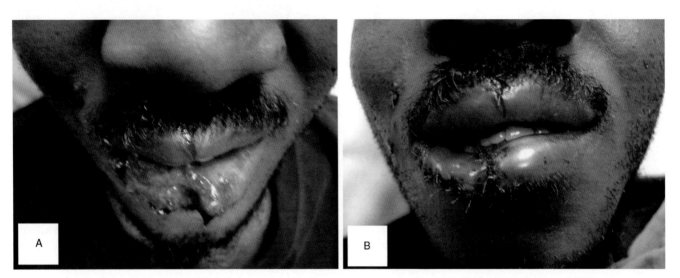

Figure 9.8 (A) Human bite of the lower lip with loss of tissue. (B) Primary repair is safe and provides good results.

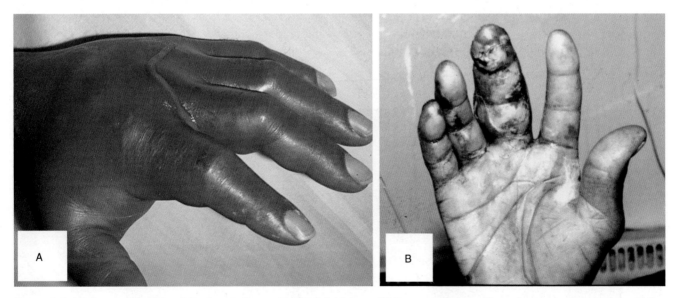

Figure 9.9 (A) Severe infection of the hand after a clenched-fist injury. (B) Severe tenosynovitis and osteomyelitis of the middle finger following a human bite. In neglected cases like this, there is a high risk for finger loss.

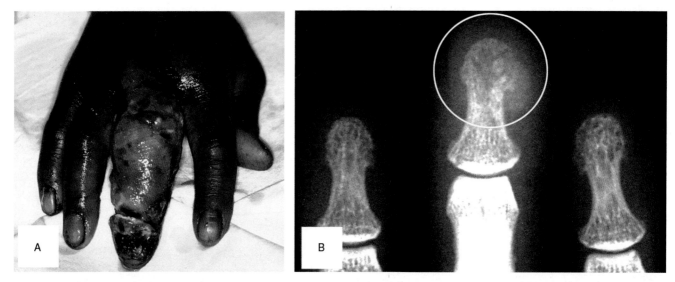

Figure 9.10 Severe tenosynovitis and osteomyelitis of the middle finger following a human bite (A). Note osteomyelitis of the distal phalanx (B).

9.4 High-Pressure Injection Injury

High-pressure injection injuries to the hand are often occupationally related and have devastating complications. These injuries are commonly the result of paint guns, grease guns, and diesel injectors. Though paint and grease are the most commonly injected chemicals, other substances may be implicated. The injury involves tremendous forces, as the injector guns use pressures of 2,000–10,000 psi, and thus direct hand contact with the paint gun is not necessary.

Physical examination may initially reveal an innocuous-looking wound, though as hours progress, a severe inflammatory process is seen. The affected digit is often swollen and may be pale from associated vascular compromise. Radiographs may reveal discrete opaque areas that can help delineate the extent of deep injury. Emergency therapy includes splinting, tetanus prophylaxis, and broad-spectrum antimicrobial coverage. These injection injuries are extremely serious and have a high rate of amputation and long-term disability. Urgent hand surgery consultation is imperative, as most patients will require emergency operative debridement and decompression.

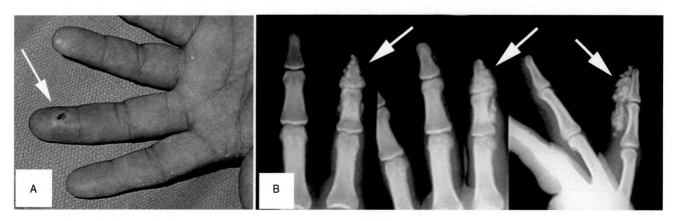

Figure 9.11 High-pressure injection injury. Despite their innocent-looking appearance they are serious injuries (A). Radiological appearance of paint injected under pressure along the flexor tendon sheath (B).

9.5 Retained Foreign Body

Retained foreign bodies in an open wound commonly cause poor wound healing and predispose to subsequent infection. Thus, all lacerations should be carefully examined to rule out the presence of a retained foreign body. If the full wound cannot be clearly visualized, plain radiographs are warranted to rule out a deep foreign body. X-rays reliably detect radiopaque material, but common objects made of wood or plastic will still be missed, and other imaging modalities such as ultrasound or MRI may be necessary in certain cases. Most authors consider glass wounds high risk, given the ability of glass to break into multiple small pieces, and thus liberal use of x-rays to detect retained glass foreign bodies is recommended.

Bullets or missile fragments are a special category of retained foreign bodies. Removal of these missiles does not reduce the risk of infection and in most cases they can be left in the body. Removal should be considered in superficially located missiles and in cases with intra-articular location or compression of major nerves or the spinal cord.

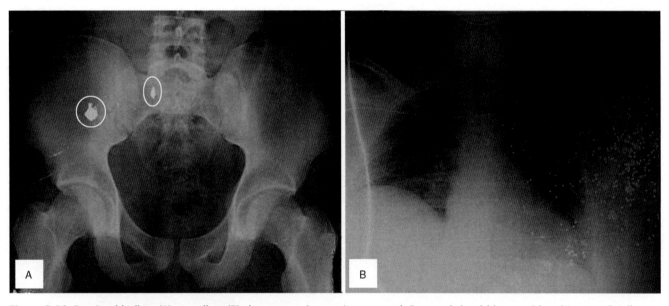

Figure 9.12 Retained bullets (A) or pellets (B) do not require routine removal. Removal should be considered in superficially located missiles and in cases with intra-articular location or compression of major nerves or the spinal cord.

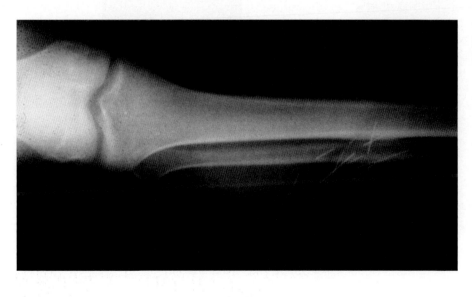

Figure 9.13 Multiple needles inserted in the subcutaneous tissue by a psychiatric patient.

Intentionally inserted sharp foreign bodies into the soft tissues, usually needles, may be found in psychiatric patients and victims of child or elderly abuse. Routine removal of these objects in asymptomatic psychiatric cases may not be advisable because these patients usually return with another self-inserted foreign object. In cases of abuse the foreign bodies should be managed case by case, based on the location of the needle and the complexity of any operation to remove them.

9.6 Extremity Compartment Syndrome

Compartment syndrome is an acute, limb-threatening emergency that occurs when the intra-compartmental pressure rises dangerously within a closed osteofascial space. Normal compartment pressure is less than 8 mm Hg. As the pressure rises, arterial perfusion diminishes and at a critical point stops completely. At an intracompartmental pressure higher than of 20–30 mm Hg, the blood flow to the muscles and nerves may be impaired resulting in ischemic damage and in neglected cases necrosis and permanent damage requiring amputation.

The lower leg is the most commonly affected site, followed by the forearm, thigh, arm, and buttocks, in that order. Causes of compartment syndrome include complex fractures, vascular injuries, hematomas, tight dressings or casts, burns, excessive exercise, infiltrated infusions, massive fluid transfusion, and prolonged immobilization or pressure on a limb.

Clinical Presentation and Investigations

Classic teaching includes evaluating for the six *P*s associated with compartment syndrome: pain, pallor, paresthesias, poikilothermia, paralysis, and pulselessness. Unfortunately, many of these signs such as pallor, paralysis, and loss of pulse are late findings, and permanent damage may already have occurred by the time these signs appear. Deep burning pain that is

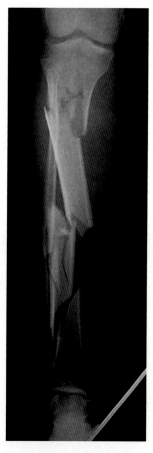

Figure 9.15 Severe communited fractures are at a high risk for compartment syndrome.

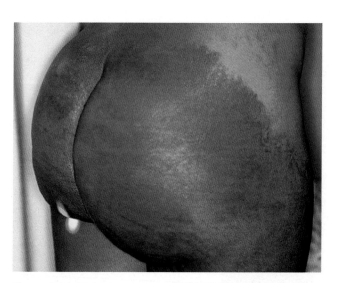

Figure 9.14 Compartment syndrome of the buttocks from a violent beating.

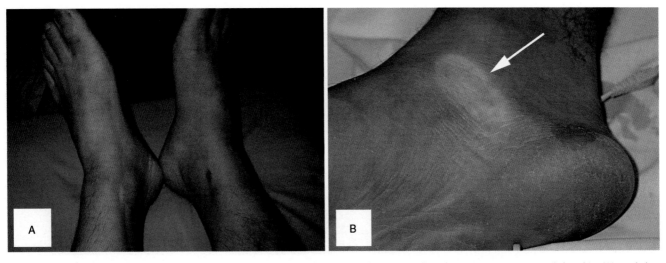

Figure 9.16 Delayed diagnosis of compartment syndrome of the right leg. Note the cyanotic appearance of the skin (A) and the delayed capillary refill of the skin (B). These are late symptoms and at this stage the limb is not salvageable.

out of proportion to the apparent injury is an important early clue to the condition, along with an increase of the pain on passive stretching of the involved muscle group. However, these useful findings cannot be detected in the unconscious or heavily sedated patient. Prompt trauma surgery or orthopedic consultation is necessary in suspected cases.

Compartment pressure measurement is a helpful adjunct in borderline cases and can easily be done by placing a needle pressure transducer within the compartment in question. When compartment syndrome is considered, the pressures of all the compartments in that extremity should be measured. Thus, in the lower leg which has four compartments, four different measurements should be obtained. Good knowledge of the anatomy of the compartments in each area is important for correct diagnosis and adequate fasciotomies. Though compartment pressures help diagnose the syndrome, the patient's clinical symptoms and signs should also be taken into account when making the diagnosis.

Pressures less than 20 mm Hg generally do not cause acute compartment syndrome but may warrant admission and serial examination. Pressures greater than 30 mm Hg are an indication for definitive therapy in the form of fasciotomy. Pressures between 20 and 30 mm Hg are considered to be in a "gray zone" area. In the presence of hypotension, these pressures can cause tissue ischemia and a fasciotomy should be considered more liberally.

Complications of compartment syndrome include muscle necrosis and infection which may result in loss of the limb. Adequate hydration is important, as

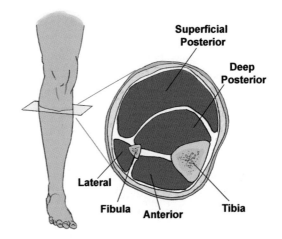

Figure 9.17 The lower leg is the most common site developing compartment syndrome. Good knowledge of the anatomy of the compartments is essential for the diagnosis and treatment of the syndrome. In assessing for compartment syndrome, pressures should be measured in all four compartments. Similarly, during fasciotomy all compartments need to be decompressed.

muscle breakdown can lead to rhabdomyolysis and myoglobinuric renal failure. In the long term, in many patients ischemic muscle is slowly converted to an elastic fibrous tissue, which leads to the development of Volkmann's contractures.

Management

Treat any treatable causes, such as by removal of tight casts, performance of escharotomy in circumferential

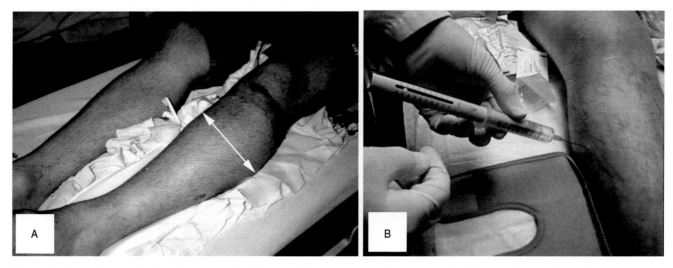

Figure 9.18 Swelling and pain of an extremity following blunt or penetrating trauma should raise the suspicion of compartment syndrome (A). Pressure measurements with one of the commercially available devices should be performed in all suspected cases (B).

burns, evacuation of any large hematomas, timely repair of arterial injuries, etc. Mannitol (0.5–1 g/kg over 20 minutes) may be helpful in borderline cases and might reduce the need for fasciotomy. Fasciotomy and decompression should be performed without delay in all cases with a confirmed diagnosis of compartment syndrome.

Common Mistakes and Pitfalls

1. Covering with bandages or casts the toes or fingers of a severely injured extremity, especially if the patient is pharmacologically sedated or paralyzed. Ischemic problems may be missed.
2. Treating persistent and disproportionate pain with higher doses of analgesics, without ruling out compartment syndrome.
3. Relying on clinical examination alone to diagnose compartment syndrome. Clinical examination can be very unreliable. In suspected cases measure the compartment pressures.
4. Technical errors in measuring the compartment pressures are common. Measurements should be performed in *ALL* compartments (i.e., four measurements in the lower leg).

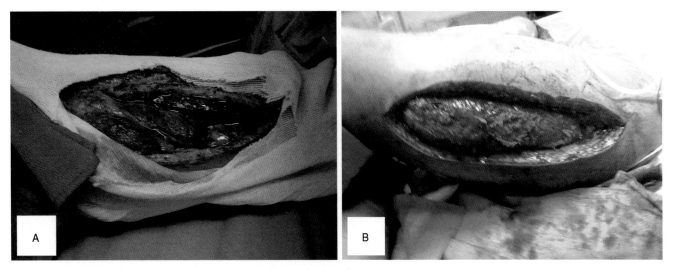

Figure 9.19 (A) Necrotic muscle of the lower leg following delayed treatment of a compartment syndrome. All dead tissues need to be excised. (B) Same patient after removal of nonviable muscle. Note the healthy color of the remaining muscle.

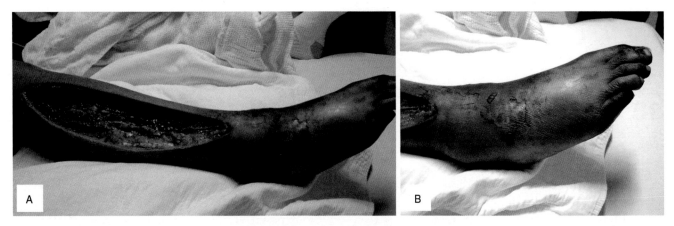

Figure 9.20 Nonsalvageable leg following delayed treatment of compartment syndrome. Note that even after extensive muscle debridement there is still a significant amount of dead tissue and exposure of the neurovascular structures (A). Note the necrotic toes and patches of dead skin (B). This patient required amputation of the leg.

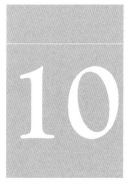

Ballistics

Ramon Cestero, David Plurad, and Demetrios Demetriades

Introduction

Firearm injuries account for nearly 860,000 admissions per year and are responsible for more than 20% of all trauma deaths in the United States. War injuries, especially due to high-velocity missiles and bomb explosions, pose special and complex problems. It is essential that surgeons and emergency physicians have a good understanding of the mechanisms of tissue damage with these injuries and have an excellent knowledge of the basic principles in the evaluation and management of these challenging traumas.

10.1 Definitions

Caliber: The caliber of a handgun or rifle is typically described as the diameter of the bore, although this can sometimes vary depending on how the diameter is measured. For example, a 0.38 bullet refers to a bullet that can be fired along a bore which measures 0.38 inches in diameter. The caliber is expressed in inches in the USA (for example 0.45 inches) or mm in other countries (for example 9 mm).

Bullet designs: Traditional bullets are made of lead, a relatively soft material which expands on impact and increases damage to the intended target as more energy is imparted. Harder bullet materials, such as lead alloy, copper, bronze, and steel limit this mushrooming effect on impact and can therefore penetrate deeper into tissues, but may not transfer as much energy if they completely traverse the target.

(a) **Jacketed Bullets:** At velocities greater than 2000 ft/sec, lead bullets begin to strip and deposit metal as they travel down the barrel, increasing the probability of jamming. To avoid this problem, a "jacket" of a harder metal such as copper or zinc can either partially or completely enclose the softer lead core. In addition the jacket provides stability to the missile and prevents fragmentation of deformation on impact. Civilian hollow-point and soft-point bullets are only partially jacketed, leaving the lead core exposed at the tip which can then flatten out or mushroom on impact. Hunting rifle bullets are not jacketed and deform or fragment on impact, causing extensive tissue damage. An unjacketed bullet can cause up to 40 times more tissue damage than a jacketed bullet. Military bullets, constrained in design by the Hague Convention, are completely surrounded by a metal jacket ("full-metal jacket"), thereby preventing deformation upon impact.

(b) **Hollow-Point Bullets:** These missiles deform on impact and increase tissue damage. They are prohibited by the Geneva Convention for military use but are common in civilian use.

(c) **Scored Bullets:** Scoring of the bullet encourages fragmentation on impact which results in increased tissue damage.

(d) **"Black Talon" Bullets:** The missile is covered with a copper jacket, which on impact peels back to form six sharp petals. These sharp edges can injure the exploring finger of the surgeon during attempts to remove the bullet.

(e) **PTFE (Teflon)-Coated Bullets:** Teflon-coated bullets are designed to reduce the wear on the barrel and to decrease the chance of ricochet, and are more likely to penetrate bullet-proof vests (popularly called "cop killers"). Armor-piercing designs, in which the bullet core is made of a hard substance such as depleted uranium or steel, are sometimes coated in Teflon and are not available for civilian use.

(f) **Explosive Bullets:** The bullet tip contains a small cavity filled with a low amount of explosive and explodes upon impacting a hard surface, such as bone. It often fails to explode and there is a risk of subsequent explosion during manipulation by the surgeon.

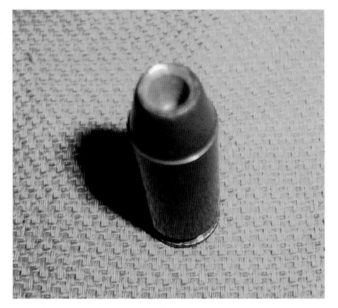

Figure 10.1 Hollow-point bullets are designed to expand on impact and transfer kinetic energy to the target.

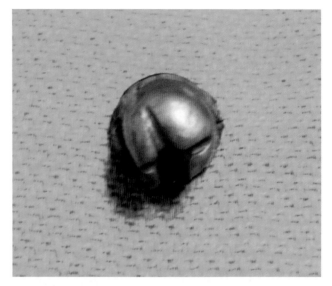

Figure 10.3 Bullet scoring promotes fragmentation on impact and increased tissue damage.

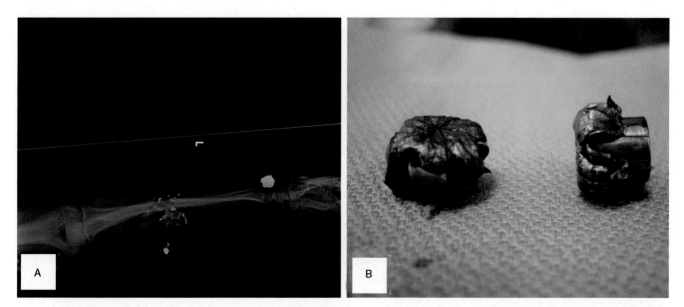

Figure 10.2 (A) Victim with gunshot wounds with "Black Talon" bullets. Left forearm x-ray with resultant fracture of radius and ulna. (B) Hollow-point "Black Talon" bullets removed from the victim. The copper jacket peels back into six sharp petals upon impacting tissue, causing more tissue damage. The sharp petals may cut the exploring finger of the surgeon during the operation.

Bullet Velocity: This refers to the velocity of the missile at the muzzle of the gun and plays a critical role in the amount of inflicted tissue damage. The kinetic energy of missiles is determined by the mass of the projectile and its velocity:

$$KE = 1/2(\text{mass})(\text{velocity})^2$$

However, the degree of tissue destruction is not always proportional to the speed of the missile. The damage is proportional to the energy released into the tissues. Often the missile passes through the tissues without any major release of energy and results in modest damage. Ballistics studies have shown that an AK-47 bullet releases its maximum energy only after traveling 25–30 cm into the tissues. If this bullet travels through a thin anatomical structure (e.g., the forearm) it might cause fairly limited damage.

10.2 Low-Velocity Projectiles

Low-velocity bullets (<1000 feet or <340 meters per second) are commonly used in civilian firearms (handgun 9 mm at 280 m/sec, handgun 0.45 inches at 255 m/sec). These bullets cause damage by direct crushing and laceration of tissues in the path of the missile. This path of destruction is referred to as the "permanent cavity." Secondary injuries can occur as the bullet fragments or impacts bone, imparting kinetic energy to these structures and converting them into secondary missiles.

The entrance wound is often characterized by an "abrasion ring" which develops at the edges of the skin defect and is typically round in appearance. This is caused as the bullet abrades the epidermis at the edges of the bullet path, leaving a reddish-brown circumferential ring on the damaged skin. This ring may develop irrespective of range but it does not appear on palms, soles, axilla, and scalp. In comparison to entrance wounds, exit wounds generally tend to be larger and more irregular in shape. As a bullet travels through the body, it tends to deform and tumble, so a larger area of the bullet is presented at the skin as it exits. This causes an irregularly shaped wound at the skin surface. However, despite entrance and exit wounds having some

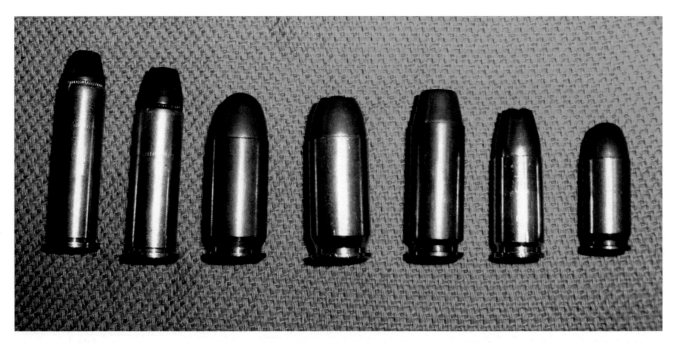

Figure 10.4 Examples of low-velocity bullets used in handguns, including hollow-point bullets.

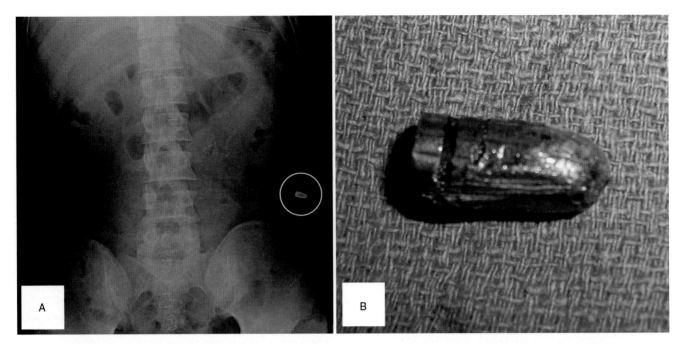

Figure 10.5 Radiological appearance (A) of non-fragmented and not deformed low-velocity bullet (B) recovered from gunshot victim.

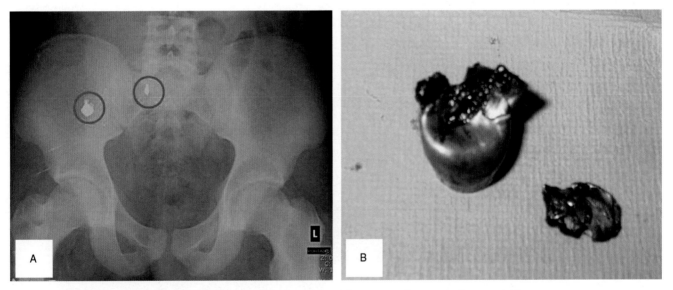

Figure 10.6 Bullet fragmentation. Radiological appearance (A) and fragments after surgical removal (B).

individual unique visual characteristics, frequently they cannot be differentiated on visual examination alone. From a medicolegal point of view the physician should describe the appearance of all wounds, ideally with photo documentation, avoiding any characterization of a wound as entry or exit.

Assessment of all missile injuries, irrespective of velocity, includes physical examination and radiologic studies (x-ray, CT scan, CT angiography, Doppler studies), in order to determine the bullet path, fragmentation, and injuries to the underlying organs, bones, or neurovascular structures. Wound management includes washout, tetanus prophylaxis, and a clean dressing. There is no need for surgical debridement and the wound should not be sutured because of the high incidence of infection.

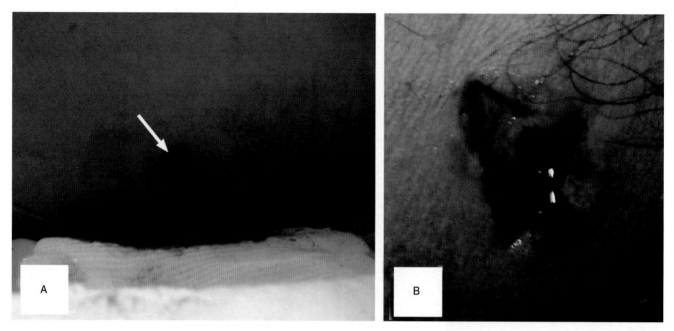

Figure 10.7 (A) Close-up image of entry site of a low-velocity gunshot wound, with erythematous abrasion ring at the edges of the circumferential wound. (B) Close-up image of the exit wound. Note the larger and irregular edges caused by the tumbling bullet.

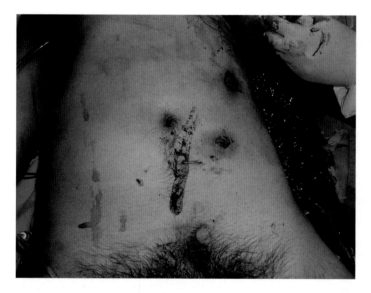

Figure 10.8 Multiple low-velocity gunshot wounds to the anterior abdomen. The wounds do not need debridement and they should not be sutured.

10.3 High-Velocity Projectiles

High-velocity missiles (>1000 ft/sec or 340 m/sec) are mainly used by the military but they are not uncommon in urban civilian injuries (AK-47 rifle at 1,130 m/sec, M-16 rifle at 1,100 m/sec, 0.347 handgun at 423 m/sec). They cause much more extensive tissue destruction than low-velocity missiles and the mechanism of injury is more complex. High-velocity bullets travel straight without any tumbling. However, some bullets (AK-47, M-16) flip once (180 degrees) once they hit the tissues and then travel backwards. This

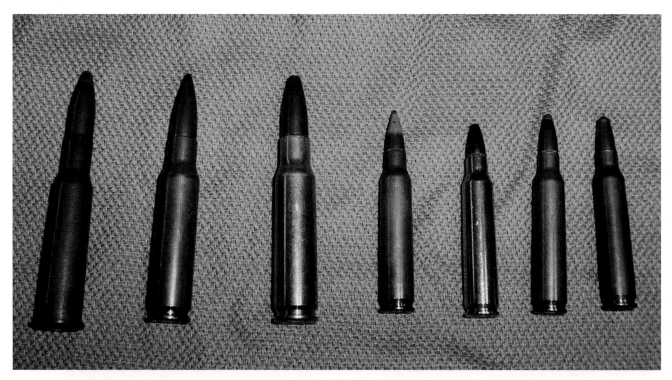

Figure 10.9 Examples of high-velocity bullets typically used in military and hunting weapons. Note the jacketing used to prevent lead stripping as the bullet travels down the barrel.

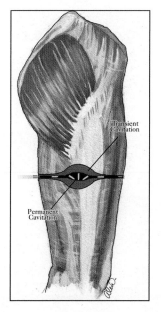

Figure 10.10 The damage in high-velocity missile injuries is proportional to the energy released into the tissues. Ballistics studies have shown that an AK-47 bullet releases its maximum energy only after traveling 25–30 cm into the tissues. If the bullet travels through a thin anatomical structure (e.g., the forearm) it might cause fairly limited damage. Note the permanent cavitation which is aggravated by the bullet tumbling. The transient cavitation is much larger than the diameter of the bullet.

tumbling increases the tissue damage. In addition to the direct crushing and laceration (as with low-velocity missiles), high-velocity missiles also cause damage laterally along their path by transient cavitation. During cavitation, tissues are essentially pushed in an outward fashion for several milliseconds as the bullet travels, causing a temporary cavity which can be up to 10 times larger than the diameter of the bullet. Solid organs, such as bone, liver, kidneys, and spleen, are more susceptible to cavitation than hollow or air-containing organs. The role of the supersonic or shock wave of the high-velocity missiles in tissue damage is not clear. As the bullet travels through tissue, rapid pressure changes are generated which can potentially damage surrounding organs. Although this is debatable, there is some evidence directly linking traumatic brain injury and pressure waves.

The management of high-velocity bullet wounds includes debridement of obviously devitalized tissue, removal of foreign material, antibiotics, and tetanus prophylaxis. Some surgeons recommend routine extensive surgical debridement while others are more conservative. The treatment should not be based exclusively on the information that a high-velocity bullet was the wounding mechanism. Even ballistic experts often cannot distinguish between low- and

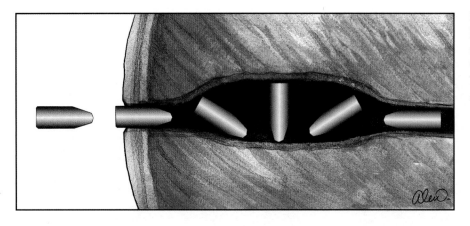

Figure 10.11 Some high-velocity bullets (AK-47, M-16) flip once (180 degrees) when they hit the tissues and then travel backwards. This tumbling increases the tissue damage.

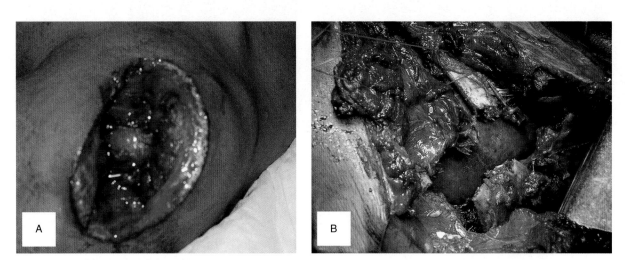

Figure 10.12 (A, B) Military high-velocity injuries caused by an AK-47 assault rifle, with extensive tissue destruction. These injuries need surgical debridement and the wound should be left open.

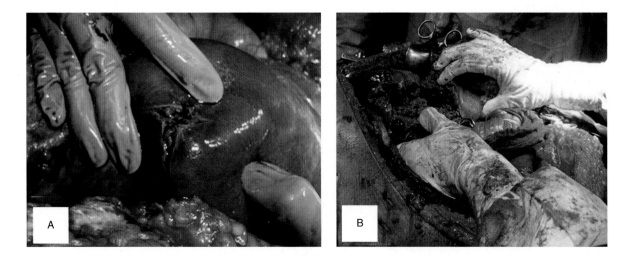

Figure 10.13 Comparison of injuries from low-velocity (A) versus high-velocity gunshot wounds (B and C) to the liver. Note the increased amount of liver damage and tissue destruction from high-velocity projectiles compared to the much less severe injury from a low-velocity bullet. Factors such as cavitation and the shock wave phenomenon are responsible for the more destructive effects of high-velocity missiles.

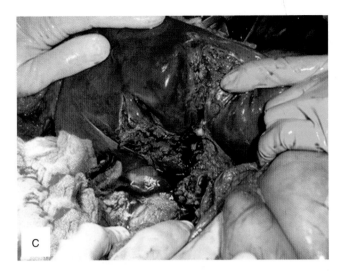

Figure 10.13 (*cont.*)

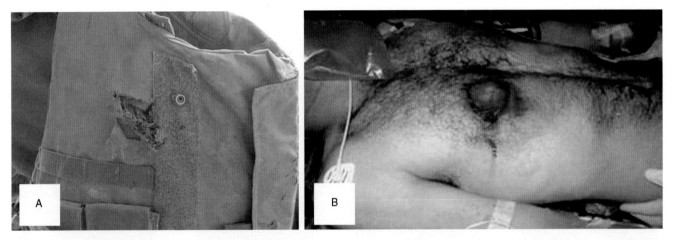

Figure 10.14 (A) Ballistic vests are made from multiple layers of strong woven fibers. The layers are designed to "catch" a bullet, thereby deforming it, and dissipating its energy to a larger area of the vest. Ceramic plates are added to ballistic vests to afford protection against high-velocity rounds. (B) Blunt injuries can occur beneath the vest as the body absorbs the remaining energy from the round.

high-velocity injuries. It is essential to individualize the care of each patient and "treat the wound, not the velocity." It is important to leave wounds open and avoid primary closure, as these wounds almost always become infected due to the amount of tissue damage. Frequent re-examination of the wound is recommended, as devitalized tissue can become infected or necrotic over the ensuing days after injury.

10.4 Shotgun Injuries

Whereas handguns and rifles fire a single bullet down a grooved (rifled) barrel, shotguns have a smooth bore and can fire up to several hundred pellets at a time.

The term "gauge" refers to the weight of a lead ball, in fractions of a pound that would have the same internal diameter of the barrel. Therefore, a 12-gauge

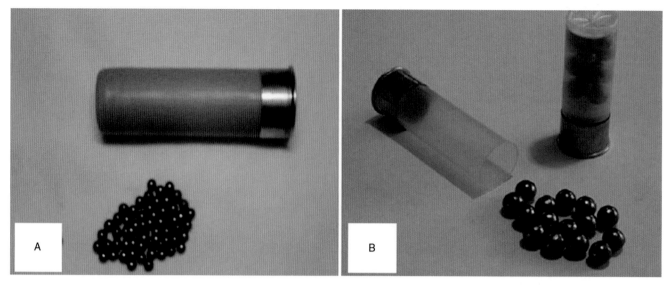

Figure 10.15 Shotgun injuries. (A) Birdshot shells. (B) Buckshot shells.

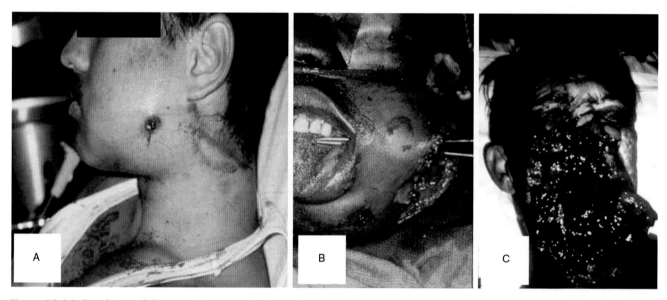

Figure 10.16 Gunshot and shotgun injuries to the face. (A) Low-velocity gunshot wound with minimal tissue damage. (B) High-velocity gunshot wound with extensive tissue damage. (C) Close-range shotgun injury with massive tissue destruction.

shotgun has an internal barrel diameter that would fit a lead sphere weighing 1/12th of a pound. Shotgun shells are constructed of a plastic case filled with primer, wadding (paper and plastic which provides a gas seal), and the corresponding shot (birdshot or buckshot). As indicated by the name of the intended target, birdshot pellets are smaller in size than buckshot pellets. Shotguns can also fire large slugs which are designed for hunting large animals.

The distance from the shotgun to the point of impact and the length of the barrel are major determinants of the magnitude of injury. Since the muzzle velocity of shotguns is close to 500 m/sec, these injuries can cause a devastating amount of tissue damage at close range. At very short distances (<2 meters), the entire shot charge (along with the wadding) is deposited into the wound, causing severe trauma and typically resulting in a single-hole wound with massive underlying destruction. Powder tattooing, in which the still-burning gunpowder embeds in the skin, may be seen around the wound edges. At ranges between 2 and 6 meters, there is still significant destruction but the degree of injury decreases as distance increases. The diameter of the circular wound

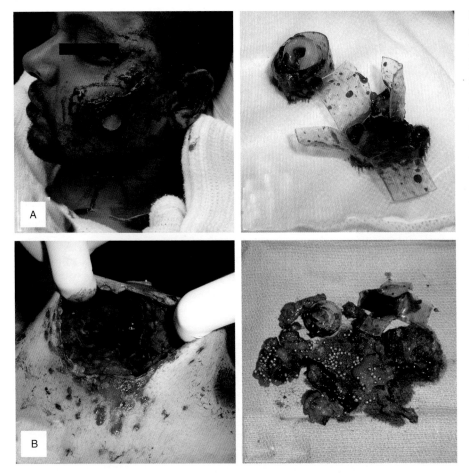

Figure 10.17 At close range (<6 meters), shotgun injuries cause massive tissue damage. In closer ranges (<2 meters) the shotgun shell and wadding may be lodged into the tissues. (A) Close-range shotgun wound to the face with wadding embedded in the soft tissues. (B) Close-range shotgun wound to the shoulder with significant tissue loss. Note the wadding and numerous pellets which were removed from the subcutaneous tissues and the underlying muscles.

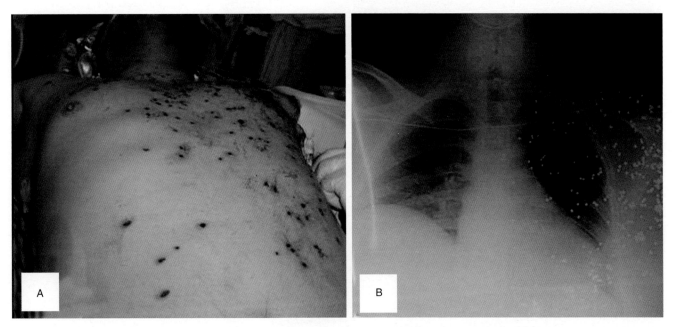

Figure 10.18 Long-distance (>6 meters) shotgun injuries cause minor or modest damage and the pellets often remain in the skin. (A) Shotgun injury to the chest and abdomen from a long distance. There is significant spread of the pellets and the damage to the tissues is superficial. (B) The chest x-ray shows the spread of the pellets. (C) The abdominal CT scan shows no intraperitoneal involvement.

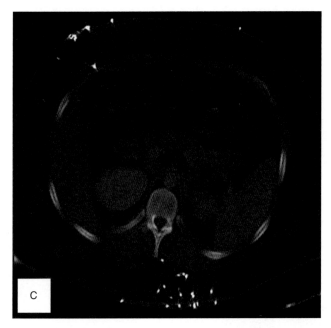

Figure 10.18 (*cont.*)

gradually enlarges until a distance is reached where individual pellets separate from the main charge and can be seen individually entering the skin. Due to a significant loss of kinetic energy at greater distances (>6 meters), shotgun injuries cause fairly limited tissue damage.

Sawn-off shotguns are often used by criminals in order to conceal the weapon. In this situation, the pellets lose most of their velocity and in distances >4 meters cause minimal damage.

Due to the multiple pellets involved, x-rays and CT angio evaluation should be part of the routine evaluation of shotgun injuries, as each missile can cause injury along its individual path. Angiographic evaluation should be considered if vascular injury is a potential concern, as in extremity or neck injuries.

Close-range wounds require extensive surgical debridement and open gauze packing. No reconstruction should be considered in the acute stage. Long-distance injuries to the soft tissues do not require any specific local treatment and no attempts should be made to remove deep-located pellets.

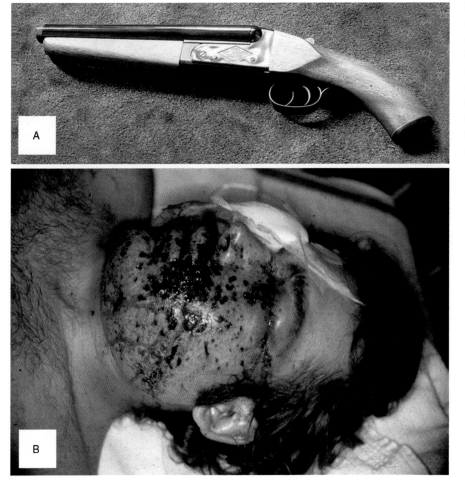

Figure 10.19 Sawn-off shotguns are often used by criminals in order to conceal the weapon. In this situation, the pellets lose most of their energy and at distances >4 meters they cause minimal damage. (A) Sawn-off shotgun. (B) Sawn-off shotgun injuries to the face from a distance of a few meters. Note the minor soft tissue damage.

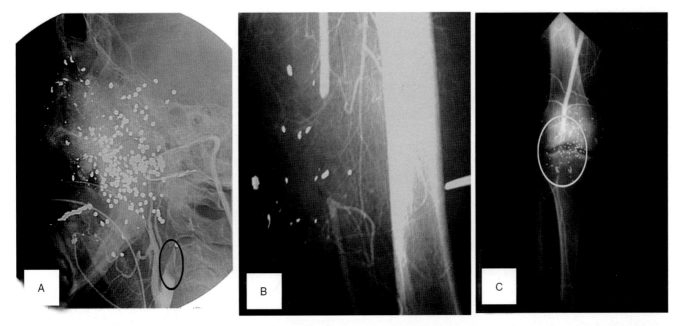

Figure 10.20 Shotgun injuries in the neck or extremities should be evaluated by formal angiography to rule out vascular trauma. (A) The angiogram shows injury and thrombosis of the left internal carotid artery. (B) Angiogram shows injury and thrombosis of the superficial femoral artery. (C) Angiogram shows injury to the popliteal artery.

10.5 Blast Injuries

Explosions have the capacity to cause a wide variety of injuries and are typically divided into five categories:

1. Direct injuries from high-velocity bomb fragments.
2. Blast wave injury which is caused by the direct wave pressure effect on tissues, affecting mainly air-filled structures. This direct-pressure effect is augmented in enclosed spaces, causing more severe injury. Ears are most often affected, followed by the lungs and gastrointestinal tract. The lung injuries are often devastating and air embolism is often a cause of death.
3. Injuries due to objects from the explosion which become missiles.
4. Tertiary blast injury, seen when individuals are thrown through the air by the explosion, striking walls and other objects, causing blunt trauma. Tertiary injuries also describe those due to structural collapse upon the patient.
5. Quaternary (or miscellaneous) blast injury is made up of all other injuries resulting from the explosion, such as burns from associated fires.

Improvised Explosive Devices

The majority of blast injuries in current military conflicts are due to improvised explosive devices (IEDs). An IED is a "homemade" explosive device designed to cause injury or death, and is commonly used in modern military conflicts by nonconventional forces. IEDs can use homemade explosives, military explosives, or commercially available agents. There are three main categories of IEDs: package type IEDs, vehicle-borne IEDs (VBIEDs), and suicide bomb IEDs. Injuries are similar to those seen in explosions, and these can be the result of both blunt and penetrating trauma. Penetrating injuries predominate due to fragmentation of the device casing itself or materials added to the device.

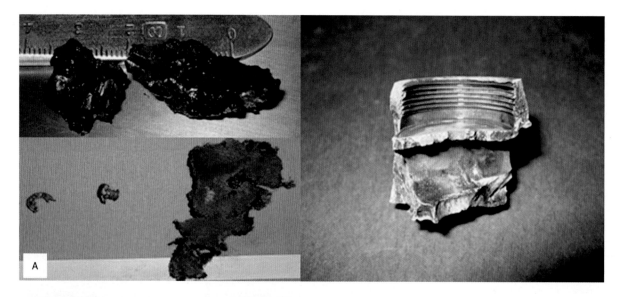

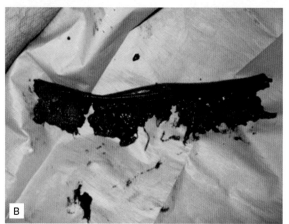

Figure 10.21 (A, B) Most injuries due to blast event are due to secondary penetrating injuries. Fragments can include parts of the blast device casing itself, materials from surrounding structures and even pieces of the vehicle in which the victim was an occupant.

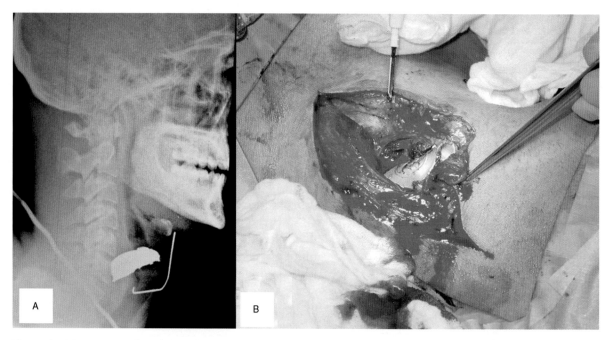

Figure 10.22 Improvised explosive device (IED) injuries. (A) Radiological appearance of a fragment in the neck following an IED injury. (B) Intraoperative appearance of an IED lodged into the neck.

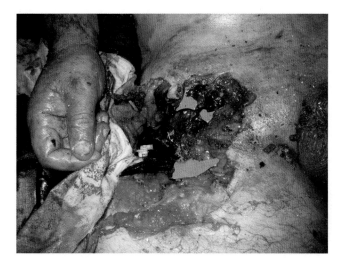

Figure 10.23 Fragmentation from IEDs cause secondary penetrating injury. Here, fragments of the device became deeply embedded into a groin wound. Unfortunately, the extremities are relatively unprotected even while wearing protective garments and vascular injury is a common cause of early death due to exsanguination.

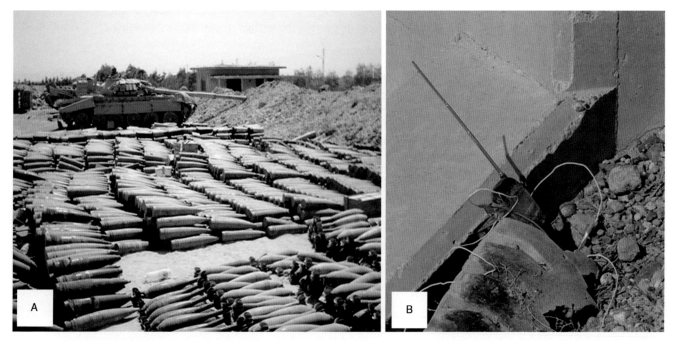

Figure 10.24 (A) Unexploded ordnance is readily available in combat zones from multiple previous conflicts and is commonly used in IEDs. (B) As commonly seen, a rudimentary cellular phone is used as part of a remote triggering mechanism.

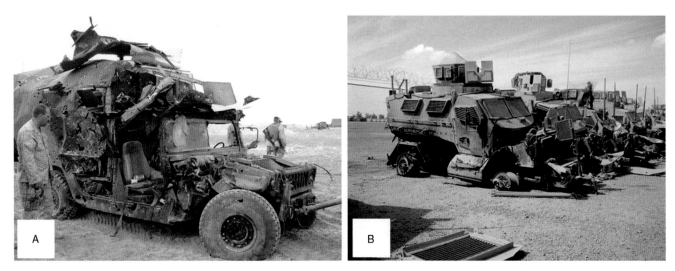

Figure 10.25 Improvised explosive device (IED) injuries. (A) Occupants of unarmored vehicles, such as this military ambulance, are essentially defenseless against the effects of a roadside IED. (B) In "Mine Resistant Ambush Protected" (MRAP) vehicles the passenger compartments remain relatively intact due to up-armoring and the blast-deflecting V-shaped undercarriage. Significant injuries from blunt trauma can still occur due to violent displacement of the occupants within the passenger compartments.

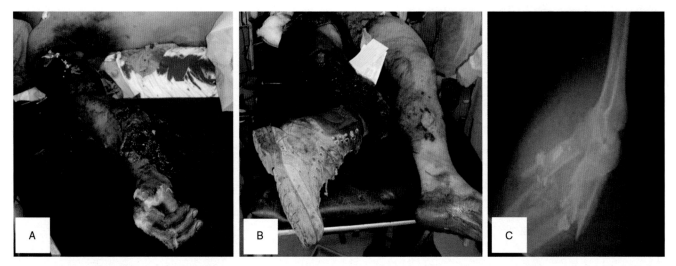

Figure 10.26 IEDs cause the majority of extremity injuries in current conflicts. These are characterized by massive soft tissue and bone disruption in association with extensive embedded fragmentation and debris. Irrigation and debridement is needed in tissue planes. Most of these injuries require amputations.

Figure 10.27 Examples of beanbag shells.

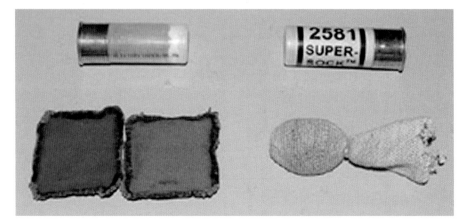

10.6 Nonlethal Weapons

Nonlethal weapons are designed to temporarily incapacitate an individual, and are commonly used by a number of police forces. These can include beanbag rounds, rubber bullets, and electroshock discharges (TASER or Stun Gun). Although less likely to be lethal than conventional weapons, these can still cause a variety of injuries including contusions, lacerations, eye injuries, fractures, and solid organ injury depending on the location of impact and the proximity to the weapon when it is fired.

Conductive energy devices (CED), such as the TASER or Stun Gun, are battery-operated hand-held units, commercially available for both law enforcement and civilian use. The most widely used device in the United States is TASER. It fires 4 mm darts attached by insulated wires up to 35 feet away. The CED works by discharging electrical bursts causing neuromuscular incapacitation. Although in healthy volunteers no significant complications have been seen, there are case reports of deaths, especially in subjects with associated medical problems or illicit drug intoxication.

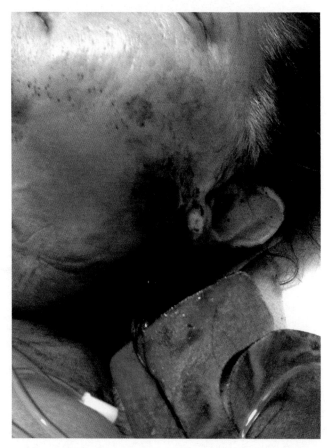

Figure 10.29 Soft tissue injury after suspect was subdued by police with beanbag missile.

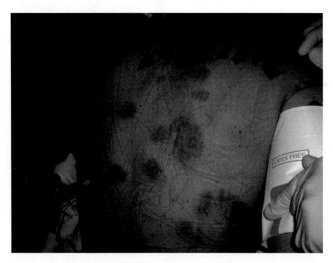

Figure 10.28 Contusions on upper and mid-back after victim was shot with beanbag missiles. At close range these injuries can cause serious injury or even death.

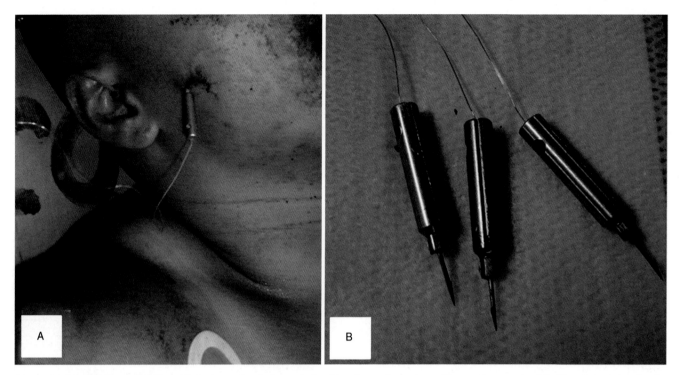

Figure 10.30 Taser gun injuries. (A) Patient after being subdued by the police using a Taser. Note embedded hook in right cheek. (B) Taser hooks removed from the same subject.

10.7 Myths and Facts about Bullets

There are many inaccuracies and myths regarding bullet properties and the care of bullet injuries.

(a) *Myth*: High-velocity bullets travel with continuous tumbling. *Fact*: Most bullets travel straight. Some bullets (AK-47, M-16) flip once (180 degrees) once they hit the tissues and then travel backwards.

(b) *Myth*: Bullets are sterile. *Fact*: Bullets are not sterile. The high temperature at the muzzle does not last long enough to sterilize the bullet.

(c) *Myth*: The tissue damage is proportional to the bullet velocity. *Fact*: The degree of tissue damage depends on the amount of energy released by the bullet. In many cases the bullet releases only a small amount of energy and exits the body without any major damage.

(d) *Myth*: Military bullets are made to inflict maximum damage. *Fact*: Military bullets are jacketed and designed not to fragment or deform on impact. Fragmentation and deformation are critical factors for extensive tissue damage.

(e) *Myth*: The appearance of the soft tissue injury can reliably distinguish between low-velocity and high-velocity bullets. *Fact*: In many cases even ballistic experts cannot reliably distinguish between low- and high-velocity injuries.

(f) *Myth*: All high-velocity injuries need extensive surgical debridement. *Fact*: A conservative debridement is more appropriate. Treat the injury, not the velocity.

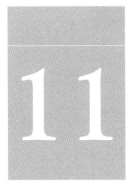

Disaster Medicine

Edward J. Newton

Introduction

Man-made and natural disasters usually occur without any warning and result in mass casualties that can overwhelm the capacity of the regional healthcare system. The most lethal natural disasters include earthquakes, hurricanes, floods, tsunamis, snowstorms, and fires. Man-made disasters include wars, building collapses, mine cave-ins, chemical and biological exposures, nuclear accidents, and civil unrest.

Each trauma system and trauma center needs to have a well-rehearsed plan for mass casualty events for different disaster scenarios (i.e., earthquakes, fires, airport accidents, different types of terrorist attack, etc.), based on the geographical site and availabilities of resources. A disaster plan should be as simple as possible and should be based on the daily working routine as much as possible.

11.1 Epidemiology of Injuries in Mass Disasters

The type and number of casualties depends on multiple factors listed in Table 11.1.

The Loma Prieta earthquake in 1989 near San Francisco and the Haiti earthquake of 2010 illustrate how these principles can result in vastly different results from similar disasters. The Loma Prieta quake was 6.9 magnitude whereas the Port-au-Prince quake was slightly larger at 7.0 magnitude. Both areas are port cities with populations of approximately 2 million. The Loma Prieta quake resulted in 63 deaths, 3,757 injuries and 3,000 to 12,000 persons homeless. The true toll of the Port-au-Prince quake may never be known but it is estimated that 230,000 persons died, 300,000 were injured, and 1 million rendered homeless. Clearly, poor construction standards; geographical isolation; poorly developed EMS, search and rescue, and medical capacity; and lack of heavy equipment and emergency planning led to the high number of casualties in the Haiti disaster.

Table 11.1 Variables affecting mortality in natural disasters

The magnitude and nature of the disaster

The density of the population in proximity to the disaster

The political and geographic accessibility of the region to adjacent areas that can provide early relief

Building construction standards

The sophistication of EMS and medical systems in the region

The functional status of EMS rescue services and healthcare facilities after the disaster

A developed disaster plan that includes emergency food, water, and medical stores as well as emergency shelters

The availability of heavy equipment and expertise to assist with rescue efforts, and to reopen roads, airports, and seaports

The pre-disaster health of the population

The relative wealth of the region

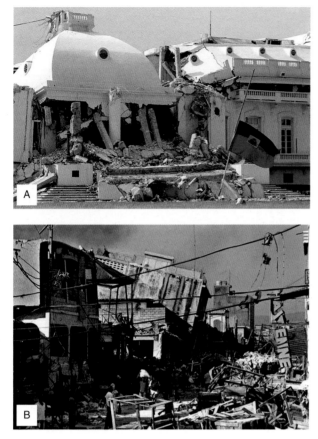

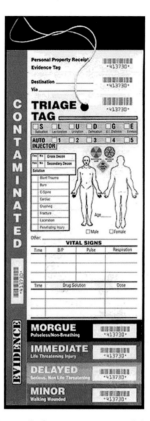

Figure 11.2 Color-coded tags are very useful in classifying the required level of medical care for each mass disaster victim.

Figure 11.1 Haiti earthquake disaster in 2010.

11.2 Triage

The success of a disaster plan depends on the ability of the team to weed out the large number of victims who will do well with minimal care from those with nonsurvivable injuries and direct the limited resources to the victims with survivable severe trauma. Effective triage at the scene and later on in the hospital is one of the most critical components for the successful management of a mass disaster incident.

The triage methods used in the field (START: Simple Triage And Rapid Transportation) which is based on mental status, ventilation, and perfusion are useful criteria for the scene triage but not reliable enough for an effective triage at the hospital. A much more detailed clinical examination by an experienced physician is needed for a more reliable triage. The triage should take place outside the emergency room (ER). The color-coded tag system is a useful way in classifying the required level of medical care (black = dead, red = immediate care,

yellow = urgent care in 1–2 hours, green = low-level care).

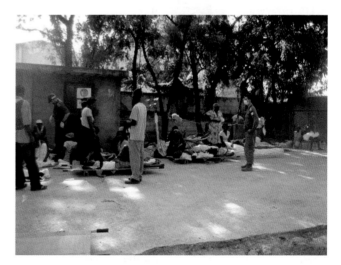

Figure 11.3 Haiti earthquake: triage in the field.

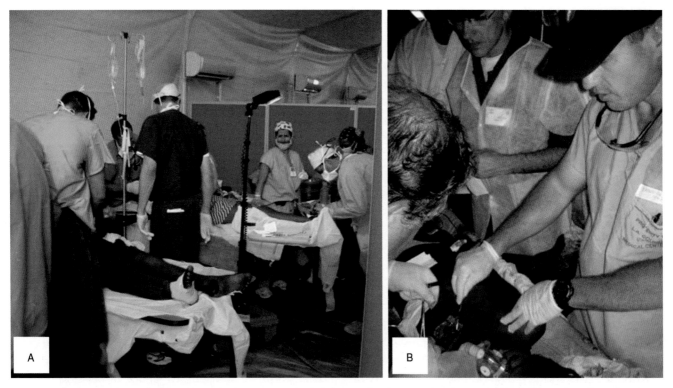

Figure 11.4 Haiti earthquake. (A, B) Medical care in makeshift hospital. Often medical care must be delivered under difficult conditions and with minimal resources.

The medical team needs to modify drastically its usual standards of care, in an attempt to preserve the available limited resources for the salvageable group of patients with severe trauma. Such changes of usual practices of care may include the following:

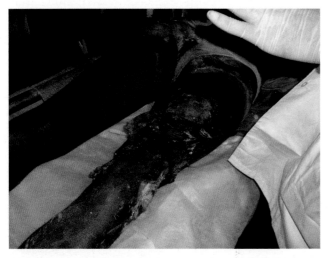

Figure 11.5 A 27-year-old woman who was pulled from the debris of her home after 6 days. There is a necrotic, infected wound of her left thigh. She succumbed to renal failure the following day. Note the proximal tourniquet on the thigh which was placed to avoid flooding the circulation with potassium and myoglobin when the leg was freed.

(a) No resources should be spent on nonsalvageable victims.

(b) Complex fractures are best stabilized by casts or external fixation rather than intramedullary rodding.

(c) Radiology, especially the CT scanner, is a major bottleneck of patient flow in mass disaster events. CT scanning and radiology in general, should be used judiciously, and certainly below the usual standards of care.

- Patients with clinical hemothorax might have a chest drain inserted without chest x-rays. Chest x-rays should be reserved for patients with certain types of trauma, such as blast injuries, missile injuries, or cases who cannot be evaluated clinically.

- Radiography for C-spine clearance or liberal pelvic x-rays are deferred for a later stage.

- Urgent CT scanning should be reserved only for selected patients with significant potentially salvageable head injuries. Minor head injuries (GCS ≥ 13) do not undergo CT scan evaluation.

- CT scanning of the chest or abdomen is deferred for a later stage. Clinical examination, Focused Assessment with Sonography for Trauma (FAST), and diagnostic peritoneal aspirate (DPA) should be the primary means of abdominal evaluation.

- Suspected extremity fractures may be splinted without radiological confirmation.
- Patients undergoing radiological investigations in the Radiology suite should not return to the ER. It is a one-way route! Failure to follow this rule may result in bottlenecks and aggravation of the ER overcrowding.

(d) Laboratory studies should be kept to a minimum. The only routine lab is Hb. Arterial blood gases, serum electrolytes, BUN, CPK, and coagulation studies are reserved only for certain victims, such as chemical terror attacks, crush injuries, and inhalation injuries.

11.3 Specific Injuries

In earthquakes and collapsed structures there are two closely related syndromes that occur in severely compressed limbs: crush syndrome and compartment syndrome. The severity of crush injury is a function of the pressure involved and time. Even a relatively light compression can cause serious problems if the pressure is sustained over a long period of time. Crush injury of the limbs ranges from near avulsion or complete "pancaking" of the limb to lesser degrees of compressive injury in which there is an opportunity to salvage the limb. The concern with crushed, entrapped limbs is that when they are released and perfusion re-established, there will be a rapid washout of lactic acid, potassium, and myoglobin into the systemic circulation. In addition, a sudden increase in blood loss from the decompressed limb may lead to hemorrhagic shock. Consequently, intravenous lines should be established before releasing the limb if possible, and many rescuers place proximal limb tourniquets to avoid further bleeding and washout of toxic metabolites.

Compartment syndrome occurs when a crushed limb or a fractured bone in the limb results in progressive edema in a soft tissue compartment that is bound by relatively inflexible fascia. As the pressure in the compartment rises, arterioles and venules are compressed causing ischemic injury to the tissues. This results in further edema until all perfusion of tissues in the affected limb ceases. At this point cells begin to break down and release their contents into the extracellular fluid. Some of these substances (potassium, phosphate, myoglobin) are toxic to other organs and result in major organ dysfunction once the compartment is reperfused and those substances enter the systemic circulation. A sudden surge in potassium can cause potentially lethal dysrhythmias. Phosphate may complex with calcium, potentiating the toxic effect of potassium on the heart. Myoglobin is filtered by the kidney and commonly results in acute renal failure as it deposits in renal tubules. Myoglobinuric renal failure is often reversible over the course of several weeks to months but requires bridging hemodialysis during this interval to sustain life. Inability to provide hemodialysis in the weeks following a disaster results in secondary potentially preventable loss of life. The ability to recognize and treat compartment syndrome by emergency fasciotomy or amputation is essential to deal with a large number of casualties with crushed limbs.

Tetanus is a concern when treating a large number of unvaccinated victims who have sustained severe wounds contaminated by soil. Given the lack of tetanus immune globulin and intensive care unit (ICU) capacity including ventilators, tetanus is an invariably fatal disease in these circumstances.

Outbreaks of infectious diseases including cholera are common after floods, tsunamis, and hurricanes but relatively uncommon after earthquakes. However,

---

Table 11.2 Indications for field amputation

Imminent danger to the patient or rescuers from impending building collapse, rising flood water, or fire

A patient with severe concomitant injuries who would not survive a lengthy extrication process

Lack of necessary equipment to extricate the patient or inability to move the equipment into position when the patient is trapped in confined quarters such as a mine or cave or on a mountain cliff

A patient who is trapped by a limb that is obviously crushed beyond hope of salvage

---

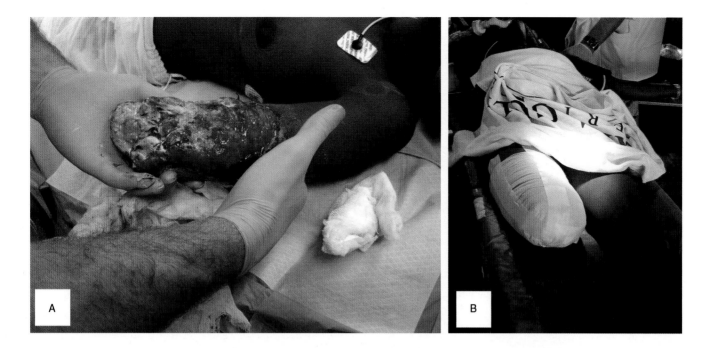

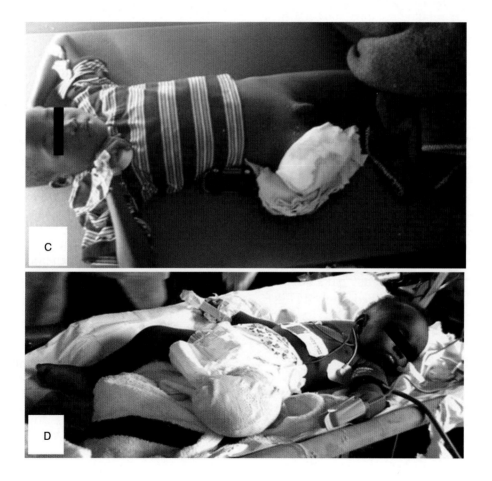

Figure 11.6 Haiti earthquake. (A, B) Amputations were the most common operations, very often because of open fractures receiving delayed or suboptimal care.

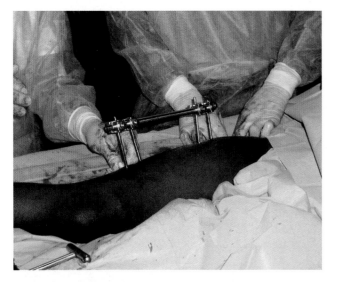

Figure 11.7 Haiti earthquake. Most severe long bone fractures were managed with external fixation because of the lack of resources and the heavily contaminated wounds.

other infections such as influenza, infectious diarrhea, hepatitis, and tuberculosis are common to all spontaneous refugee camps because of lack of hygiene and overcrowding.

Dead bodies are often disposed of hastily in disasters without adequate methods of identification or notification of relatives. Victims should be photographed before burial or cremation for later identification.

Many survivors suffer from severe post-traumatic stress disorder after losing multiple family members, their homes, employment, and all of their possessions. Psychiatric support services are typically not available in the acute phase of a disaster and often are limited by language and cultural barriers, but community-based support services should be organized early in the course of the recovery and have proven effective.

11.4 Guidelines for Rescue Efforts

Rescue efforts are often uncoordinated initially. A central command structure to direct resources to areas with the greatest need is highly desirable but depends on the cooperation of multiple NGOs to be effective. The United Nations High Commission for Refugees (UNHCR) has published a list of priorities to be established during disaster relief and a group of humanitarian NGOs has published the SPHERE Humanitarian Charter and Minimum Standards in Disaster Response which are guidelines for the construction of refugee camps. Both of these are useful to guide relief efforts.

Relief efforts must transition from the acute phase where the focus is on rescue and individual patient care to the subacute phase (14 days–months) where the focus is on caring for the whole population. In this

Table 11.3 Timeline for disaster relief efforts

Week1	Week2	Week3	Week4	Month2	Month3	Ongoing
Acute rescue operations						
Acute surgical care						
Establish water supply						
Orthopedics, renal failure, compartment syndrome, limb amputation, hemodialysis						
Establish emergency shelters						
Resume treatment of chronic medical problems						
Establish food supply						
Rehabilitation, occupational therapy						
Permanent shelters						

Table 11.4 SPHERE minimum standards for refugee camps

- 45 m²/person in camps
- Water: 15 L/person per day
- Latrines: 20 persons/toilet; within 500 m of dwellings
- Health workers: <50 patients/8 hrs
- Syndromic surveillance for infectious diseases

phase the priorities are establishing shelters, providing clean food and water supplies, reuniting families, ensuring security, treating infectious diseases that emerge, controlling insect disease vectors, vaccinations, re-establishing medical care for chronic medical problems, and providing rehabilitation and psychiatric support services. Restoring communications, road access, and electricity are also high priorities.

Index

abdominal injury 119–157
  bladder 135
  blunt 122–142
  clinical examination 119
  colorectal 141, 152
  duodenum 139
  hematoperitoneum 123
  investigations 119–120
  kidneys 133–135, 150
  liver 127, 146
  management 120
  mistakes and pitfalls 120
  pancreas 131–133, 150
  penetrating 121–122, 142–149
    clinical examination 121
    investigations 121, 144
    management 121
    mechanism of injury 142
    mistakes and pitfalls 122
  pregnancy 154–159
    cesarean section 159
    clinical examination and
      investigations 155
    management 157
    pregnancy-related complications
      156
  small bowel 140
  spleen 125–127, 149
  urethra 137
  vascular 153
acute respiratory distress syndrome 263
advanced trauma life support
  burn injuries 253
  head injury 3
  neck injury 50, 51
  thoracic injury 75
airway
  intubation See intubation
  neck injury 65
  spinal injury 210
airway pressure release ventilation 90
amniotic fluid embolization 157

amoxicillin–clavulanic acid 274, 276
amputations 168–169, 272
  field 304
amylase 120, 139
angioembolization 101, 131
  liver injury 146
  pelvic fracture 191, 193
angiography
  abdominal injury 120, 121
  cerebral 2
  CT See CT angiography
  neck injury 51
    penetrating 60
  pelvic fractures 191
  thoracic injury 76
ankle dislocation 201
ankle fracture 200
ankle–brachial index 160
anterior cord syndrome 216
antibiotic prophylaxis
  dog bites 274
  human bites 276
anticonvulsants 19
antiplatelet therapy 74
aorta
  blunt injury 101–102
  traumatic rupture 77
aortography 101
arterial blood gases 76, 254
arteriovenous malformation 16
asphyxia, traumatic 117
atlantoaxial dislocation 218
atlanto-occipital dislocation 217
atlas fracture 222
autotransfusion in thoracic injury 88
avulsion injuries 271
axillary nerve injury 176
axonotmesis 174

Bacteroides spp. 274
ballistics 300
  blast injuries 295

bullet velocity 286
bullets See bullets
  caliber 284
  gunshot wounds See gunshot wounds
  high-velocity missiles 288–291
  improvised explosive devices 295
  low-velocity projectiles 286
  nonlethal weapons 299
Barton fracture 181
Battle's sign 1, 5, 8, 31
beanbag rounds 299
Beck's triad 92
Bennett's fracture 178
berry aneurysm 16
bladder injuries 135
blast injuries 295
blowout fracture 31
blunt trauma
  abdominal 122–142
  cardiac 100
  diaphragm 110
  ear 32
  head 1
  laryngotracheal 74
  neck 71–74
Bohler's angle 206
bone scan 160
boxer's fractures 177
brachial–brachial index 54, 59
bronchoscopy
  aerodigestive tract injuries 76
  burn injuries 254
Brown-Séquard syndrome 208, 215
bulbocavernosus reflex 208
bullets 279
  black talon 284
  design 284
  explosive 285
  hollow-point 284
  jacketed 284
  myths and facts 300
  rubber 299

scored 284
Teflon-coated 285
velocity 286
   high-velocity 288–291
   low-velocity 286
wounds *See* gunshot wounds
burn injuries 269
  abdominal compartment syndrome
    264
  chemical burns 267
  circumferential burns 265
  clinical examination 253–254
  electrical burns 268
  extent of 256–262
  first-degree 256
  fourth-degree 262
  inhalation injury 263–264
  investigations 254
  Lund–Browder chart 253
  management 254–255
  mistakes and pitfalls 255
  outcome 269
  Rule of Nines 253
  scalds 266
  second-degree 257
    deep 258
    superficial 257
  third-degree 261
  transfer criteria 254

C-1 burst fracture 222
C-1 on C-2 rotatory subluxation 219
C-2 fracture 224
C-7 fracture 232
calcaneal fracture 205, 211
caliber (of guns) 284
canthotomy 36
carbon monoxide poisoning 254
carboxyhemoglobin 254, 263
cardiac injury
  blunt 100
  diagnosis 95
  penetrating 92–99
    late sequelae 99
    retained missiles 96
cardiac rupture 100
cardiac tamponade 92
carotid artery
  penetrating trauma 68
cat bites 275–276
cellulitis 276
central cord syndrome 208, 210, 213
central herniation 24
cerebellar tonsillar herniation 24
cerebral angiography 2
cerebral blood flow 25

cerebral contusion 19
  seizures 19
cerebral edema 26
cerebral perfusion pressure 3
cerebrospinal fluid *See* CSF
cervical spine injury 2
cervicothoracic spinal injury 237
cesarean section, perimortem 159
Chance fracture 245
chemical burns 267
chemosis 36
chest trauma *See* thoracic injury
chest wall injuries 78
chest x-ray 75
  abdominal injury 119, 121
  burn injuries 254
child abuse 27
  head injury 4
  shaken baby syndrome 13, 27
children
  concussion 28
  dog bites 273
  epiphyseal injuries 165
  fractures 166
    forearm 181
    hip 195
  head injury 27–28
  skull fracture 5
  spinal injury 248
cholera 304
cingulate gyrus herniation 24
circumflex nerve injury 176
clavicle fractures 187
clay shoveler's fracture 232
clindamycin 274, 276
coagulopathy 4, 19, 23
Colles' fracture 180
color flow Doppler
  neck injury 51
    blunt 72
    penetrating 60
  thoracic injury 76
  thoracic outlet injuries 105
colorectal injuries 141
  penetrating 152
compartment syndrome 161, 174, 254,
    255, 280–282
  abdominal 264
  causes 280
  clinical presentation and investigations
    280
  complications, 281
  disaster medicine 304
  management 281
  mistakes and pitfalls 282
computerized tomography *See* CT

concussion 1
  children 28
conductive energy devices 299
corneal abrasion 33
coup–contrecoup injury 19
cranial nerve injury 8, 32 *See also individual*
    cranial nerves
cricothyroidotomy 32, 42, 44, 51, 52
crush syndrome 304
crystalloid hydration 255
CSF
  drainage 3
  leaks 3
  otorrhea *See* otorrhea
  rhinorrhea *See* rhinorrhea
C-spine collars 51
CT
  abdominal injury 120, 121
  brain scan 58
  epidural hematoma 11
  facial injury 31
  head injury 2
  musculoskeletal injury 160
  neck injury 51
  pelvic fractures 191
  penetrating facial injury 43
  skull fracture 5, 8
  spinal injury 208
  subdural hematoma 14
  thoracic injury 76
CT angiography
  musculoskeletal injury 160
  neck injury 51
    blunt 72
    penetrating 58
  thoracic injury 76

dancer's fractures 204
degloving injuries 271
dens fracture 224
diaphragmatic hernia, traumatic 111
diaphragmatic injuries 109–114
  blunt 110
  penetrating 109, 122
diffuse axonal injury 28
dinner fork deformity 180
diplopia 37, 39
disaster medicine 307
  compartment syndrome
    See compartment syndrome
  crush syndrome 304
  injury epidemiology 301
  mortality 301
  post-traumatic stress disorder 306
  rescue guidelines 306
  triage 302–304

disaster relief efforts 306
dislocations
    ankle 201
    elbow 183
    facet 234
    hip 193
    knee 198–199
    lunate and perilunate 179
    scapholunate 179
    shoulder 185–186
    sternoclavicular 188
    subtalar 202
    upper cervical spine 216–222
disseminated intravascular coagulopathy 4, 19, 272
dog bites 273–275
Doppler stethoscope 254
doxycycline 274, 276
drooling 39
duodenal injuries 139
dysarthria 39

ear
    blunt trauma 32
    examination 31
    penetrating trauma 32
ECG
    cardiac injury 95, 100
    thoracic injury 75
    transmediastinal gunshot wounds 63
elbow dislocation 183
electrical burns 268
electrocardiogram See ECG
embolization
    amniotic fluid 157
    neck injury 60
    vertebral artery trauma 69
emphysema, subcutaneous 50, 54, 63, 90
endoscopic retrograde cholangiopancreatography 131
endoscopy
    neck injury 51, 63
    thoracic injury 76
endotracheal intubation 32
enophthalmos 31, 34, 39
epidural hematoma 1, 3, 11
epilepsy, post-traumatic 19
epiphyseal injuries 165
    Salter–Harris classification 165
erythroblastosis fetalis 156
escharotomy 265
esophageal trauma 50, 114
esophagography 51, 63
esophagoscopy 51
etomidate 25
exophthalmos 31

extradural hematoma in children 28
eye examination 30–31
eye injuries 32, 33–37
    corneal abrasion 33
    foreign body 33
    hyphema 33
    orbital blowout fracture 37
    periorbital lacerations 37
    retrobulbar hematoma 36
    ruptured globe 34
eyebrow, laceration of 37
eyelid, laceration of 30, 32

face
    examination 30
    zones of 42
facet dislocation 234
facial fractures 37–41
    Le Fort See Le Fort fractures
    mandible 39
    orbital blowout 37
facial injury 30–48
    examination 30–31
    eye See eye injuries
    investigation 31–32
    management 32
    mistakes and pitfalls 32
    nose 42
    oromaxillofacial trauma 44–46
    parotid gland 48
    penetrating 42–43
    zygoma fractures 40
facial nerve injury 47
FAST 75
    hemoperitoneum 123
    pelvic fractures 191
    pericardial 95
    thoracic injury 77
    transmediastinal gunshot wounds 107
femoral nerve injury 176
femoral shaft fracture 196
fetal mortality 157
fetomaternal bleeding 156
flail chest 77, 80
Focused Assessment with Sonography for Trauma See FAST
forearm fractures 181
foreign body
    eye 33
    impaled thoracic 118
    retained 279
Fox shield 32
fractures 161–168, 177–206
    angulation 162

cervical spine 222–234 See also individual fractures
classification 161
    greenstick fractures 166
    supracondylar fractures 167
    torus fractures 166
displacement 162
epiphyseal injuries 165
facial 37–41
Gustilo classification 162
lumbar spine 242–247 See also individual fractures
mangled extremity 163
open (compound) 162
open joint injuries 164 See also individual fractures
fungal enophthalmitis 33
furosemide 3
Fusobacterium spp. 274

Galeazzi fracture complex 182
Glasgow Coma Scale 1, 50
globe (of eye), rupture 34
glycemic control in burn injuries 254
greenstick fractures 166
gunshot wounds
    abrasion ring 286
    assessment 287
    ballistics See ballistics
    head 1, 23
    neck 54
    permanent cavity 286
    shotgun injuries 291–295
    transmediastinal 107
    transpelvic 145
Gustilo classification 162

hangman's fracture 226
head injury 1–29
    blunt 1
    children 27–28
    clinical examination 1–2
    gunshot wounds 1, 20–24
    investigation 2
    management 3
    mild 1
    mistakes and pitfalls 3–4
    moderate 1
    penetrating 20–24
    scalp 4 See also individual injuries
hematemesis 51
hematuria 120
hemiparesis 72
hemiplegia 72
hemoperitoneum 123
hemopneumothorax 81–88

hemoptysis 50, 54, 63
hemothorax 57, 83
hemotympanum 1, 8, 31
high-frequency percussive
ventilation 90
high-pressure injection injury 278
hip dislocation 193
hip fractures 195–196
hoarseness 50, 54, 63
Horner's syndrome 50
human bites 276–278
disease transmission 276
human immunodeficiency virus
(HIV), transmission by bites
277
humeral shaft fractures 184
hydrofluoric acid 268
hypercapnia 254
hypercarbia 3
hyperkalemia 272
hyperphosphatemia 272
hyperthermia 3
hyperventilation 3
hyphema 33
hypocalcemia 272
hypotension 3, 77
hypovolemic shock 272
hypoxia 3, 254

impalement injuries
head 20
thoracic foreign body 118
improvised explosive devices 295
independent lung ventilation 90
infant concussion syndrome 28
inhalation injury 263–264
intracranial hematoma 11–16
epidural See epidural hematoma
subdural See subdural hematoma
intracranial pressure, raised 2, 3
intraocular pressure 36, 37
intraparenchymal hemorrhage 18
intravenous pyelogram 120, 133
intraventricular hemorrhage 3, 17
intubation
endotracheal 32
nasotracheal 32, 51
orotracheal 44, 65
rapid sequence 25

Jefferson fracture 222
joint injuries
open 164 See also individual joints

Kernohan's notch phenomenon 24
knee dislocation 198–199

laminar fracture 233
laparoscopy
abdominal injury 121, 144
thoracic injury 76
laryngoscopy 51
burn injuries 254
laryngotracheal hematoma 51
laryngotracheal trauma 50, 63
blunt 74
lateral masses, fracture of 234
lateral popliteal nerve injury 176
Le Fort fractures 30, 32, 40
type I 40
type II 40
type III 41
leptomeningeal cyst 5
lipase 120
lips, laceration of 47
Lisfranc fracture 203
liver injury 127
penetrating 146
Loma Prieta earthquake 301
lunate dislocation 179
Lund–Browder chart 253
lung contusion 89
luxatio erecta 185

mafenide acetate 255, 260
magnetic resonance imaging See MRI
Maisonneuve fracture complex 200
mandible fracture 39
mangled extremity 163, 272
Mangled Extremity Severity Score
(MESS) 164
mannitol 3, 28
mean arterial pressure 25
medial popliteal nerve injury 176
median nerve injury 175
mediastinum, widened 77
metacarpal fractures 177
classification 177
first metacarpal 178
metatarsal base fractures 204
methylprednisolone 210
metronizadole 274
Monteggia fracture complex 182
Morexella spp. 274
mouth, examination of 31
MR cholangiopancreatography
120, 131
MRI
head injury 2
musculoskeletal injury 160
spinal injury 208
MRSA 162
musculocutaneous nerve injury 176

musculoskeletal injury 205
amputations 168–169
clinical examination 160
fractures See fractures
investigations 160
management 160–161
mistakes and pitfalls 161
peripheral nerve injuries
174–177
peripheral vascular injury 170
tendon injury 170
myoglobin 304
myoglobinemia 272
myoglobinuria 272

nasal injury 42
nasotracheal intubation 32, 51
neck injury 50
blunt 71–74
vascular injuries 72
examination 50–51
investigation 51
management 51–52
mistakes and pitfalls 52
penetrating 52–71
aerodigestive tract evaluation 63
airway establishment 65
bleeding control 66
epidemiology 54
evaluation 56
physical examination 54
radiological investigations
57–58
vascular evaluation 59–63
neck, anatomical zones 52
nerve injuries
peripheral 174–177 See also individual
nerves
neurogenic shock 208, 210, 211
neuropraxia 174
neurotmesis 174
nightstick fractures 183
nimodipine 3
nonlethal weapons 299
nose, examination of 31

odontoid fracture 224
odynophagia 50, 51, 54
ophthalmoplegia 36
oral trauma 47
orbital blowout fracture 37
oromaxillofacial trauma 44–46
orotracheal intubation 44, 65
osmotic diuresis 3
osteomyelitis 162
otorrhea 1, 3, 8, 31

pancreatic injury 131–133
 penetrating 150
pancreaticoduodenal injuries 120, 121
pancreatoduodenectomy 150
Parkland formula 255
parotid duct laceration 31, 48
parotid gland injury 48
partial cord syndromes 210
Pasteurella spp. 274
patellar fracture 197
pedicles, fracture of 233
pelvic binders 191
pelvic fractures 189–193
 classification 189
 clinical examination 191
 investigations 191
 management 191
pelvic x-ray 119
penetrating injuries
 abdominal 121–122, 142–149
 cardiac 92–99
 colorectal 152
 diaphragm 109
 ear 32
 face 43
 head 20–24
 liver 146
 neck 52–71
 pancreas 150
 renal 150
 spinal cord 250
 spleen 149
 thoracic outlet 105
pentobarbital 25
pericardiocentesis 76, 95
perilunate dislocation 179
periorbital lacerations 37
peritoneal aspirate, diagnostic 120, 191,
 303
peritoneal lavage, diagnostic 120, 140
phenytoin 19
piece of pie sign 180
placental abruption 156
pneumocephalus 7
pneumoperitoneum 120
pneumothorax 57, 81
 tension 77, 81
post-traumatic stress disorder 306
pregnancy
 abdominal injury 154–159
 anatomical and physiological changes
 154
premature rupture of membranes 157
priapism 208
propofol 25
proptosis 36

pseudoaneurysm 174
pseudoeschar 255
ptosis, ipsilateral 2, 24
pulse oximetry 254
pulsus paradoxus 92

rabies 275
raccoon eyes 1, 8
radial head fractures 183
radial nerve injury 175, 184
radiography
 chest x-ray 75, 119, 121, 254
 mandible fracture 39
 musculoskeletal injury 160
 neck injury 51
  penetrating 57
 pelvic fractures 191
 pelvic x-ray 119
 skull 2
 skull fracture 5
renal artery thrombosis 135
renal injury 133–135
 penetrating 150
retained foreign body 279
retrobulbar hematoma 36
retro-orbital hematoma 31
rhinorrhea 1, 3, 8
rib fractures 78–81
 flail chest *See* flail chest
 lower ribs 80
 middle ribs 79
 upper ribs 78
Rolando's fracture 178
Rule of Nines 253

saddle-nose deformity 42
saline, hypertonic 3
Salter–Harris classification 165
scalds 266
scalp injuries 4
scaphoid fracture 178
scapholunate dislocation 179
scapula fracture 188
sciatic nerve injury 176
SCIWORA 208, 248
scoop and run principle
 neck injury 51
 thoracic injury 77
seatbelt marks
 abdomen 120, 123
 chest 78
 neck 50, 72
Seidel's test 31
seizures 3
 cerebral contusion 19
 depressed skull fracture 6

Seldinger guidewire 86
shaken baby syndrome 13, 27
shotgun injuries 291–295
shoulder dislocation 185
Siedel's test 36
silver sulfadiazine 255, 260
Simple Triage And Rapid Transportation
 (START) 302
skull fracture 4–8
 basilar 3, 8
 children 5
 closed 3
 depressed 3, 6
 linear 5–6
 open 7
skull x-rays 2
small-bowel perforation 140
Smith fracture 180
soft tissue injuries 282
 cat bites 275–276
 dog bites 273–275
 face *See* facial injury
 high-pressure injection injury 278
 human bites 276–278
 major 271–273
  complications 272
  investigations 272
  management 272
 retained foreign body 279
SPHERE Humanitarian Charter and
 Minimum Standards in Disaster
 Response 306, 307
spilled teacup sign 180
spinal cord injuries 211–216
 anterior cord syndrome 216
 Brown-Séquard syndrome 215
 central cord syndrome 208, 210, 213
 complete transection 211–212
 penetrating 250
spinal injury 250
 cervical spine 207
  evaluation 209
  fractures 222–234
 cervicothoracic spine 237
 children 248
 clinical examination 207–208
 facet dislocation 234
 investigations 208
 lumbar spine
  fracture-dislocation 247
  fractures 242–247
 management 210
 mistakes and pitfalls 210–211
 thoracic spine 239
 upper cervical spine dislocations
  216–222

spinal shock 211, 212
splenic injury 125–127
   penetrating 149
stab wounds *See* penetrating injuries
Staphylococcus aureus, osteomyelitis 162
Staphylococcus spp. 274, 276
stenting in neck injury 60
sternoclavicular dislocation 188
Streptococcus spp. 274, 276
stun guns 299
subarachnoid hemorrhage 1, 3, 16–17
subclavian vascular trauma 70
subcutaneous emphysema *See* emphysema,
     subcutaneous
subdural hematoma 1, 3, 13–16
   acute 13
   chronic 13, 16
subtalar dislocation 202
subxiphoid pericardial window 76, 95
supracondylar fractures 167
Swischuk's line 248

Tasers 299
teardrop fracture
   extension 229
   flexion 229
teeth, missing 47
temporomandibular joint trauma 39
tendon injury 170
tension pneumothorax 77, 81
tetanus 304
thoracic duct injury 116
thoracic injury 75–118
   autotransfusion 88

blunt aortic trauma 101–102
cardiac injury
   blunt 100
   penetrating 92–99
chest wall 78
diaphragm 109–114
esophagus 50, 114
examination 75
hemopneumothorax 81–88
impaled thoracic foreign bodies 118
investigations 75–77
lung contusion 89
management 77
   thoracotomy 77
mistakes and pitfalls 77
rib fractures 78–81
subcutaneous emphysema
     See emphysema, subcutaneous
transmediastinal gunshot wounds
     107
thoracic outlet injuries 105
thoracic spinal injury 239
thoracoscopy 76
thoracostomy tube insertion 83, 84
thoracotomy 77
   emergency department 97
tibial plateau fracture 198
tongue, laceration of 47
torus fractures 166
tracheoscopy 51
transtentorial herniation 3, 11, 19,
   24–26
Trendelenburg position 51
triage 302–304

trimethoprim–sulfamethoxazole 274, 276
troponin, serum levels 76, 100
tylenol 3

ulnar nerve injury 175
ulnar shaft fractures 183
ultrasound
   abdominal injury 119, 121
   FAST *See* FAST
   musculoskeletal injury 160
uncal herniation 24
urethral injuries 137
urinalysis 120
uterine rupture 157

vascular injuries
   abdominal 153
   neck 72
   peripheral 170
ventilation *See* various types
ventriculostomy 3, 25, 26
vertebral artery, penetrating trauma 69
vertebral body fracture 228, 231–232
Volkmann's contractures 281

Whipple's pancreatoduodenectomy 132
wrist fractures 180
   Barton's 181
   Colles' 180
   Smith's 180

x-rays *See* radiography

zygoma fractures 40